History and Pathology of Vaccination

HISTORY AND PATHOLOGY

OF

VACCINATION

HISTORY AND PATHOLOGY

OF

VACCINATION

VOL. II.

SELECTED ESSAYS

EDITED BY

EDGAR M. CROOKSHANK, M.B.

PROFESSOR OF COMPARATIVE PATHOLOGY AND BACTERIOLOGY, AND FELLOW OF KING'S COLLEGE, LONDON,

AUTHOR OF PAPERS ON THE ETIOLOGY OF SCARLET FEVER; ANTHRAX IN SWINE; TUBERCULOSIS AND THE PUBLIC MILK SUPPLY; AND THE HISTORY AND PATHOLOGY OF ACTINOMYCOSIS; IN REPORTS OF THE AGRICULTURAL DEPARTMENT OF THE PRIVY COUNCIL.

AUTHOR OF "A MANUAL OF BACTERIOLOGY," ETC.

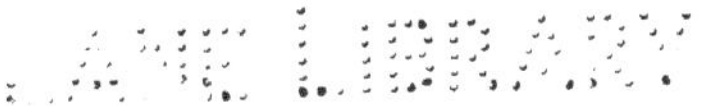

LONDON

H. K. LEWIS, 136, GOWER STREET, W.C.

1889.

CONTENTS.

PAGE

An Inquiry into the Causes and Effects of the Variolæ Vaccinæ.—EDWARD JENNER 1

An Inquiry Concerning the History of the Cow Pox.—GEORGE PEARSON, M.D., F.R.S. 35

Reports of a Series of Inoculations for the Variolæ Vaccinæ, or Cow-Pox.—WILLIAM WOODVILLE, M.D., F.R.S. 93

Further Observations on the Variolæ Vaccinæ, or Cow Pox.—EDWARD JENNER, M.D., F.R.S., F.L.S., &c. . . 155

An Address to the Public on the Advantages of Vaccine Inoculation.—HENRY JENNER, Surgeon, F L S., &c. . 191

A Conscious View of Circumstances and Proceedings respecting Vaccine Inoculation.—ANONYMOUS . . 203

A Continuation of Facts and Observations relative to the Variolæ Vaccinæ.—EDWARD JENNER, M.D., F.R.S,, &c. 247

The Origin of the Vaccine Inoculation.—EDWARD JENNER, M.D., F.R.S., &c. 267

An Account of some Experiments on the Origin of the Cow-Pox.—JOHN G. LOY, M.D. 275

An Examination of that Part of the Evidence relative to Cow-Pox, &c.—W. R. ROGERS 287

A Letter occasioned by the Many Failures of Cow-Pox.—JOHN BIRCH, Esq. 303

PAGE

On Cow Pox discovered at Passy (near Paris)—M. BOUSQUET 311

Account of a Supply of Fresh Vaccine Virus from the Cow.—ESTLIN 323

Observations on the Variolæ Vaccinæ.—CEELY . . . 363

Report of the Vaccination Section of the Provincial Medical and Surgical Association 449

Further Observations on the Variolæ Vaccinæ.—CEELY 469

A Detail of Experiments confirming the Power of Cow Pox to protect the Constitution from a Subsequent attack of Small Pox, by proving the Identity of the Two Diseases.—JOHN BADCOCK 513

Correspondence from Members of the Medical Profession, relative to Recent Supplies of Variolæ Vaccinæ, or Modified Small Pox 528

Small Pox and Cow Pox.—AUZIAS-TURENNE 543

Cow Pox at Eysines (Laforêt) (First Outbreak), 1881.—DUBREUILH 563

Cow Pox at Eysines (Second Outbreak), 1883. And at Cérons, 1884.—LAYET 575

Outbreak of Cow Pox near Cricklade (Wiltshire), 1887.—CROOKSHANK 591

AN

INQUIRY

INTO

THE CAUSES AND EFFECTS

OF

THE VARIOLÆ VACCINÆ.

[*Reprinted from the First Edition* (1798). *The readings in the MS. of the Original Paper, and the corrections in the Third Edition* (1801) *will be found in foot-notes.*—E.M.C.]

[TITLE OF ORIGINAL PAPER, MS.]

AN

INQUIRY

INTO

THE NATURAL HISTORY

OF

A DISEASE

KNOWN IN

GLOSTERSHIRE

BY THE NAME OF

THE COW-POX.

[*From the Manuscript of the Original Paper in the Library of the Royal College of Surgeons, London.*—E.M.C.]

[*REDUCED FACSIMILE OF THE TITLE PAGE OF THE FIRST EDITION.*]

AN

INQUIRY

INTO

THE CAUSES AND EFFECTS

OF

THE VARIOLÆ VACCINÆ,

A DISEASE,

DISCOVERED IN SOME OF THE WESTERN COUNTIES OF ENGLAND,

PARTICULARLY

GLOUCESTERSHIRE,

AND KNOWN BY THE NAME OF

THE COW POX.

BY EDWARD JENNER, M. D. F R.S. &c.

——QUID NOBIS CERTIUS IPSIS
SENSIBUS ESSE POTEST, QUO VERA AC FALSA NOTEMUS

LUCRETIUS.

London:

PRINTED, FOR THE AUTHOR,

BY SAMPSON LOW, Nº 7, BERWICK STREET, SOHO

AND SOLD BY LAW, AVE-MARIA LANE; AND MURRAY AND HIGHLEY, FLEET STREET

1798

*TO

C. H. PARRY, M.D.

AT BATH.

MY DEAR FRIEND,

IN the present age of scientific investigation, it is remarkable that a disease of so peculiar a nature as the Cow Pox, which has appeared in this and some of the neighbouring counties for such a series of years, should so long have escaped particular attention. Finding the prevailing notions on the subject, both among men of our profession and others, extremely vague and indeterminate, and conceiving that facts might appear at once both curious and useful, I have instituted as strict an inquiry into the causes and effects of this singular malady as local circumstances would admit.

The following pages are the result, which, from motives of the most affectionate regard, are dedicated to you, by

Your sincere Friend,

EDWARD JENNER.

Berkeley, Gloucestershire,
June 21st, 1798.

---

* For the dedication of the Second Edition, see next page.—E.M.C.

*TO

THE KING.

SIR,

WHEN I first addressed the Public on a Physiological subject, which I conceived to be of the utmost importance to the future welfare of the human race, I could not presume in that early stage of the investigation to lay the result of my Inquiries at your Majesty's feet.

Subsequent experiments, instituted not only by myself, but by men of the first rank in the medical profession, have now confirmed the truth of the theory which I first made known to the world.

Highly honoured by the permission to dedicate the result of my Inquiries to your Majesty, I am emboldened to solicit your gracious patronage of a discovery which reason fully authorises me to suppose will prove peculiarly conducive to the preservation of the loss of mankind.

To a Monarch no less justly than emphatically styled the Father of his People, this Treatise is inscribed with perfect propriety; for, conspicuous as your Majesty's patronage has been of Arts, of Sciences, and of Commerce, yet the most distinguished feature of your character is your paternal care for the dearer interests of humanity.

I am,

SIR,

With the most profound respect,

Your Majesty's most devoted Subject and Servant,

EDWARD JENNER.

Berkeley, Gloucestershire,
Dec. 20, 1799.

[* Dedication of the Second Edition of the "Inquiry."—E.M.C.]

AN

INQUIRY,

&c. &c.

THE [1]deviation" of Man from the state in which he was originally placed by Nature [2]seems" to have proved to him a prolific source of Diseases. From the love of splendour, from the indulgences of luxury, and from his fondness for amusement, he has familiarised himself with a great number of animals, which may not originally have been intended for his associates.

The Wolf, disarmed of ferocity, is now pillowed in the lady's lap.* The Cat, the little Tyger of our island, whose natural home is the forest, is equally domesticated and caressed. The Cow, the Hog, the Sheep, and the Horse, are all, for a variety of purposes, brought under his care and dominion.

There is a disease to which the Horse, from his state of domestication, is frequently subject. The Farriers have termed it *the Grease*. It is an inflammation and swelling in the heel, [3]—" from which issues [4]matter" possessing properties of a very peculiar kind[5], which seems" capable of generating a disease in the Human Body (after it has undergone the modification [6]which" I shall presently speak of), which bears so strong a resemblance to the Small Pox, that I think it highly probable it may be the source of that disease.

In this Dairy Country a great number of Cows are kept[7], and the

* The late Mr. John Hunter proved, by experiments, that the Dog is the Wolf in a degenerated state.

---

[1] "*deviations.*" MS. [2] "*seem.*" MS. [3] "*accompanied at its commencement with small cracks or fissures.*" 3rd ed. [4] "*a limpid fluid.*" 3rd ed. [5] ". *It is*" (MS.), or ". *This fluid seems*" (3rd ed.). [6] Omit. 3rd ed. [7] ". *The office of milking is here.*" MS.

office of milking is" performed indiscriminately by [1]—" Men and Maid Servants. One of the former having [2]—" been appointed to apply dressings to the heels of a Horse affected with *the* [3]*Grease*," and not paying due attention to cleanliness, incautiously bears his part in milking the Cows, with some particles of the infectious matter adhering to his fingers. [4]When this is the case," it [5]commonly" happens that a disease is communicated to the Cows, and from the Cows to the Dairy-maids, which [6]—" spreads [7]through the farm" until most of the cattle and domestics [8]—" feel its unpleasant consequences. [9]This disease has obtained the name of the Cow Pox." It [10]—" appears on the nipples of the Cows in the form of [11]irregular" pustules. [12]At their first appearance they are" commonly of a palish blue, or rather of a colour somewhat approaching to livid, and are [13]— surrounded by [14]—" an [15]erysipelatous" inflammation. These pustules, unless a timely remedy be applied, [16]frequently" degenerate into phagedenic ulcers, which prove extremely troublesome.* The animals become indisposed, and the secretion of milk is much lessened. [17]Inflamed spots now begin to appear" on different parts of the hands of the domestics employed in milking, and sometimes on the wrists, which [18]quickly" run on to suppuration, first assuming the appearance of the small vesications produced by a burn. Most commonly they appear [19]about" the joint of the fingers, and at their extremities; but whatever parts are affected, if the situation will admit, these superficial suppurations put on a circular form, with their edges more elevated than their centre, and of a colour distantly approaching to blue. Absorption takes place, and tumours appear in each axilla. The system becomes affected—the pulse is [20]—" quickened; [21]and shiverings, with" general lassitude and pains about the loins and limbs, with vomiting, come on. The head is painful, and the patient is now and then even affected with delirium. [22]—" These

* They who attend sick cattle in this country find a speedy remedy for stopping the progress of this complaint in those applications which act chemically upon the morbid matter, such as the solutions of the Vitriolum Zinci, the Vitriolum Cupri, etc. [23]—"

---

[1] "*both.*" MS. [2] "*perhaps.*" MS. [3] "*malady I have mentioned.*" 3rd ed. [4] "*Should this be the case.*" MS. [5] "*frequently.*" 3rd ed. [6] "*pretty rapidly.*" MS. [7] Omit. MS. [8] "*of the farm.*" MS. [9] Omit. MS. [10] "*first.*" MS. [11] "*distinct.*" MS. [12] "*They are seldom white, but more.*" MS. [13] "*generally.*" MS. [14] "*more or less of.*" MS. [15] Omit. 3rd ed. [16] "*are much disposed to.*" MS. [17] "*Several inflamed spots appear.*" MS. [18] Omit. 3rd ed. [19] "*on.*" MS. [20] "*much.*" MS. [21] "*shiverings succeeded by heat.*" 3rd ed. [22] "*It will appear in the sequel that these symptoms arise principally from the irritation of the sores, and not from the primary action of the vaccine virus upon the constitution.*" Foot-note 3rd ed. [23] [The foot-note commencing on page 9 is a continuation, in the MS., of this foot-note.—E.M.C.]

symptoms, varying in their degrees of violence, [1]—" generally continue from one day to three or four, leaving ulcerated sores about the hands, which, from the sensibility of the parts, are very troublesome, and [2]commonly heal slowly," frequently becoming phagedenic, like those from whence they sprung. [3]The" lips, nostrils, eyelids, and other parts of the body, are sometimes affected with sores; but these [4]evidently" arise from their being [5]needlessly" rubbed or scratched with the patient's infected fingers. No eruptions on the skin have followed the decline of the feverish symptoms in any instance that has come under my inspection, one only excepted, and in this [6]case" a very few appeared on the arms: they were [7]very minute," of a vivid red colour, and soon died away without advancing to maturation; so that I cannot determine whether they had any connection with the preceding symptoms. [8]—"

Thus the disease makes its progress from the Horse [9]—" to the nipple of the Cow, and from the Cow to the Human Subject.

Morbid matter of various kinds, when absorbed into the system, may produce effects in some degree similar; but what renders the Cow-pox virus so extremely singular, is, that the person who has been thus affected is for ever after secure from the infection of the Small Pox; neither exposure to the variolous effluvia, nor the insertion of the matter into the skin, producing this [10]distemper."

In support of [11]so extraordinary a fact, I shall lay before my Reader a great number of instances." *

* [12]It" is [13]necessary to observe, that pustulous sores frequently appear spontaneously" on the nipples of [14]—" Cows, and instances have occurred, though [15]very" rarely, of the hands of the servants employed in milking being affected with sores in consequence, and even of their feeling an indisposition from absorption. [16]—" [17]These pustules are of a much milder nature than those which arise from that contagion which constitutes the true Cow Pox. They are always free from the bluish or livid tint so conspicuous in the pustules in that disease. No erysipelas attends them, nor do they shew any phagedenic disposition as in the other case, but quickly terminate in a scab without creating any apparent disorder in the Cow." This complaint appears at various seasons of the year, but most commonly in the Spring, when the Cows are first taken from their winter food and fed with grass. It is very

---

[1] "(*for they rarely attack so severely*)." MS. [2] Read after *sprung*. MS. [3] "*During the progress of the disease, the.*" 3rd ed. [4] Omit. MS. [5] "*heedlessly.*" MS., and Corrigenda of 1st ed. [6] Omit. MS. [7] Read after *colour*. MS. [8] "*but am induced to think they had not.*" MS. [9] "*as I conceive.*" 3rd ed. [10] "*malady.*" MS. [11] "*this assertion I shall produce many instances. I* could *produce a great number more, but the following, I presume, will be fully sufficient to establish the fact very satisfactorily.*" [The words "*very satisfactorily*" are added in a different handwriting, and "*to the satisfaction of this very learned body*" deleted.—E.M.C.] MS. [12] "*But first it.*" 3rd ed. [This foot-note is incorporated in the text.—E.M.C.] [13] "*of importance to remark that there are other causes besides contagious matter which produce pustules and sometimes ulcerations.*" MS. [14] "*the.*" MS., and 3rd ed. [15] Omit: *though rarely* is deleted. MS. [16] "*But instances are very rare.*" MS. [17] Omit. MS.

CASE I.

JOSEPH MERRET, now an Under Gardener to the Earl of Berkeley, lived as a Servant with a Farmer near [1]this place" in the year 1770, and occasionally assisted in milking his master's cows. Several horses belonging to the farm began to have sore heels, which Merret frequently attended. The cows [2]soon" became affected with the Cow Pox, and [3]soon" after several sores [4]appeared on" his hands. Swellings and stiffness in each axilla followed, and he was so much indisposed for several days as to be incapable of pursuing his ordinary employment. [5]Previously to the appearance of the distemper among the cows there was no fresh cow brought into the farm, nor any servant employed who was affected with the Cow Pox."

In April, 1795, a general inoculation taking place here, Merret was inoculated with his family; so that a period of twenty-five years had elapsed from his having the Cow Pox to this time. However, though the variolous matter was repeatedly inserted into his arm, [6]I found it impracticable to infect him" with it; an efflorescence only, taking on an erysipelatous look about the centre, appearing on the skin near the punctured parts. During the whole time that his family had the Small Pox, one of whom had it very full, he remained in the house with them, but received no injury from exposure to the contagion.

It [7]is" necessary to observe, [8]that the utmost care was taken to ascertain, with the most scrupulous precision, that no one whose case is here adduced had gone through the Small Pox previous to these attempts to produce that disease."

[9]Had these experiments been conducted in a large city, or in a populous neighbourhood, some doubts might have been entertained; but here, where population is thin, and where such an event as a person's having had the Small Pox is always

apt to appear also when they are suckling their young. But this disease is not to be considered as [10]similar in any respect to" that of which I am treating, as it is incapable of producing any specific effects on the human Constitution. [11]However, it is of the greatest consequence to point it out here, lest the want of discrimination should" occasion an idea of security from the infection of the Small Pox, which [12]might" prove delusive.

---

[1] or "*Berkeley.*" MS. [2] or "*presently.*" MS. [3] or "*presently.*" [4] "*began to appear upon.*" [5] Omit. MS. [6] "*he could not be infected.*" MS. [7] "*may be.*" MS. [8] "*it was clearly ascertained previous to this attempt to produce the disease, that neither this patient or any other whose case is here represented ever had the Small Pox.*" MS. [9] Omit. MS. [10] "*as having any kind of connection with.*" MS. [11] "*This distinction between the two diseases becomes the more important as the want of it might.*" MS. [12] "*would.*" MS.

faithfully recorded, no risk of inaccuracy in this particular can arise."

CASE II.

SARAH PORTLOCK, of this place, was infected with the Cow Pox, when a Servant at a Farmer's in the neighbourhood, twenty-seven years ago.*

In the year 1792, conceiving herself, from this circumstance, secure from the infection of the Small Pox, she nursed one of her own children who had accidentally caught the disease, but no indisposition ensued [1]—".—During the time she remained in the infected room, variolous matter was inserted into both her arms, but without any further effect than in the preceding case.

CASE III.

JOHN PHILLIPS, a Tradesman of this town, had the Cow Pox at so early a period as nine years of age. At the age of sixty-two I inoculated him, and was very careful in selecting matter in its most active state. [2]—" It was taken from the arm of a boy just before the commencement of the eruptive fever, and instantly inserted. It very speedily produced a sting-like feel in the part. An efflorescence appeared, which on the fourth day was rather extensive, and some degree of pain and stiffness were felt about the shoulder; but on the fifth day these symptoms began to disappear, and in a day or two after went entirely off, without producing any effect on the system.

CASE IV.

MARY BARGE, of Woodford, in this parish, was inoculated with variolous matter in the year 1791. An efflorescence of a palish red colour soon appeared about the parts where the matter

* [3]I have purposely selected several cases in which the disease had appeared at a very distant period previous to the experiments made with variolous matter, to shew that the change produced in the constitution is not affected by time."

---

[1] "*in consequence*." [2] [The paragraph beginning *I have often* (p. 28) . . . . down to *skin* (p. 29) is a foot-note in the MS., which is referred to after the word *state*.—E.M.C.] [3] Omit. MS.

was inserted, and spread itself rather extensively, but died away in a few days without producing any variolous symptoms.* She has since been repeatedly employed as a nurse to Small-pox patients, without experiencing any ill consequences. This woman had the Cow Pox when she lived in the service of a Farmer [1]in this parish" thirty-one years before.

[2]—" CASE V.

MRS. H——, a respectable Gentlewoman of this town, had the [3]Cow Pox" when very young. [4]She received the infection in [5]rather an uncommon manner": it was given by means of her handling some of the same utensils † which were in use among the servants of the family, who had the disease from milking infected cows." [6]Her hands had many of the Cow-pox sores upon them, and they were communicated to her nose, which became inflamed and very much swoln." Soon after this event Mrs. H—— was exposed to the contagion of the Small Pox, where it was scarcely possible for her to have escaped, [7]—" had she been susceptible of it, as she regularly attended a relative who had the disease in so violent a degree that it proved fatal to him.

In the year 1778 the Small Pox [8]prevailed" very much at Berkeley, and Mrs. H—— not feeling perfectly satisfied respecting her safety (no indisposition having followed her exposure to the Small Pox) I inoculated her with active variolous matter. The same appearance followed as in the preceding cases—an efflorescence on the arm without any effect on the constitution.

* It is remarkable that variolous matter, when the system is disposed to reject it, should [9]excite" inflammation on the part to which it is applied more speedily than when it produces the Small Pox. Indeed it becomes almost a criterion by which we can determine whether the infection will be received or not. It seems as if a change, which endures through life, had been produced in the action, or disposition to action, in the vessels of the skin; and it is remarkable too, that whether this change has been effected by the Small Pox, or [10]—" the Cow Pox, [11]that" the disposition to sudden cuticular inflammation is the same on the application of variolous matter.

† [12]When the Cow Pox has prevailed in the dairy, it has often been communicated to those who have not milked the cows, by the handle of the milk pail.

---

[1] Omit. MS. [2] "*I believe it to be very rare for one individual accidentally to communicate Cow Pox to another. My notes furnish me with one instance only.*" MS. [3] "*complaint*" or "*disease.*" MS. [4] Omit. MS. [5] Omit. 3rd ed. [6] "*Her hands were extremely sore, and her nose was inflamed and very much swoln. It was communicated by some of the servants of the Family (who were infected by Cows), and certainly by contact, probably by her handling some of the same family utensils.*" MS. [7] "*it.*" MS. [8] "*prevailing.*" MS. [9] "*incite.*" MS. [10] "*by.*" MS. [11] Omit. MS. [12] Omit. MS.

CASE VI.

IT is a fact so well known among our Dairy Farmers, that those who have had the Small Pox either escape the Cow Pox or are disposed to have it slightly; that as soon as the complaint shews itself among the cattle, assistants are procured, if possible, [1]who are thus rendered less susceptible of it," otherwise the business of the farm could scarcely go forward.

In the month of May, 1796, the Cow Pox broke out at Mr. Baker's, a Farmer who lives near this place. The disease was communicated by means of a cow which was purchased in an infected state at a neighbouring fair, and not one of the Farmer's cows (consisting of thirty) which [2]were" at that time milked escaped the contagion. The family consisted of a man servant, two dairymaids, and a servant boy, who, with the Farmer himself, were twice a day employed in milking the cattle. The whole of this family, except Sarah Wynne, one of the dairymaids, had gone through the Small Pox. The consequence was, that the Farmer and the servant boy escaped the infection of the Cow Pox entirely, and the servant man and one of the [3]maid servants" had each of them nothing more than a sore on one of their fingers, which [4]produced no" disorder in the system. But the other dairymaid, Sarah Wynne, who never had the Small Pox, did not escape in [5]so easy a" manner. She caught the complaint from the cows, and was affected with [6]the symptoms described in the 8th page" in so violent a degree, that she was [7]confined to her bed, and rendered incapable for several days of pursuing her ordinary vocations in the farm."

March 28th, 1797, I inoculated this girl, [8]and carefully rubbed" the variolous matter into two slight incisions made upon the left arm. A little inflammation appeared in the usual manner around the parts where the matter was inserted, but so early as the fifth day it vanished entirely without producing any effect on the system.

CASE VII.

ALTHOUGH the preceding history pretty clearly evinces that the constitution is far less susceptible of the contagion of the Cow Pox after it has felt that of the Small Pox, and although in general,

---

[1] "*who are in that situation.*" MS. [2] "*was.*" MS. [3] "*maids.*" MS. [4] "*did not produce the least.*" MS. [5] "*this easy.*" MS. [6] "*it.*" MS. [7] "*incapable of doing any work for the space of ten days.*" MS. [8] "*by carefully rubbing.*" MS

as I have observed, they who have had the Small Pox, and [1]are employed in milking" cows which are infected with the Cow Pox, either escape [2]the disorder," or have sores on the hands [3]—" without feeling any general indisposition, yet [4]—" the animal economy is subject to some variation in this respect[5], which the following relation will point out:"

In the summer of the year 1796 the Cow Pox appeared at the Farm of Mr. Andrews, a considerable dairy adjoining to the town of Berkeley. It was communicated, as in the preceding instance, by an infected cow purchased at a fair in the neighbourhood. The family consisted of the Farmer, his wife, two sons, a man and a maid servant; all of whom, except the Farmer (who was fearful of the [6]consequences"), bore a part in milking the cows. The whole of them, exclusive of the man servant, had regularly gone through the Small Pox; but in this case no one who milked the cows escaped the [7]contagion." All of them had sores upon their hands, and some degree of general indisposition, preceded by [8]pains" and tumours in the axillæ: but there was no comparison in the severity of the disease as it was felt by the servant man, who had escaped the Small Pox, and by those of the family who had not, for, while he was confined to his bed, they were able, without much inconvenience, to [9]follow" their ordinary business.

February the 13th, 1797, I availed myself of an opportunity of inoculating William Rodway, the servant man above alluded to. Variolous matter was inserted into both his arms; in the right by means of [10]superficial incisions," and into the left by [11]slight punctures into the cutis." Both were perceptibly inflamed on the third day. After this the inflammation about the punctures soon died away, but a small appearance of erysipelas was manifest about the edges of the [12]incisions" till the eighth day, when a little uneasiness was felt for the space of half an hour in the [13]right axilla." The inflammation then hastily disappeared without producing the most distant mark of affection of the system.

CASE VIII.

ELIZABETH WYNNE, aged fifty-seven, lived as a servant with a neighbouring Farmer thirty-eight years ago. She was then

---

[1] "*milk.*" MS. [2] "*disorder.*" MS. [3] "*only.*" MS. [4] "*the following narration is inserted to shew that.*" MS. [5]. and omit. MS. [6] "*consequence.*" MS. [7] "*infection.*" MS. [8] "*pair.*" MS. [9] "*pursue.*" MS. [10] "*a slight incision.*" MS. [11] "*punctures.*" MS. [12] "*incision.*" MS. [13] "*axilla.**

* Foot-note.—*Variolous matter inserted into the arms of those who have had the Small Pox will often produce sudden inflammation, with a little pain and stiffness in the axilla.*" MS.

a dairymaid, and the Cow Pox broke out among the cows. She caught the disease with the rest of the family, but, compared with them, had it in a very slight degree, one very small sore only breaking out [1]on" the little finger of her [2]left hand," and scarcely any perceptible indisposition following [3]it."

As the malady had shewn itself in so slight a manner, and as it had taken place at so distant a period of her life, I was happy with the opportunity of trying the effects of variolous matter upon her constitution, and on the 28th of March, 1797, I inoculated her by making two superficial incisions on the left arm, on which the matter was cautiously rubbed. A little efflorescence soon appeared, and a tingling sensation was felt about the parts [4]where the matter was inserted" until the third day, when both began to subside, and so early as the fifth day it was evident that no indisposition would follow.

CASE IX.

ALTHOUGH the Cow Pox shields the constitution from the Small Pox, and the Small Pox proves a protection against its own future poison, yet it appears that the human body is again and again susceptible of the infectious matter of the Cow Pox, as the following history will demonstrate:

William Smith, of Pyrton in this parish, contracted this disease when he lived with a neighbouring Farmer in the year 1780. One of the horses belonging to the farm had sore heels, and it fell to [5]his" lot to attend him. By these means the infection was carried to the cows, and from the cows it was communicated to Smith. [6]On one" of his hands [7]were" several ulcerated sores, and [8]he was affected" with such symptoms as have been before described.

In the year 1791 the Cow Pox broke out at another farm where he then lived [9]as a servant," and he became affected with it a second time; and in the year 1794 he was so unfortunate as to catch it again. The disease was equally as severe the second and third time as it was on the first.*

In the spring of the year 1795 he was twice inoculated, but no

* This is not the case in general—a second attack is commonly very slight, and so, I am informed, it is among the cows. [10]—"

[1] "*upon.*" MS. [2] "*hand.*" MS. [3] Omit. MS. [4] Omit. MS. [5] "*Smith's.*" MS. [6] "*One.*" MS. [7] "*had.*" MS. [8] "*he became very ill.*" MS. [9] Omit. MS. [10] "*The reader will find further observations on this subject in the sequel. These repeated indispositions must have arisen from the local irritation, and not from the specific action of the vaccine virus.*" 3rd ed.

affection of the system could be produced from the variolous matter; and he has since associated with those who had the Small Pox in its most contagious state without feeling any effect from it.

CASE X.

[illegible] lived as a servant with Mr. Bromedge, [illegible] on his own farm[illegible] in this parish, in the [illegible] was employed in applying dressings to the sore [illegible] of his master's horses, and at the same time assisted [illegible] The cows became affected in consequence, but [illegible] shew itself on their nipples till several weeks [illegible] to dress the horse. He quitted Mr. Bromedge's [illegible] another farm without any sores upon him: [illegible] began to be affected in the common way, [illegible] indisposed with the usual symptoms. Con-[illegible] of the malady from Mr. Cole, his new master, [illegible] employed in milking, the Cow Pox was [illegible] the cows.

[illegible] Nichols was employed in a farm where [illegible], [illegible] I inoculated him with several [illegible] he continued during the whole time of [illegible] arm was inflamed, but neither the inflam-[illegible] with the inoculated family produced the [illegible]

CASE XI.

[illegible] was a fellow servant with Nichols [illegible] at the time the cattle had the Cow Pox, [illegible] infected by them. His left hand was [illegible] several corroding ulcers, and a tumour [illegible] appeared in the axilla of that side. His [illegible] small sore upon it, and no [illegible]sore[illegible] [illegible] corresponding axilla.

[illegible] was inoculated with variolous [illegible] ensued beyond a little inflamma-[illegible] A large party were inoculated [illegible] whom had the disease in a more [illegible] commonly seen from inoculation. He [illegible] but could not receive the Small

[illegible] "hand," MS. [illegible] "The." MS.
[illegible] paper, but were inserted afterwards.—

During the sickening of some of his companions, their symptoms so strongly recalled to his mind his own state when sickening with the Cow Pox, that he very pertinently remarked their striking similarity.

CASE XII.

THE Paupers of the village of Tortworth, in this county, were inoculated by Mr. Henry Jenner, Surgeon, of Berkeley, in the year 1795. Among them, eight patients presented themselves who had at different periods of their lives had the Cow Pox. One of them, Hester Walkley, I attended with that disease when she lived in the service of a Farmer in the same village in the year 1782; but neither this woman, nor any other of the patients who had gone through the Cow Pox, received the variolous infection either from the arm or from mixing in the society of the other patients who were inoculated at the same time. This state of security proved a fortunate circumstance, as many of the poor women were at the same time in a state of pregnancy.]

[1]CASE XIII.

One instance has occurred to me of the system being affected from the matter issuing from the heels of horses, and of its remaining afterwards unsusceptible of the variolous contagion; another, where the Small Pox [2]appeared obscurely"; and a third, in which its complete existence was positively ascertained.

First, THOMAS PEARCE, [3]is" the son of a Smith and Farrier near to this place. He never had the Cow Pox; but, in consequence of dressing horses with sore heels at his father's, when a lad, he had sores on his fingers which suppurated, and which occasioned a pretty severe indisposition. Six years afterwards I inserted variolous matter into his arm repeatedly, without being able to produce anything more than slight inflammation, which appeared very soon after the matter was applied, and afterwards I exposed him to the contagion of the Small Pox with as little effect.*

[4]CASE XIV.

Secondly, Mr. JAMES COLE, a Farmer in this parish, had a disease from the same source as related in the preceding case, and

* It is a remarkable fact, and well known to many, that we are frequently foiled in our endeavours to communicate the Small Pox by inoculation to blacksmiths, [5]who in the country are" farriers. They often, as in the above instance, either resist the contagion entirely, or have the disease anomalously. [6]Shall we not" be able [7]now" to account for this on a rational principle[8]?"

[1] [Case XI. in the original paper.—E.M.C.] [2] "*obscurely appeared.*" MS. [3] "*was.*" MS. [4] [Case XII. in the original paper.—E.M.C.] [5] "*and.*" MS. [6] "*We shall now, I presume.*" MS. [7] Omit. MS. [8] ". " MS

some years after was inoculated with variolous matter. He had a little pain in the axilla, and felt a slight indisposition for three or four hours. A few eruptions shewed themselves on the forehead, but they very soon disappeared without advancing [1]"to" maturation.

[2]CASE XV.

Although in the two former instances the system seemed to be secured, or nearly so, from variolous infection, by the absorption of matter from sores produced by the diseased heels of horses, yet the following case [3]"decisively proves" that this cannot be entirely relied upon, until a disease has been generated by the morbid matter from the horse on the nipple of the cow, and passed through that medium to the human subject. [4]–"

Mr. ABRAHAM RIDDIFORD, a Farmer at Stone in this parish, in consequence of dressing a mare that had sore heels, was affected with very painful sores in both [5]–" his hands, tumours in each axilla, and severe and general indisposition. A Surgeon in the neighbourhood attended him, who[6], knowing the similarity between the appearance of the sores upon his hands and those produced by the Cow Pox, and being acquainted also with the effects of that disease on the human constitution," [7] assured him that he [8]–" never need to fear the infection of the Small Pox; but this assertion proved fallacious, for, on being exposed to the infection upwards of twenty years afterwards, he caught the disease, which took its regular course in a very mild way. There certainly was a difference perceptible, although [9]"it is" not easy to describe [10]"it," in the general appearance of the pustules from that which we commonly see. Other practitioners, [10]"who visited the patient at my request," agreed with me in this point, though there was no room left for suspicion as to the reality of the disease, as I inoculated some of his family from the pustules, who had the Small Pox, [11]"with its usual appearances," in consequence.

[12]CASE XVI.

SARAH NELMES, a dairymaid at a Farmer's near this place, was infected with the Cow Pox from her master's cows in May, 1796. She received the infection on a part of the hand which

[1] "towards." MS. [2] (Case XIII in the original paper.—E.M.C.) [3] "renders it probable" 3rd ed. [4] Footnote.—"The succeeding part will give further explanations of this subject." 3rd ed. [5] "of" MS. [6] Omit. MS. [7] "would derive one great benefit from his present situation that he." MS. [8] Omit. MS. [9] Omit. MS. [10] "whom I requested to visit the Patient with me." MS. [11] Omit. MS. [12] (The case of Sarah Nelmes is only alluded to, but not described, in the original paper.—E.M.C.)

had been previously in a slight degree injured by a scratch from a thorn. A large pustulous sore and the usual symptoms accompanying the disease were produced in consequence. The pustule was so expressive of the true character of the Cow Pox, as it commonly appears upon the hand, that I have given a representation of it in the annexed plate. The two small pustules on the wrists arose also from the application of the virus to some minute abrasions of the cuticle, but the livid tint, if they ever had any, was not conspicuous at the time I saw the patient. The pustule on the forefinger shews the disease in an earlier stage. It did not actually appear on the hand of this young woman, but was taken from that of another, and is annexed for the purpose of representing the malady after it has newly appeared.]

[1]CASE XVII.

THE more accurately to observe the progress of the infection, I selected a healthy boy,[2] about eight years old, for [3]the purpose of inoculation for the Cow Pox." The matter was taken from a [4]—" sore on the hand of a dairymaid,* who was infected by her master's cows, and it was inserted, on the 14th of May, 1796, into the arm of the boy by means of two superficial incisions, [5]barely penetrating the cutis, each about half an inch long."

On the seventh day he complained of uneasiness in the axilla, and on the ninth he became a little chilly, lost his appetite, and had a slight head-ach. During the whole of this day he was perceptibly indisposed, and [6]spent the night with some degree of restlessness," but on the day following he was perfectly well.

The appearance [7]of the incisions in their progress" to a state of maturation were [8]—" much the same as when produced in a similar manner by variolous matter. [9]—" The only difference which I perceived was, [10]in the state of the limpid fluid arising from the action of the virus, which" assumed rather a darker hue, and [11]in that of" the efflorescence spreading round the incisions, [12]which had more" of an erysipelatous look than we commonly

* From the sore on the hand of Sarah Nelmes.—See the preceding case and the plate.*

[1] [Case XIV. in the original paper.—E.M.C.] [2] [James Phipps. Baron's *Life of Jenner*, vol. i., p. 137.—E.M.C.] [3] "*INOCULATION OF THE COW POX.*" 3rd ed. [4] "*suppurated.*" MS. [5] "*each about three-quarters of an inch long.*" MS. [6] "*had rather a restless night.*" MS. [7] "*and progress of the incisions.*" MS. [8] "*pretty.*" MS. [9] "*This appearance was in great measure new to me, and I ever shall recollect the pleasing sensations it excited; as, from its similarity to the pustule produced by variolous inoculation, it incontestably pointed out the close connection between the two diseases, and almost anticipated the result of my future experiments.*" Foot-note in 3rd ed. [10] "*that the edges.*" MS. [11] "*that.*" MS. [12] "*took on rather more.*" MS. * [Vol. I., Plate II.]

[illegible]

[illegible]

[illegible]

[illegible]

with that malady. Wherret never had had the Small-pox. Haynes was daily employed as one of the milkers at the farm, and the disease began to shew itself among the cows about ten days after he first assisted in washing the mare's heels. Their nipples became sore in the usual way, with bluish pustules; but as remedies were early applied they did not ulcerate to any extent.

CASE XVIII.

JOHN BAKER, a child of five years old, was inoculated March 16, 1798, with matter taken from a pustule on the hand of Thomas Virgoe, one of the servants who had been infected from the mare's heels. He became ill on the sixth day with symptoms similar to those excited by Cow-pox matter. On the 8th day he was free from indisposition.

There was some variation in the appearance of the pustule on the arm. Although it somewhat resembled a Small-pox pustule, yet its similitude was not so conspicuous as when excited by matter from the nipple of the cow, or when the matter has passed from thence through the medium of the human subject.—(See Vol. I., Plate IV.)

This experiment was made to ascertain the progress and subsequent effects of the disease when thus propagated. We have seen that the virus from the horse, when it proves infectious to the human subject, is not to be relied upon as rendering the system secure from variolous infection, but that the matter produced by it upon the nipple of the cow is perfectly so. Whether its passing from the horse through the human constitution, as in the present instance, will produce a similar effect, remains to be decided. This would now have been effected, but the boy was rendered unfit for inoculation from having felt the effects of a contagious fever in a work-house, soon after this experiment was made.[1]

CASE XIX.

WILLIAM SUMMERS, a child of five years and a half old, was inoculated the same day with Baker, with matter taken from the nipples of one of the infected cows, at the farm alluded to in page 20. He became indisposed on the 6th day, vomited once, and felt the usual slight symptoms till the 8th day, when he appeared perfectly well. The progress of the pustule formed by the infection of the virus was similar to that noticed in Case XVII., with this exception, its being free from the livid tint observed in that instance.

CASE XX.

FROM William Summers the disease was transferred to William Pead, a boy of eight years old, who was inoculated March 28th. On the 6th day he complained of pain in the

[1] [See foot-note on p. 169.—E.M.C.]

axilla, and on the 9th was affected with the common symptoms of a patient sickening with the Small-pox from inoculation, which did not terminate till the 3d day after the seizure. So perfect was the similarity to the variolous fever that I was induced to examine the skin, conceiving there might have been some eruptions, but none appeared. The efflorescent blush around the part punctured in the boy's arm was so truly characteristic of that which appears on variolous inoculation, that I have given a representation of it. The drawing was made when the pustule was beginning to die away, and the "areola"[1] retiring from the centre.—See Vol. I., Plate V.

CASE XXI.

APRIL 5th. Several children and adults were inoculated from the arm of William Pead. The greater part of them sickened on the 6th day, and were well on the 7th, but in three of the number a secondary indisposition arose in consequence of an extensive erysipelatous inflammation which appeared on the inoculated arms. It seemed to arise from the state of the pustule, which spread out, accompanied with some degree of pain, to about half the diameter of a six-pence. One of these patients was an infant of half a year old. By the application of mercurial ointment to the inflamed parts (a treatment recommended under similar circumstances in the inoculated Small-pox) the complaint subsided without giving much trouble.

HANNAH EXCELL an healthy girl of seven years old, and one of the patients above mentioned, received the infection from the insertion of the virus under the cuticle of the arm in three distinct points.[2] The pustules which arose in consequence, so much resembled, on the 12th day, those appearing from the insertion of variolous matter, that an experienced Inoculator would scarcely have discovered a shade of difference at that period. Experience now tells me that almost the only variation which follows consists in the pustulous fluids remaining limpid nearly to the time of its total disappearance; and not, as in the direct Small-pox, becoming purulent.—(See Vol. I., Plate VI.)

CASE XXII.

FROM the arm of this girl matter was taken and inserted April 12th into the arms of John Marklove, one year and a half old,

Robert F. Jenner, eleven months old,
Mary Pead, 5 years old, and
Mary James, 6 years old.

Among these Robert F. Jenner did not receive the infection. The arms of the other three inflamed properly and began to affect the system in the usual manner; but being under some

[1] "*areola*" [italics]. 3rd ed. [2] "*This was not done intentionally, but from the accidental touch of the point of the lancet, one puncture being always sufficient.*" Footnote 3rd ed.

apprehensions from the preceding Cases that a troublesome erysipelas might arise, I determined on making an experiment with the view of cutting off its source. Accordingly [1]—' after the patients had felt an indisposition [2]—" of about twelve hours, I applied in two of these Cases out of the three, on the vesicle formed by the virus, a little mild caustic, composed of equal parts of quick-lime and soap, and suffered it to remain on the part six hours.* It seemed to give the children but little uneasiness, and effectually answered my intention in preventing the appearance of erysipelas. Indeed it seemed to do more, for in half an hour after its application, the indisposition of the children ceased.† These precautions were perhaps unnecessary, as the arm of the third child, Mary Pead, which was suffered to take its common course, scabbed quickly, without any erysipelas. [3]—"

CASE XXIII.

FROM this child's arm matter was taken and transferred to that of J. Barge, a boy of seven years old. He sickened on the 8th day, went through the disease with the usual slight symptoms, and without any inflammation on the arm beyond the common efflorescence surrounding the pustule, an appearance so often seen in inoculated Small-pox.

After the many fruitless attempts to give the Small-pox to those who had had the Cow-pox, it did not appear necessary, nor was it convenient to me, to inoculate the whole of those who had been the subjects of these late trials; yet I thought it right to see the effects of variolous matter on some of them, particularly William Summers, the first of these patients who had been infected with matter taken from the cow. He was therefore inoculated with variolous matter from a fresh pustule; but, as in the preceding Cases, the system did not feel the effects of it in the smallest degree. I had an opportunity also of having this boy [4]—" and William Pead inoculated by my Nephew, Mr. Henry Jenner, whose report to me is as follows: "I have inoculated Pead and Barge, two of the boys whom you lately infected with the Cow-pox. On the 2d day the incisions were inflamed and there was a pale inflammatory stain around them. On the 3d day these appearances were still increasing and their arms itched considerably. On the 4th day, the inflammation was evidently subsiding, and on the 6th it was scarcely perceptible. No symptom of indisposition followed.

* Perhaps a few touches with the lapis septicus would have proved equally efficacious.

† What effect would a similar treatment produce in inoculation for the Small-pox?

---

[1] "*on the eighth day.*" [2] "*that was just perceptible.*" [3] "*The subsequent part of this treatise will sufficiently show the proper practice in cases of inoculation of the inoculated arm.*" Foot-note 3rd ed. [4] "(*Barge*)." 3rd ed.

To convince myself that the variolous matter made use of was in a perfect state, I at the same time inoculated a patient with some of it who never had gone through the Cow-pox, and it produced the Small-pox in the usual regular manner."

These experiments afforded me much satisfaction; they proved that the matter in passing from one human subject to another, through five gradations, lost none of its original properties, J. Barge being the fifth who received the infection successively from William Summers, the boy to whom it was communicated from the cow.

[1]I shall now conclude this Inquiry with some general observations on the subject and on some others which are interwoven with it.]

Although I presume it may be unnecessary[2] to produce further testimony in support of my assertion "that the Cow-pox protects the human constitution from the infection of the Small-pox," [3]yet it affords me considerable satisfaction to say, that Lord Somerville, the President of the Board of Agriculture, to whom this paper was shewn by Sir Joseph Banks, has found upon inquiry that the statements were confirmed by the concurring testimony of Mr. Dolland, a surgeon, who resides in a dairy country remote from this, in which these observations were made. With respect to the opinion adduced "that the source of the infection is a peculiar morbid matter arising in the horse," although I have not been able to prove it from actual experiments conducted immediately under my own eye, yet the evidence I have adduced appears sufficient to establish it."

They who are not in the habit of conducting experiments may not be aware of the coincidence of circumstances necessary for their being managed so as to prove [3]perfectly" decisive; nor how often men engaged in professional [4]pursuits" are liable to interruptions which disappoint them almost at the instant of [5]their being accomplished."

[[6]However, I feel no room for hesitation respecting the common origin of the disease, being well convinced that it never appears among the cows (except it can be traced to a cow introduced among the general herd which has been previously infected, or to an infected servant), unless they have been milked by some one who, at the same time, has the care of a horse affected with diseased heels.

[1] "*I presume it would be swelling this paper to an unnecessary bulk were I.*" MS.
[2] "*I shall proceed then to offer a few general remarks upon the subject, and some others which are connected with it. Though I am myself perfectly convinced, from a great number of instances which have presented themselves, that the source of the Cow Pox is the morbid matter issuing from the newly diseased heels of horses, yet I could have wished, had circumstances allowed me, to have impressed this fact more strongly on the minds of my readers* ["*of this Society*" deleted.—E.M.C.] *by experiments.*" MS.
[3] Omit. MS. [4] "*employments.*" [5] "*completion.*" [6] Omit. MS.

> The spring of the year 1797, which I intended particularly to have devoted to the completion of this investigation, proved, from its dryness, remarkably adverse to my wishes; for it frequently happens, while the farmers' horses are exposed to the cold rains which fall at that season that their heels become diseased, and no Cow-pox then appeared in the neighbourhood."]

The active quality of the virus from the horses' heels is greatly increased after it has acted on the [1]nipples" of the cow, as it rarely happens that the horse affects his dresser with sores, and as rarely that a milk-maid escapes the infection when she milks infected cows. It is most active at the commencement of the disease, [2]even" before [3]it has acquired" a pus-like appearance; [4]—" [5]indeed I am not confident whether this property in the matter does not entirely cease as soon as it is secreted in the form of pus. I am induced to think it does cease,* and that it is the thin darkish-looking fluid only, oozing from the newly-formed cracks in the heels, similar to what sometimes appears from erysipelatous blisters, which gives the disease. Nor am I certain that the nipples of the cows are at all times in a state to receive the infection. The appearance of the disease in the spring and the early part of the summer, when they are disposed to be affected with spontaneous eruptions so much more frequently than at other seasons, induces me to think, that the virus from the horse must be received upon them when they are in this state, in order to produce effects: experiments, however, must determine these points. But it is clear that when the Cow-pox virus is once generated, that the cows cannot resist the contagion, in whatever state their nipples may chance to be, if they are milked with an infected hand."

Whether the matter, either from the cow or the horse, will affect the sound skin [6]of the human body, I cannot positively determine; probably it will not, unless on those parts" where the cuticle is extremely thin, as on the lips [7]for example. I have known an instance of a poor girl who produced an ulceration on her lip by frequently holding her finger to her mouth to cool the raging of a Cow-pox sore by blowing upon it. The

* It is very easy to procure pus from old sores on the heels of horses. This I have often inserted into scratches made with a lancet, on the sound nipples of cows, and have seen no other effects from it than simple inflammation.

[1] "*nipple.*" MS. [2] Deleted. MS. [3] "*it acquires.*" [4] "*After the disease has been of long continuance the matter ceases to produce specific effects.*" [5] Omit. MS. [6] "*I cannot determine, but am inclined to think it will not, excepting.*" MS. [7] ". *The hands of the farmers' servants in this neighbourhood, from the nature of their employments, are constantly exposed to those injuries which occasion abrasions of the cuticle, to punctures from thorns and such like accidents.*" MS.

hands of the farmers' servants here, from the nature of their employments, are constantly exposed to those injuries which occasion abrasions of the cuticle, to punctures from thorns and such like accidents; so that they are always in a state to feel the consequences of exposure to infectious matter."

[[1]It is singular to observe that the Cow-pox virus, although it renders the constitution unsusceptible of the variolous, should, nevertheless, leave it unchanged with respect to its own action. I have already produced an instance* to point out this, and shall now corroborate it with another.

Elizabeth Wynne, who had the Cow-pox in the year 1759, was inoculated with variolous matter, without effect, in the year 1797, and again caught the Cow-pox in the year 1798. When I saw her, which was on the 8th day after she received the infection, I found her affected with general lassitude, shiverings, alternating with heat, coldness of the extremities, and a quick and irregular pulse. These symptoms were preceded by a pain in the axilla. On her hand was one large pustulous sore, which resembled that delineated in Plate II." [2]—"]

It is curious [3]also" to observe, [4]that the virus, which with respect to its effects is undetermined and uncertain previously to its passing from the horse through the medium of the cow, [5]—" should then not only become more active, but should invariably and completely possess those specific properties" which induce in the human constitution symptoms similar to those of the variolous fever, and effect in it that peculiar change which for ever renders it unsusceptible of the variolous contagion.

May [6]it not, then, be reasonably conjectured, that the source of the Small Pox is morbid matter of a peculiar kind, generated by a disease in the horse," and that accidental circumstances may have again and again arisen, still working new changes upon it, until it has acquired the contagious and malignant form under which we now commonly see it making its devastations amongst us? And, from a consideration of the change which the infectious matter [7]undergoes from producing" a disease on the cow, may we not conceive that many contagious

* See Case IX.

[1] Omit. MS. [2] "*As I have before observed, these symptoms probably arose from the irritation of the sore, which was very painful.*" Foot-note, 3rd ed. [3] Omit. MS. [4] "*that this matter acquires new properties by passing from the horse through another medium, that of the cow; not only is its activity hereby increased, but those specific properties become unvariable.*" MS. [5] "*Further explanations will be adduced on this subject.*" Foot-note, 3rd ed. [6] "*we not then reasonably infer that the source of the Small Pox is the matter generated in the diseased foot of a Horse.*" MS. [7] "*from the Horse has undergone after it has produced.*" MS.

diseases, now prevalent among us, may owe their present appearance not to a simple, but to a compound origin? For example, is it [1]difficult″ to imagine that the measles, the scarlet fever, and the ulcerous sore throat with a spotted skin, have [2]all″ sprung from the same source, assuming some variety in their forms according to the nature of their new combinations? The same question will apply respecting the [3]origin of many other contagious diseases, which bear a strong analogy to each other.″

There [4]are″ certainly more forms than one, [5]without considering the common variation between the confluent and distinct,″ in which the Small-pox appears in what is called the natural way.—About seven years ago a species of Small-pox spread through [6]many″ of the towns and villages of this part of Gloucestershire: it was of so mild a nature, that a fatal instance was scarcely ever heard of, and consequently so little dreaded by [7]the lower orders″ of the community, that they scrupled not to hold the same intercourse with each other as if no infectious disease had been present among them. I never saw nor heard of an instance of its being confluent. [8]—″ The most accurate manner, perhaps, in which I can convey an idea of it is, by saying, that had fifty individuals been taken promiscuously and infected by exposure to this contagion, they would have had as mild and light a disease as if they had been inoculated with variolous matter in the usual way. The harmless manner in which it shewed itself could not arise from any peculiarity either in the season or the weather, for I watched its progress upwards of a year without perceiving any variation in its general appearance. I consider it then as a *variety* of the Small-pox.[9]*

[[10]In some of the preceding cases I have noticed the attention that was paid to the state of the variolous matter previous to the experiment of inserting it into the arms of those who had gone through the Cow-pox. This I conceived to be of great importance in conducting these experiments, and were it always properly attended to by those who inoculate for the Small-pox, it might prevent much subsequent mischief and confusion. With the view of enforcing so necessary a precaution, I shall

* [11]My friend Dr. Hicks, of Bristol, who during the prevalence of this distemper was resident at Gloucester, and Physician to the Hospital there, (where it was seen soon after its first appearance in this country) had opportunities of making numerous observations upon it, which it is his intention to communicate to the Public.

[1] "*hard.*" MS. [2] Omit. MS. [3] "*Yaws and the Syphilis, and indeed many other diseases.*" MS. [4] "*is.*" MS. [5] Omit. MS. [6] "*most.*" MS. [7] "*most.*" MS. [8] "*It obtained the name among the Nurses and the Common People (I know not why) of the* Swine or Pig Pox." [9] [For continuation of the original paper turn to p. 30.—E.M.C.] [10] Omit. MS. [11] Omit. MS.

take the liberty of digressing so far as to point out some unpleasant facts, relative to mismanagement in this particular, which have fallen under my own observation."]

[1]—"

A Medical Gentleman (now no more), [2]who for many years inoculated" in this neighbourhood, frequently preserved [3]the variolous" matter [4]intended for his use," on a piece of lint or cotton, which, in its [5]fluid" state was put into a vial, corked, [6]—" and conveyed into a warm pocket; a situation certainly favourable for [7]speedily" producing putrefaction in it. In this state (not unfrequently after it had been taken several days from the pustules) it was inserted into the arms of his patients, and brought on inflammation [8]of" the incised parts, swellings of the axillary glands, fever, and [9]sometimes eruptions." But what was this disease? Certainly not the Small-pox; for the matter having from putrefaction lost, [10]or suffered a derangement in" its specific properties, was no longer capable of producing that malady, [11]those" who had been inoculated in this manner [12]being" as much subject to the contagion of the Small-pox, as if they had never been under the influence of this artificial disease; and many, unfortunately, fell victims to it, who thought themselves in perfect security. The same unfortunate circumstance of giving a disease, supposed to be the Small-pox, with inefficaceous variolous matter, having occurred under the direction of some other practitioners [13]within my knowledge," and probably from the same incautious method of securing the variolous matter, I avail myself of this opportunity of mentioning what I conceive [14]to be" of great importance; and, as a further cautionary hint, I shall [15]again digress so far as to add" another observation on the subject of Inoculation.

Whether it be yet ascertained by experiment, that the quantity of variolous matter inserted into the skin makes any difference with respect to the subsequent mildness or violence of the disease, I know not; but I have the strongest reason for supposing that if either the punctures or incisions be made so deep as to go *through* it, and wound the adipose [16]membrane," that the risk of bringing on a violent disease is greatly increased. I have known an inoculator, whose practice was "to [17]cut" deep enough (to use

[1] "*I have often been a witness to very direful effects arising from the improper management of the variolous matter previous to its being used for the purpose of inoculation.*" Foot-note on folio 12. MS. [2] "*who inoculated great numbers.*" MS. [3] "*his.*" MS. [4] Omit. MS. [5] "*wet.*" MS. [6] "*up.*" MS. [7] Omit. MS. [8] "*in the.*" MS. [9] "*as I have been informed by the Patients themselves, eruptions.*" MS. [10] Omit. MS. [11] "*and they.*" MS. [12] "*were.*" MS. [13] Omit. MS. [14] "*as.*" MS. [15] "*take the liberty of adding.*" MS. [16] "*covering beneath.*" MS. [17] "*go.*" MS.

his own expression) to see a bit of fat," and there to lodge the matter. The great number of bad Cases, [1]independent of inflammations and abscesses on the arms," and the fatality which attended this practice was almost inconceivable; and I cannot account for it on any other principle than that of the matter being placed in this situation instead of the skin. [2]—"

[[3]It was the practice of another, whom I well remember, to pinch up a small portion of the skin on the arms of his patients and to pass through it a needle, with a thread attached to it previously dipped in variolous matter. The thread was lodged in the perforated part, and consequently left in contact with the cellular membrane. This practice was attended with the same ill success as the former. Although it is very improbable that any one would now inoculate in this rude way by design, yet these observations may tend to place a double guard over the lancet, when infants, whose skins are comparatively so very thin, fall under the care of the inoculator.

A very respectable friend of mine, Dr. Hardwicke, of Sodbury in this county, inoculated great numbers of patients previous to the introduction of the more [4]moderate" method by Sutton, and with such success, that a fatal instance occurred as rarely as since that method has been adopted. It was the doctor's practice to make as slight an incision as possible *upon* the skin, and there to lodge a thread saturated with the variolous matter. When his patients became indisposed, agreeably to the custom then prevailing, they were directed to go to bed and were kept moderately warm. Is it not probable then, that the success of the modern practice may depend more upon the method of invariably depositing the virus in or upon the skin, than on the subsequent treatment of the disease?

I do not mean to insinuate that exposure to cool air, and suffering the patient to drink cold water when hot and thirsty, may not moderate the eruptive symptoms and lessen the number of pustules; yet, to repeat my former observation, I cannot account for the uninterrupted success, or nearly so, of one practitioner, and the wretched state of the patients under the care of another, where, in both instances, the general treatment did not differ essentially, without conceiving it to arise from the different modes of inserting the matter for the purpose of producing the disease. As it is not the identical matter inserted which is absorbed into the constitution, but that which is, by some peculiar process in the animal economy, generated by it, is it not probable that different parts of the

---

[1] Omit. MS. [2] "*for let it be recollected that it is only from a different mode of receiving the infectious particles that the difference between inoculation and the natural Small Pox arises. Though it is very improbable that any one would inoculate in this way by design, yet this observation may tend to place a double guard over the Lance. when infants fall under the care of the inoculator, as the skin is comparatively so very thin. Query. In what manner is the Small Pox communicated in what is called the natural way?*" MS. [3] Omit. MS. [4] "*modern.*" Corrigenda, 1st ed.

human body may prepare or modify the virus differently? Although the skin, for example, adipose membrane, or mucous membranes are all capable of producing the variolous virus by the stimulus given by the particles originally deposited upon them, yet I am induced to conceive that each of these parts is capable of producing some variation in the qualities of the matter previous to its affecting the constitution. What else can constitute the difference between the Small-pox when communicated casually or in what has been termed the natural way, or when brought on artificially through the medium of the skin? After all, are the variolous particles, possessing their true specific and contagious principles, ever taken up and conveyed by the lymphatics unchanged into the blood vessels? I imagine not. Were this the case, should we not find the blood sufficiently loaded with them in some stages of the Small Pox to communicate the disease by inserting it under the cuticle, or by spreading it on the surface of an ulcer? Yet experiments have determined the impracticability of its being given in this way; although it has been proved that variolous matter when much diluted with water, and applied to the skin in the usual manner, will produce the disease. But it would be digressing beyond a proper boundary, to go minutely into this subject here."]

At what period the Cow-pox was first noticed here is not upon record. [1]Our oldest farmers were not unacquainted with it in their earliest days, when it appeared among their farms without any deviation from the phænomena which it now exhibits. Its connection with the Small-pox seems to have been unknown to them. Probably the general introduction of inoculation first occasioned the discovery.

Its" rise in this country may not have been of very remote date, as the practice of milking cows might formerly have been in the hands of women only; which I believe is the case now in some other dairy countries, and, consequently that the cows might not in former times have been exposed to the contagious matter brought by the men servants from the heels of horses.* Indeed [2]a knowledge of the source of the infection" is new in the minds of most of the farmers in this neighbourhood, but it has

* I have been informed from respectable authority that in Ireland, although dairies abound in many parts of the Island, the disease is entirely unknown. The reason seems obvious. The business of the dairy is conducted by women only. Were the meanest vassal among the men employed there as a milker at a dairy, he would feel his situation unpleasant beyond all endurance. [This foot-note is omitted from the 3rd ed.—E.M.C.]

[1] "*The oldest inhabitants among the farmers were not unacquainted with it in their earliest days, and have heard their forefathers speak of it, yet it is probable that its.*' MS. [2] "*the fact itself is that it.*" MS.

at length produced [1]good consequences; and it seems probable″ from the precautions they [2]are now″ disposed to adopt, [3]—″ that the appearance of the Cow-pox here may either be entirely extinguished or become extremely rare.

Should it be asked whether this [4]investigation″ [5]is″ a matter of mere curiosity, or whether it [6]tends″ to any beneficial purpose? I should answer, that notwithstanding the happy effects of Inoculation, with all the improvements which the practice has received since its [7]first″ introduction into this country, [8]it not very unfrequently produces deformity of the skin, and sometimes, under the best management, proves fatal.

These circumstances must naturally create in every instance some degree of painful solicitude for its consequences. But as I have never known fatal effects″ arise from the Cow-pox, even when impressed in the most unfavourable manner, [9]producing″ extensive inflammations and suppurations on the hands; and as it clearly appears that this disease leaves the constitution in a state of perfect security from the infection of the Small-pox, may we not infer that a mode of Inoculation [10]may″ be introduced preferable to that at present adopted, especially among those families, which, from previous circumstances, we may judge to be predisposed to have the disease unfavourably? It is an excess in the number of pustules which we chiefly dread in the Small-pox; but, in the Cow-pox, no pustules appear, nor does it seem possible for the contagious matter to produce the disease [11]from″ effluvia, or by any other means [12]than contact, and that probably not simply between the virus and the cuticle;″ so that a single individual in a family might at any time receive it without the risk of infecting the rest, or of spreading a [13]distemper″ that fills a country with terror.[14]—″

[1] "*conviction and probably.*" [2] "*now seem.*" MS. [3] ("*for a Farmer is not the most flexible of human beings.*") [4] "*Investigation, discovery.*" MS. [The word "investigation" is written over the word "discovery" in a different handwriting (Woodville's?).—E.M.C.] [5] "*be.*" 3rd ed. [6] "*tend.*" 3rd ed. [7] Omit. MS. [8] "*we sometimes observe it to prove fatal, and from this circumstance we feel at all times somewhat alarmed for its consequences. But as fatal effects have never been known to.*" MS. [9] "*that is, when it has accidentally produced.*" MS. [10] "*might.*" MS. [11] "*by.*" MS. [12] "*as I have before observed, than* contact." MS. [13] "*disease.*" MS. [14] "*Without further research I should therefore not in the least hesitate to inoculate Adults, and Children not very young, with the matter of Cow Pox in preference to common variolous matter. How far it may be admissible on the tender skins of infants further experiments must determine. I have no other scruples than such as arise from the darkish appearance of the edges of the incisions in the arm of the Boy whom I inoculated with this matter* (see p. 19), *the only experiment I had an opportunity of making in that way. But in this case the incisions, though perfectly superficial, were made to a much greater extent than was necessary for communicating the infection to the system. However, it proved of no consequence, as the arm never became painful, nor required any application. I shall endeavour still further to prosecute this Inquiry, an Inquiry I trust not merely speculative, but of sufficient moment to inspire the pleasing hope of its becoming essentially beneficial to Mankind.*" MS. [*End of the original paper.*—E.M.C.]

[Several instances have come under my observation which justify the assertion that the disease cannot be propagated by effluvia. The first boy whom I inoculated with the matter of Cow-pox, slept in a bed, while the experiment was going forward, with two children who never had gone through either that disease or the Small-pox, without infecting either of them.

A young woman who had the Cow-pox to a great extent, several sores which maturated having appeared on the hands and wrists, slept in the same bed with a fellow-dairymaid who never had been infected with either the Cow-pox or the Small-pox, but no indisposition followed.

Another instance has occurred of a young woman on whose hands were several large suppurations from the Cow Pox, who was at the same time a daily nurse to an infant, but the complaint was not communicated to the child.

In some other points of view, the inoculation of this disease appears preferable to the variolous inoculation.

In constitutions predisposed to scrophula, how frequently we see the inoculated Small-pox rouse into activity that distressful malady. This circumstance does not seem to depend on the manner in which the distemper has shewn itself, for it has as frequently happened among those who have had it mildly, as when it has appeared in the contrary way. There are many, who from some peculiarity in the habit resist the common effects of variolous matter inserted into the skin, and who are in consequence haunted through life with the distressing idea of being insecure from subsequent infection. A ready mode of dissipating anxiety originating from such a cause must now appear obvious. And, as we have seen that the constitution may at any time be made to feel the febrile attack of Cow Pox, might it not, in many chronic diseases, be introduced into the system, with the probability of affording relief, upon well-known physiological principles? [1]—"

Although I say the system may at any time be made to feel the febrile attack of Cow-pox, yet I have a single instance before me where the virus acted locally only, but it is not in the least probable that the same person would resist the action both of the Cow-pox virus and the variolous.

Elizabeth Sarsenet lived as a dairy maid at Newpark farm, in this parish. All the cows and the servants employed in milking had the Cow-pox; but this woman, though she had several sores upon her fingers, felt no tumours in the axillæ, nor any general indisposition. On being afterwards casually exposed to variolous infection, she had the Small-pox in a mild way. [2]—" —Hannah Pick, another of the dairy maids who was a fellow-servant with Elizabeth Sarsenet when the distemper broke out at the farm, was at the same time infected; but this young woman had not only sores upon her hands, but felt

[1] "*Inoculation, in a common way, upon the arm will seldom produce this effect. When the disease takes place among the dairy people, the virus comes in contact with pre-existing sores, which does not fail to produce an irritation that affects the system generally.*" Foot-note, 3rd ed. [2] "*This will be more satisfactorily explained in the sequel.*" Foot-note, 3rd ed.

herself also much indisposed for a day or two. After this, I made several attempts to give her the Small-pox by inoculation, but they all proved fruitless. From the former Case then we see that the animal economy is subject to the same laws in one disease as the other.

The following Case which has very lately occurred renders it highly probable that not only the heels of the horse, but other parts of the body of that animal, are capable of generating the virus which produces the Cow-pox.

An extensive inflammation of the erysipelatous kind, appeared without any apparent cause upon the upper part of the thigh of a sucking colt, the property of Mr. Millet, a farmer at Rockhampton, a village near Berkeley. The inflammation continued several weeks, and at length terminated in the formation of three or four small abscesses. The inflamed parts were fomented, and dressings were applied by some of the same persons who were employed in milking the cows. The number of cows milked was twenty-four, and the whole of them had the Cow-pox. The milkers, consisting of the farmer's wife, a man and a maid servant, were infected by the cows. The man servant had previously gone through the Small-pox, and felt but little of the Cow-pox. The servant maid had some years before been infected with the Cow-pox, and she also felt it now in a slight degree: But the farmer's wife, who never had gone through either of these diseases, felt its effects very severely.

That the disease produced upon the cows by the colt and from thence conveyed to those who milked them was the *true* and not the *spurious* Cow-pox,* there can be scarcely any room for suspicion; yet it would have been more completely satisfactory, had the effects of variolous matter been ascertained on the farmer's wife, but there was a peculiarity in her situation which prevented my making the experiment.

Thus far have I proceeded in an inquiry, founded, as it must appear, on the basis of experiment; in which, however, conjecture has been occasionally admitted in order to present to persons well situated for such discussions, objects for a more minute investigation. In the mean time I shall myself continue to prosecute this inquiry, encouraged by the [1]—" hope of its becoming essentially beneficial to mankind.]

* See Note in Page 9.

[1] "*pleasing.*" 3rd ed.

AN INQUIRY

CONCERNING

THE HISTORY

OF THE

COW POX.

PRINCIPALLY WITH A VIEW TO

SUPERSEDE AND EXTINGUISH

THE

SMALL POX.

By GEORGE PEARSON, M.D., F.R.S.,

PHYSICIAN TO ST. GEORGE'S HOSPITAL,

OF THE COLLEGE OF PHYSICIANS, ETC.

FELICIORES INSERIT.—*Hor.*

LONDON:

PRINTED FOR J. JOHNSON, No. 72, ST. PAUL'S CHURCHYARD

1798.

INQUIRIES

CONCERNING THE

COW POX.

THE curiosity of the public has been lately gratified by the publication of the long-expected treatise of Dr. Jenner,* on an epizootic disease, commonly known to dairy farmers by the name of the *Cow Pox*. This distemper of Cows has been noticed, time immemorial, in many provincial situations, where it has been also observed to have been communicated from these diseased animals to the persons who milk them. In the work just spoken of several facts are related, which seem to let new light into the nature of the animal œconomy, and to exhibit a near prospect of most important benefits in the practice of physic. But as some of these facts do not accord, nay, as they are at variance in essential particulars with those to which they are nearest related, the truth of them is rather invalidated than confirmed by analogy; hence the testimony of a single observer, however experienced, and worthy to be credited, it is apprehended is insufficient for procuring such facts a general acceptance. But granting that the facts should be generally admitted, without hesitation, to be true in the instances which have fallen under the notice of the writer of the above work, the more judicious part of the medical profession will require the observations to be derived from much more extensive and varied experience, in order to appreciate, justly, the value of the practical conclusions. Hence there appears but little likelihood of improvements in practice being made, unless the subject be investigated by many inquirers, and the attention of the public at large be kept excited. I do not think that it is necessary for me to explain the various modes, and point out the situations in which inquiries may be prosecuted. These I suppose will, without difficulty, be understood by perusing Dr. Jenner's

* *An Inquiry into the Causes and Effects of the Variolæ vaccinæ, etc., or the Cow Pox*, by Edward Jenner, M.D., F.R.S., etc., 4to, London, 1798.

treatise. I hope I shall not be considered as assuming too much in recommending, not only those of the profession of physic, but dairy farmers, and others who reside in the country, to collect the facts on the subject, which have hitherto fallen under notice only in a casual way. From such a procedure, it is reasonable to calculate that the acquisition of established truths will be greatly accelerated, or error will be exploded.

Agreeably to the preceding representation, I go forward to examine the evidence of the principal facts asserted in the publication on the Cow Pox; and to state what farther evidence I have derived from my own experience, and from the communications of a number of professional gentlemen, of unsuspected veracity and undoubted accuracy.

Perhaps it may be right to declare, that I entertain not the most distant expectation of participating the smallest share of honour, on the score of discovery of facts. The honour on this account, by the justest title, belongs exclusively to Dr. Jenner; and I would not pluck a sprig of laurel from the wreath that decorates his brow.

This declaration I can prove to demonstration * is utterly superfluous for this gentleman himself, but I am not confident that it is altogether without use, to exempt me from the suspicions which certain members of the profession (with whom I will have no fellowship) would be anxious to excite.

The first fact in order which I shall examine may be stated in the following terms:

I. *Persons who have undergone the SPECIFIC FEVER and LOCAL DISEASE, occasioned by the Cow Pox infection, communicated in the accidental way (who had not undergone the Small Pox), are thereby rendered unsusceptible of the Small Pox.*

To establish this important fact, Dr. Jenner has related (pp. 9-26) about twenty instances of inoculation of the Small Pox, of persons who were known to have gone through the Cow Pox, but not one of them took the Small Pox in this way; nor by associating afterwards with patients labouring under this disease. The permanency of the inexcitability of the constitution to the Small Pox was manifested by some of the instances being persons who had been affected with the Cow Pox twenty, thirty, forty, and even fifty-three years before. It must not be supposed that the

* On showing to Dr. Jenner the original paper which I read, as a lecture on the Cow Pox, and which furnishes the principal materials of this dissertation, he seemed only anxious that I should not think it important enough for publication.

fact is supported by merely these twenty instances, which were selected for illustration; for Dr. Jenner, having resided in Gloucestershire twenty years, in which county the Cow Pox is frequently epizootic, several hundred instances must have fallen under his own observation, or that of his acquaintance, of persons not taking the Small Pox, who had gone through the Cow Pox. Dr. Jenner appears to have been occupied for a long time in ascertaining this fact. And to prove that he has an extraordinary claim to credit on that account, I will mention the following occurrence. When I was in company with the late Mr. John Hunter, about nine years ago, I heard him communicate the information he had received from Dr. Jenner, that in Gloucestershire an infectious disorder frequently prevailed among the Milch Cows, named the Cow Pox, in which there was an eruption on their teats—that those who milked such Cows were liable to be affected with pustulous eruptions on their hands, which were also called the Cow Pox—that such persons as had undergone this disease could not be infected by the variolous poison, and that as no patient had been known to die of the Cow Pox, the practice of inoculation of the poison of this disease, to supersede the Small Pox, might be found, on experience, to be a great improvement in physic.

I noted these observations, and constantly related them, when on the subject of the Small Pox, in every course of lectures which I have given since that time.

This fact has been mentioned in two publications: namely, by Mr. Adams,* in his book on morbid poison, etc., in 1795; and by Dr. Woodville, in his *History of Inoculation*, in 1796.†

On conversing with *Sir George Baker, Bart.*, concerning the Cow Pox rendering people unsusceptible of the variolous disease, Sir George observed, he had been informed of the fact, in some papers on the Cow Pox, communicated to him many years ago; but that as the statement did not then obtain credit, it was not published. After a fruitless search for these papers, Sir George, whose zeal for the improvement of Physic did not forsake him on this occasion, authorized me to write to his relative, the

* "The Cow Pox is a disease well known to the dairy farmers in Gloucestershire. What is extraordinary, as far as facts have hitherto been ascertained, the person who has been infected is rendered insensible to the variolous poison."—ADAMS, *On Morbid Poisons*, 8vo, 1795, p. 156.

† "It has been conjectured that the Small Pox might have been derived from some disease of brute animals; and if it be true that the mange, affecting dogs, can communicate a species of itch to man; or that a person, having received a certain disorder from handling the teats of cows, is thereby rendered insensible to variolous infection ever afterwards, as some have asserted; then indeed the conjecture is not improbable."—WOODVILLE, p. 3.

Rev. Herman Drewe, of Abbotts. From this gentleman, who had availed himself of great opportunities of inquiring into the nature of the Cow Pox, when he resided in Dorsetshire, I immediately received answers in a very polite letter, to all the queries which I took the liberty of proposing. With regard to the fact under examination, the information received from this gentleman is in these terms: "Mr. Bragge,* who inoculated my parish, rejoiced at having an opportunity of ascertaining the fact. Three women had had the Cow Pox; he therefore charged them with a superabundance of matter, but to no purpose; all his other patients, more than fifty, took the infection, but the three women were not in the least disordered, even though they associated constantly with those who were infected. Thirteen similar instances I at that time, in that neighbourhood, ascertained." Mr. Drewe observes, that the disorder "is epizootic in Devonshire, Dorsetshire, and Somersetshire, and there is no doubt that it is to be met with elsewhere, under the name of Cow Pox, or some other denomination. When I made inquiries about the Cow Pox I resided in Dorsetshire, and gained all my information from a Mr. Downe, Surgeon of Bridport, a Mr. Bragge, Surgeon of Axminster, and a Mr. Barnes, of Colyton (since dead). I have not thought of the matter since, and as my letters on the subject have escaped Sir George Baker's search, so many particulars have my recollection."

Dr. Pulteney† *of Blandford*, who did me the honour to answer the question which I troubled him with, informs me "that the disease is well known in Hampshire, Dorsetshire, Somersetshire, and Devonshire. That it is not uncommon in Leicestershire and other midland counties, but dairymen keep it a secret as much as possible, as it is disreputable to the cleanliness of the produce. An intelligent and respectable inoculator in this country informed me, that of several hundreds whom he had inoculated for the Small Pox, who had previously had the Cow Pox, very few took the infection; and such as did he had great room to believe were themselves deceived, in regard to their having had the Cow Pox."

I am deeply indebted for several letters on the subject to the *Rev. Henry Jerome de Salis, D.D.*‡ "I have heard," says he, "a good deal of the Cow Pox in this country. I have given a copy of your questions to Mr. Heurtley, and another to Sir William Lee, and I daresay, after a time, this country will produce much in-

* Mr. Drewe's Letter, Abbotts, July 5th, 1798.
† Dr. Pulteney's Letter, Blandford, July 14th, 1798.
‡ Dr de Salis' Letters, Wing, Bucks, July 20th, 25th, and 29th, 1798.

formation relative to the Cow Pox. I have found that in this parish (Wing) this disorder raged in one farm, but did not get beyond it, three years ago. A man who now works with me was employed with three others in milking the Cows. None but himself had had the Small Pox, all three had the Cow Pox, but he quite escaped it. One of these three is now in the parish, and I will have him inoculated for the Small Pox. He was much struck with the resemblance of the symptoms to those he had lately experienced in the Small Pox. Mr. Thomas Rhodes, a respectable farmer and dairyman at Abbots-Aston (a parish adjoining to this) had the Cow Pox when he was a boy, and was afterwards inoculated for the Small Pox, without effect. As this is a case quite in point, and as I know the man perfectly well, and also know the inoculator, I will have all the particulars drawn up in the manner you may direct, and authenticated in the course of a few days. I have the name of a servant of his father's who had the Cow Pox at the same time that he had it. This man lives in the adjoining parish of Soulbury, and if he has not had the Small Pox since I will have him inoculated after harvest.

"In the dairy farm above mentioned, in which the Cow Pox raged three years ago, it had not appeared for the preceding fourteen or fifteen years. Two men were then infected, one of whom lives now at Aylesbury, and the other at Bushey. For reasons which I will hereafter give you, I shall inquire after the man at Aylesbury."

From *Mr. Downe,* Surgeon of Bridport,* I have received some important information.

"The Cow Pox is a disorder in Devonshire as well as Dorsetshire, but it so rarely occurs that the sources of information are very scanty. A few years ago, when I inoculated a great number for the Small Pox, I remarked that I could not, by any means, infect one or two of them, and on inquiry, I was informed they had previously been infected with the Cow Pox. Some few families who had been infected with the Cow Pox were repeatedly inoculated with the matter of the Small Pox, and without effect. I know that a medical man in this part of the country was injured in his practice, by a prejudice raised unjustly, that he intended to substitute the Cow Pox for the Small Pox. So great an enemy to improvement are the prejudices of the public in the country, that I think experiments of importance can only be made in hospitals.

"A farmer's† wife in this neighbourhood, her daughter, and two

* Mr. Downe's Letter, Bridport, August 1st, 1798.

† Mr. Downe's Second Letter, Bridport, August 25th, 1798.

sons, were all employed in milking the Cows when this disorder prevailed among them. The mother had gone through the Small Pox in the natural way, but the others had never had the Small Pox. The latter, viz., the two sons and daughter, were infected from the Cows, and the mother continued to milk them the whole time, without the least inconvenience. The daughter and two sons had a slight fever, and afterwards eruptions on the hands, by which they were much relieved of their fever. I had this account from one of the parties infected, and it may be depended upon.

"About three years since I inoculated between six and seven hundred, and I recollect one or two of the number who could not be infected. On inquiry I found they had previously had the Cow Pox."

The *Rev. John Smith, of Wendover*, to whom I owe many thanks for very willingly, at my request, taking upon himself the trouble of making inquiries in his neighbourhood, informs me* "that the high land of his parish does not admit of dairying upon it, and the dairy farmers here know nothing of the Cow Pox. But Mr. Henderson, the surgeon in the parish, whose practice takes him a little into the vale, tells me that he has met with the disease, and that a few years ago he three times endeavoured to inoculate a lad, who had been used to milking, but could only excite inflammation upon the arm, without any pustulous appearance. And upon inquiry, he found the lad had previously been affected with the Cow Pox. Mr. Woodman, a surgeon at Aylesbury, had met with the disease among the Cow boys in the vale. Mr. Grey, a surgeon of Buckingham, says the disorder is common among the milkers in his neighbourhood. He had not been led to consider, particularly, the effects of the disease, but he remembers one boy possessed of the idea that he could not take the Small Pox by inoculation, because he had had the Cow Pox, and that he could only excite redness upon the boy's arm. He thinks he recollects cases of boys having had the Small Pox, after having had the Cow Pox. The disease is not very notorious, for I passed some days last week with two intelligent farmers; one of them had kept seventy Milch Cows for many years past, but knew nothing of the Cow Pox among his servants. The other knew as little."

Mr. Giffard,† *Surgeon of Gillingham, near Shaftesbury*, has been so good as to write to me on the subject of the Cow Pox; he informs me that "it is a disease more known in Dorsetshire than

* Mr. Smith's Letter, Vicarage, Wendover, August 5th, 1798.
† Mr. Giffard's Letter, Gillingham, August 9th, 1798.

in most other counties." "I last winter," says he, "inoculated three parishes, and some of the subjects told me they had had the Cow Pox, and that they should not take the Small Pox, but I desired to inoculate them. I did so two or three times, but without effect." "Persons never take the Small Pox after they have had the Cow Pox."

On Thursday, June 14th last, happening, with Mr. Lucas, Apothecary, to be on professional business at Mr. Wilan's farm, adjoining to the New Road, Marybone—which farm is appropriated entirely for the support of from 800 to 1,000 Milch Cows—I availed myself of that opportunity to make inquiry concerning the Cow Pox. I was told it was a pretty frequent disease among the Cows of that farm, especially in winter. That it was supposed to arise from sudden change from poor to rich food. It was also well known to the servants, some of whom had been affected with that malady, from milking the diseased Cows. On inquiry, I found three of the men servants, namely, Thomas Edinburgh, Thomas Grimshaw, and John Clarke, had been affected with the Cow Pox, but not with Small Pox. I induced them to be inoculated for the Small Pox: and, with the view of ascertaining the efficacy of the variolous infection employed, William Kent and Thomas East, neither of whom had either the Cow Pox or the Small Pox, were also inoculated.

Three of these men, viz., Edinburgh, East, and Kent, were inoculated in each arm with perhaps a larger incision, and more matter, than usual, on Sunday, June 17th, by Mr. Lucas; and Dr. Woodville and myself were present. The matter was taken from a boy present, who had been inoculated fourteen days before this time, and who was obligingly provided by Dr. Woodville.

CASE I.

Thomas Edinburgh, aged twenty-six years, had lived at the farm the last seven years. Had never had the Small Pox, nor Chicken Pox, nor any eruption resembling these diseases but the Cow Pox, which he was certainly affected with six years ago. He was so lame from the eruption on the palm of the hands as to leave his employ, in order to be for some time in a public hospital; and he testified that his fellow-servant, Grimshaw, was at the same time ill with the same disorder. A cicatrix was seen on the palm of the hands, but none on any other part. He said that for three days in the disease he suffered from pain in the axillæ, which were swollen and sore to the touch. According to the patient's description, the disease was uncommonly painful and of long continuance; whether on account of the unusual thickness of the skin, which was perceived by the lancet in inoculation, future observations may determine.

THIRD DAY.—*Tuesday, June 19th.*

A slight elevation appeared on the parts inoculated. No disorder was perceived of the constitution, nor complaint made.

FIFTH DAY.—*Thursday, 21st.*

The appearance on the part inoculated of the left arm was like that of a gnat bite, and Mr. Wacksel, Apothecary to the Small Pox Hospital, observed that the inflammation seemed too rapid for that of the variolous infection, when it produces the Small Pox. On the other arm there had been a little scab, which was rubbed off, leaving only a just visible red mark. No complaint was made.

EIGHTH DAY.—*Sunday, 24th.*

The inflammation on the left arm had subsided, and there was in place of it a little scab. The right arm as before. Has remained quite well.

Sent the patient with Mr. Wacksel to the Small Pox Hospital, where he was inoculated a second time with matter from a person present, who then laboured under the Small Pox.

FOURTH DAY.—*After Second Inoculation, Wednesday, 27th.*

A little inflammation appeared on the part inoculated of one arm, but none of that of the other. Except some slight pains and headach on Monday last, had remained quite well.

EIGHTH DAY.—*After Second Inoculation, Sunday, July 1st.*

A little dry scab was upon each part inoculated. No symptoms of disorder had appeared.

CASE II.

Thomas Grimshaw, aged about thirty years. Had lived in town, at the farm only seven weeks, but six years ago also lived at this place, when he was affected with the Cow Pox; and he testified that his fellow-servant, Edinburgh, was at the same time ill of the same disease. Grimshaw said he had pains and soreness on touching the axillæ during that illness, but he got much sooner well than Edinburgh.

On Tuesday, the 19th June, Grimshaw was inoculated in both arms at the Small Pox Hospital, from a patient then ill of the Small Pox.

THIRD DAY.—*Thursday, 21st.*

A little inflammation and fluid appeared under a lens in the parts inoculated, as if the infection had taken effect. Remained quite well.

SIXTH DAY.—*Sunday, 24th.*

Inflammation, which had spread near the parts inoculated, has disappeared; and now nothing was seen but a dry scab on them. Had not been at all disordered. He was inoculated this day a second time, as before, at the Small Pox Hospital.

FOURTH DAY.—*Second Inoculation, Wednesday, June 27th.*

Not the least inflammation from the last inoculation, nor any complaint.

EIGHTH DAY.—*Second Inoculation, Sunday, July 1st.*

Not the smallest inflammation from the inoculation. Had remained quite well.

CASE III.

John Clarke, twenty-six years of age, had the Cow Pox ten years ago at Abingdon, where he was under the care of a medical practitioner of that place. He was inoculated by Mr. Wacksel at the Small Pox Hospital, on Tuesday, June 29th, from a patient affected with the Small Pox.

THIRD DAY.—*Thursday, June 21st.*

There was inflammation and a fluid in the parts inoculated; but these appearances were judged to be premature with respect to the Small Pox.

SIXTH DAY.—*Sunday, June 24th.*

The appearances of inflammation and fluid in the right arm were such as to make it doubtful whether or not the variolous infection had taken effect; but there was no such appearance on the left arm, the inflammation being gone.

He was this day inoculated a second time at the Small Pox Hospital, from a patient.

EIGHTH DAY.—*After Second Inoculation, Sunday, July 1st.*

No effect but inflammation, and afterwards festering, from the second inoculation.

The inflammation on the right arm, from the first inoculation, went off in a day or two after the last report. He had remained quite well in all respects.

CASE IV.

William Kent, thirty years of age, had lived at Mr. Wilan's farm about eight weeks. Had never laboured under the Small Pox, but said he had gone through the Chickenpox; and he had been told that he had been affected with a disorder, which was supposed to be the Cow Pox, when he was four years of age. He was inoculated under the same circumstances as Thomas Edinburgh by Mr. Lucas, on Sunday, June 17th.

THIRD DAY.—*Tuesday, 19th.*

The parts inoculated were scarcely red, yet their appearance was such, when viewed under a lens, as to render it probable the Small Pox would take place. Remained quite well.

FIFTH DAY.—*Thursday, 21st.*

The inoculated part of the left arm appeared red; and on viewing it with a magnifier a little bladder was seen in the middle. The same was the state of the right arm, but less evidently. Continued free from illness. Pulse 94 after walking two miles on a very hot day.

EIGHTH DAY.—*Sunday, 24th.*

The left arm was more inflamed, and a small flat vesication appeared in the middle of the inflamed part. The right arm was affected in the same manner, but in a less degree. It was not doubted that he was infected with the variolous disease, especially as he complained of soreness of the armpits, and he had been very much disordered the two last nights, having had pain of his bones in general, and headach, and had felt very hot, but not chilly. Pulse was only eighty, and his tongue had the healthy appearance; nor was he thirsty.

ELEVENTH DAY.—*Wednesday, 27th.*

Variolous eruptions in number perhaps twenty or thirty had made their appearance.

FIFTEENTH DAY.—*Sunday, July 1st.*

Eruptions are in a suppurated state. Had been quite well, and he has continued his employ during the present hot week.

CASE V.

Thomas East, aged twenty-one years. He believed he had never been affected with the Small Pox, and certainly not with the Cow Pox. There were several cicatrices, however, on his arms, exactly like those from the Small Pox, and if the inoculation had not succeeded I should have been disposed to conclude that he had already gone through that disease.

He was inoculated by Mr. Lucas on Sunday, 17th June, at the same time and under the same circumstances as Thomas Edinburgh and William Kent.

THIRD DAY.—*Tuesday, June 19th.*

Only a just visible scab on the parts inoculated, and it was thought the infection had not taken effect. Remained well.

Went to the Small Pox Hospital and was inoculated a second time.

FIFTH DAY.—*Thursday, June 21st.*

Redness appears now in the parts inoculated, as if both the first and second inoculation had taken effect.

EIGHTH DAY.—*Sunday, June 24th.*

All the four parts inoculated were so much inflamed that it seemed now doubtful whether the Small Pox would come on. Parts first inoculated less inflamed than those of the second inoculation; and the right arm more inflamed than the left. Pains of the axillæ were complained of, which were a little swelled and sore to the touch. There were no symptoms of fever.

ELEVENTH DAY.—*Wednesday, June 27th.*

About a dozen variolous eruptions were now out. No complaints were made.

FIFTEENTH DAY.—*Sunday, July 1st.*

Variolous eruptions were in a state of suppuration. There was a suppuration of the parts inoculated pretty much alike, from both the first and second inoculation.

It was thought the second inoculation had excited inflammation in the parts first inoculated, which otherwise might not have taken place so soon, or not at all.

Notwithstanding the hot weather for the last fortnight, the temperature being generally 68° to 78° of Fahrenheit's thermometer, the patients who took the Small Pox were so little disordered that they continued their daily work.

No treatment was prescribed previously to inoculation, all the men being in health; but every other day after it, for a fortnight, they were purged with salts, and directed to abstain from strong liquors and to eat very little animal food.

I did not require any farther evidence than what I have already procured in my own practice to satisfy me that the quantity of variolous matter does not influence the disease; but on account of some late assertions, that the disorder is rendered milder by using a smaller quantity of matter in the above cases, a larger quantity was purposely inserted; yet milder cases than the above could not be desired.

It should also be noticed that the three patients above mentioned, who did not take the infection on inoculation for the Small Pox, had their children soon afterwards inoculated, who all took the Small Pox. These men lived in the same apartments with their children during the illness of the Small Pox, but not one of them was infected.

We have seen in the above cases five persons inoculated for the Small Pox, under the most favourable circumstances for the efficaciousness of the infection; two of them took the disease from once inserting variolous matter, but the other three were uninfected, although the matter was twice inserted, and although they were exposed to infection by living with their children while they were suffering under the Small Pox.

The three patients who did not take the Small Pox gave strong circumstantial evidence that they had been affected with the Cow Pox, but not with the Small Pox. The other two patients who were infected with the Small Pox, there is no reason to doubt, were as credible persons as the former, and they attested that they had not had the Small Pox, which attestation being verified by their taking the disease, it would be injustice to question the other part of their evidence that they had not laboured under the Cow Pox. For as to the mere traditionary story of William Kent having the Cow Pox, no circumstance supported the truth of it against the extreme improbability of a boy, of four years of age or under, suffering a disease which is contracted by handling the teats of Cows in milking, when they are so difficult to manage that male instead of female servants must then generally be employed. In some places, it seems, the eruptive disease, which is known to medical men by the name of the Chicken or Swine Pox, is called by the lower orders of people Cow Pox. Mr. Giffard takes notice that "there are two kinds of Cow Pox." The one is attended with eruptions of the skin in general, and sometimes produces pits; but the other is a disease confined to the hands. It is most probable that Kent's eruptive disease, when a child, was the Chicken Pox, if he really had an eruptive disease. One of three reasons may be assigned for the above three patients not taking the Small Pox, viz.: 1. That they had already suffered the Small Pox. 2. That they had not had this disease, and that their constitutions were not excitable at the time they were inoculated; for one can scarce suspect the failure to be from the mode of inserting the matter. 3. That they were not capable of infection with the Small Pox poison, because they had undergone the Cow Pox. In respect of the first assignable reason, it must be allowed that a person may go through the Small Pox and the disease be so slight that it is neither noticed by the patient nor by his friends. But such unobserved cases are extremely rare, and they bear so very small a proportion to the others, that for three such cases to occur together on the present occasion seems to be barely a possibility.

With regard to the second assigned reason, probably about one out of fifty persons does not take the Small Pox by inoculation of the same matter, and in the same manner; and perhaps not more than one out of fifty of those who are not infected by a first inoculation fail to be infected on a second inoculation. According to this representation, then, it appears to be a mere possibility that the Small Pox poison should not take effect for the second assignable reason, namely, a peculiar disposition; especially as the patients were subsequently under very favourable circumstances for being affected with variolous effluvia.

With regard to the third assignable reason, as in so many instances now recorded, it appears that persons who have undergone the Cow Pox are not susceptible to the Small Pox; and as the failure of the inoculation cannot be imputed with justice to the two other causes above mentioned, it seems most reasonable to impute the inefficacy of the variolous poison in the above three instances to a state of inexcitability produced by the Cow Pox poison.

On making inquiries at *Mr. Kendal's* farm for Milch Cows, on the New Road, Marybone, a female servant informed me that she laboured under the Cow Pox many years ago, when she lived in Suffolk, where this disease prevails. From her description I could not doubt that she had really been affected with the Cow Pox. After this she took what she believed to be the Small Pox from an infant, which was nourished by her breasts. A fever preceded the eruptions, which were only about fifty in number, and they disappeared in a few days after they came out. If the latter part of this testimony is accurate, one cannot admit this case to be an example of the Small Pox taking place in a constitution which had previously been affected with the Cow Pox.

At this farm a Cow was shown to me which was said to be affected with the Cow Pox; on examination the disorder appeared to be in its last stage of desiccation. However, eight persons who had not undergone the Small Pox were inoculated with the scabs of this disorder, but no disease ensued.

On calling at *Mr. Rhodes'* milk farm on the Hampstead Road, where there is a very large stock of Cows, I found the Cow Pox had not fallen under his observation; but two of the male servants were well acquainted with some parts of its history. It appeared also, on inquiry, that one of the Cows had really laboured under the disease two months before, namely, in May last, but the milker was not infected, because, he said, there were no cuts on his hands, or abrasion of the cuticle. It was described very clearly to be a different disease from the common inflammations and eruptions which produce scabbed nipples. One of the male servants had often seen the disease in Wiltshire and Gloucestershire. The milkers, he said, were sometimes so ill as to lie in bed for several days, and there was a fever at the beginning, as in the Small Pox, but that no one ever died of it. He had known many persons who had laboured under the Cow Pox, but who had never suffered the Small Pox, although it prevailed in their own families; except in one instance, in which he was told that the person who took the Small Pox had gone through the Cow Pox when a child. The same servant said it was a common opinion that people who have been affected with the Cow Pox, to use his own words, are "hard to take the Small Pox."

Mr. Francis, who keeps a farm for Milch Cows on the road to Somers' Town, had seen the disease several times in the autumn among his cattle, and he knew that it was very apt to produce painful sores on the hands of the milkers; but he had never heard, or observed, that it prevented persons from having the Small Pox.

He said that three years ago, in the spring, the disease prevailed at several farms on the New Road.

A male servant of Mr. Francis, who has a good understanding, and is a man of veracity, and had lived in dairy farms all his life, stated, that he had seen the Cow Pox thirty-five years ago at King's Wood, in Somersetshire, and frequently there and in London since that time. The disease, he said, was then vulgarly called the Cow Pox; it appeared on their teats and udders with fiery or flame-like eruptions—was very infectious among the Cows and the milkers; but never knew either human creature or beast die of it. It affects the hands and arms of the milkers with painful sores, as large as a sixpence, which last for a month or more, so as to disable the sufferers from continuing their employment. The disease breaks out especially in the spring, but occasionally at other times of the year. Most of the Cows in his master's, Mr. Francis', farm, were infected three years ago in the spring, at which times many of the milkers were also infected. A new Cow is very liable to take the disease. He had always understood that a person who had had the Cow Pox could not take the Small Pox, and never knew in the course of his life an instance of the Small Pox in such persons.

The following instances fell under his own observation: a fellow male and a female servant were affected with the Cow Pox; some time after this, the parish in which they lived were in general inoculated for the Small Pox, but these two persons, who had never laboured under the Small Pox, could not be infected with this disease: nor did they take it, although they subsequently lived with their children while they were suffering the Small Pox. He also believed, and it was a common opinion in many parts of the country, that persons who have undergone the Small Pox cannot take the Cow Pox. He himself laboured under the inoculated Small Pox when seventeen years of age, but never took the Cow Pox, although he had milked a great number of Cows labouring under the disease, and by which other milkers were affected. He had never known either a human creature, or Cow, have the disease more than once. He had the Measles previously to the Small Pox, as well as the Hooping Cough.

At some other farms near London, where Milch Cows are kept, I found the disorder was not known either to the masters or servants.

Dr. Haygarth very kindly wrote me a letter from Bath, on the 30th of August last, in which he says, "To none of your questions, concerning the Cow Pox, can I give any answer from my own knowledge. Of such a distemper I never heard among the Cheshire or Welsh farmers. My first intelligence upon this subject came from my friend Dr. Worthington, of Ross, some time ago. He, as well as another friend, Dr. Percival, speak very favourably of Dr. Jenner, on whose testimony the extraordinary facts he has published at present principally depend."

I feel most sensibly the great favour shown to me by *Professor Wall*, of Oxford. Although this gentleman's zeal and ability in promoting useful inquiries are acknowledged, I cannot but attribute the great pains which he bestowed to procure answers to my queries in so short a time as I required, in part, to the friendship founded in the days of academical studies: to use this amiable gentleman's own words—"those days of free, manly, and liberal conversation which I reflect on with infinite pleasure."

The information belonging to this place, from Professor Wall,* is the answer to the question whether there is sufficient evidence that the Small Pox cannot infect a person who has once had the Cow Pox, attended with fever: and if there has been a local affection without fever, is such person still capable of taking the Small Pox?

"I receive but one answer to the two different modes of the question, which is, that any person who has ever had the Cow Pox, has never been known to have the Small Pox."

A servant who has kept the Cows of a considerable dairy-farm in this neighbourhood a great many years, told me that he had the Cow Pox early in life. Yet about six or seven years ago he wished, for security, to be inoculated for the Small Pox; the operation was performed three several times, but no disorder nor eruption ensued; the Surgeon, a gentleman of great eminence in this place, asked him if he had ever had the Cow Pox; upon his answering yes, the surgeon replied, "Then it is useless to make any farther trial." This servant, the next year, had several children inoculated by Sutton. He was with them all the time till their recovery, but did not receive the infection. A servant-girl at another considerable farm told me she had the Cow Pox early in life; several years after she was inoculated, but nothing took place, except the appearance of red blush round the incision similar, I suppose, to what Dr. Jenner mentions.

This red suffusion has been hastily, by some inoculators, regarded as a proof that the system has been infected with the virus of the Small Pox; but neither this appearance, nor even a much more considerable affection of the arm, is always sufficient security against future infection, unless there has been some eruption.—See *Memoirs of the Medical Society*.

* See Dr. Wall's Letter, Oxford, September 3rd, 1798.

From *Mr. Dolling*, an Inoculator at *Blandford*, I have received important intelligence, for which I am under further obligations to the Rev. Herman Drewe.* "Mr. Dolling has inoculated for the Small Pox a great number of persons, who said they had been affected with the Cow Pox, and very few of them took the infection, to produce the Small Pox, and he is of opinion that those who took the Small Pox were mistaken in supposing they had really laboured under the Cow Pox. In one family five out of seven children took the Cow Pox, by handling the teats of a cow affected with the Cow Pox ; these seven children were inoculated for the Small Pox, but none took the infection, except the two who had not laboured under the Cow Pox.

Dr. Croft tells me, that in Staffordshire, to his knowledge, the fact has been long known, of the Cow Pox, which prevails in that county, affording an exemption of the human subject from the Small Pox. This gentleman affords me an unequivocal proof of his conviction of the safety and efficacy of the inoculated Cow Pox, by his application to me for matter, in order to inoculate one of his own children.

My honourable friend, Mr. Edward Howard, has been assured on very good authority—that of a relation, who is an officer in the Oxfordshire Militia—that it is a received opinion among the soldiers that it is unnecessary to be inoculated for the Small Pox if they have already laboured under the Cow Pox, as many of them have done.

Dr. Redfearn, of *Lynn*,† informs me, that "the Cow Pox is a common disease among the cattle in this part, and the farmers have made use of the appellation Cow Pox for near thirty years, although totally ignorant of the disease existing in the West of England." But,

Dr. Alderson, of *Norwich*,‡ acquaints me that there is reason to believe the disease is not known in his neighbourhood.

My correspondents in the North and East Ridings of Yorkshire, in Durham, in Lincolnshire, and in the neighbourhood of Windsor, acquaint me that the Cow Pox is not known in those parts. But from the success which I have had in discovering the disease, by making a strict inquiry in farms where it was believed not to exist, I can scarce doubt that it breaks out occasionally in every part where a number of Cows are kept, and that the infection is widely disseminated.

* The Rev. H. Drewe's Second Letter, September 17th, 1798.
† Dr. Redfearn's Letter, September 15th, 1798.
‡ Dr. Alderson's Letter, Norwich, September 16th, 1798.

I do not find that the Cow Pox is known in Lancashire. *Dr. Currie,** of *Liverpool*, obligingly answers my letter; he says, "I have made inquiries among the farmers, but I have not been able to find one who is acquainted with the disease. Of course I cannot answer any of your queries. My friend Dr. Percival, of Manchester, who is now here, never heard of the Cow Pox in this county, any more than myself."

II. *Persons who have been affected with the specific fever, and peculiar local disease, by INOCULATION OF THE COW POX INFECTION, who had not previously undergone the Small Pox, are thereby rendered unsusceptible of the Small Pox.*

The first set of evidences of this fact are those of Dr. Jenner, in the Cases xvii., xix., xx., xxi., xxii., xxiii. They are instances of inoculation of the Cow Pox as in the Small Pox, with matter taken from the teats of cows. A fever like that of the Small Pox arose in six to nine days after the incision, but scarce of more than twenty-four hours' duration; attended with an inflammatory appearance, or erythematous efflorescence around the parts inoculated, and pustulous sores of those parts; which do not suppurate, but remain limpid till they disappear; and there is no eruption of other parts of the skin, as in the Small Pox.

In the cases of inoculation under *Dr. Jenner*, the local affection was commonly as slight as in the inoculated Small Pox, but sometimes there appeared a disposition to a more extensive inflammation of the skin around the parts in which the matter was inserted. "It seemed to arise from the state of the pustule, which spread out, accompanied with some degree of pain, to about half the diameter of a sixpence. By the application of mercurial ointment to the inflamed parts (as is practised in the inoculated Small Pox), the complaint soon subsided. To prevent inflammation of the skin, caustic was also applied to the vesicle of the inoculated part, to excite a different kind of inflammation; but the precaution was perhaps unnecessary, as a third patient had nothing applied, and he also mended quickly, without any erysipelas.

One of these patients inoculated with the Cow Pox was only six months old, and who took the disease. In none of the above cases, after the Cow Pox, could the Small Pox be excited, by repeated inoculation. The confidence of Dr. Jenner in the safety and efficacy of the inoculation of the Cow Pox is unequivocally evinced by the inoculation of his own son, R. F. Jenner, aged

* Dr. Currie's Letter, Liverpool, September 8th, 1798.

eleven months; although the poison did not take effect in this instance. The project of inoculation of the Cow Pox occurred to other practitioners, antecedently to Dr. Jenner's experiments.

Mr. Drewe, in his letter above cited, speaks of the practice. He says, "Mr. Bragge and I endeavoured to try the experiment of inoculating with the matter of the Cow Pox, but from the scarceness of the disease, and unwillingness of patients, we were disappointed."

Dr. Pulteney informs me, that "a very respectable practitioner acquainted him that of seven children whom he had inoculated for the Small Pox, five had been previously *infected with the Cow Pox purposely*, by being made to handle the teats and udders of infected Cows; in consequence of which they suffered the distemper. These five, after inoculation for the Small Pox, did not sicken; the other two took the distemper."

Farther, "A farmer in this country inoculated his wife and children with matter taken from the teat of a Cow. At the end of a week the arms inflamed, and the patients were so far affected as to alarm the farmer, although unnecessarily, and incline him to call in medical assistance. They all soon got well, and were afterwards inoculated for the Small Pox, but no disease followed. I was not applied to in this case, but the fact is sufficiently ascertained."

Mr. Downe furnishes me* with important information on the present fact. "R. F., near Bridport, when about twenty years of age, was at a farm house when the dairy was infected with the Cow Pox. It being suggested to him that it would be the means of preserving him from the Small Pox, which he had never taken, if he would submit to be inoculated with the Cow Pox, he gave his consent; he was infected in two or three places in his hand with a needle. He felt no inconvenience till about a week, when the parts began to inflame and his hand to swell, his head to ach, and many other symptoms of fever came on. He was recommended to keep much in the open air, which he did, and in four or five days the symptoms of fever went off, as the maturation of the hand advanced. The parts soon healed, leaving permanent scars. He was afterwards inoculated twice by my grandfather, and a considerable time after twice by my father, but without any other effect than a slight irritation of the part, such as is occasioned in the arms of persons who have already had the Small Pox. It was not expected at the time that the Small Pox

* See Mr. Downe's Letter of August 25th, 1798.

[illegible] it was inserted, partly by way of [illegible] of precaution, the Small Pox being [illegible] Small Pox has been repeated since in his [illegible] avoided it, being confident that it was [illegible] with this disease." The next case by [illegible] defective evidence, is not useless. [illegible] a person who was, in play, inocu- [illegible] Cow Pox matter. The wounds [illegible] and then inflamed. He had a [illegible] headach, sickness, and slight fever. [illegible] there was no inflammation at the [illegible] related by *Dr. Jenner*, in the Cases xix. to xxiii., pp. 21 to 23. Hence, according to these instances, the poison of the Cow Pox has the same properties, as appears from its effects on the human constitution, whether it be generated by the Cow or by the human animal; and these properties are the same, however remote from the origin of the poison in the Cow. But it has not been determined, by inoculating the teats of Cows with the matter taken from the Cow, and with that taken from the human creature, that the properties of the poison from this latter source are the same with regard to the brute as those of the matter from the Cow with regard to the same animal.

I apprehend that the Cow Pox is the only example at present known, of a permanent specific infectious disease in the human constitution, produced by matter from a different species of animal; but it has been often conjectured that many of the infectious diseases of the human species are derived from brutes.

IV. *A person having been affected with the Specific Fever, and Local Disease, produced by the Cow Pox poison, is liable to be again affected as before by the same poison; and yet such person is not susceptible of the Small Pox.*

I find that most part of professional men are extremely reluctant in yielding their assent to this fact. Some, indeed, reject it in the most unqualified terms. They are not averse from admitting the evidence that the Cow Pox may affect the same constitution repeatedly; or even that a person, having had this disease, is unsusceptible of the Small Pox; but that the constitution having suffered the Cow Pox should still be susceptible of this disease, and not be susceptible of the Small Pox, is an assertion with regard to which they demur to acquiesce. The unfavourable reception of the evidence for this fact does not seem to arise so much from the observations in support of it being suspected to be inaccurate, or sufficiently full and complete, as from its appearing, as they say, absurd and inconceivable. On inquiring why the fact appears in this light, we find it is because there is no support from any other analogous fact. There is, in reality, no analogous fact. We have facts which show that a person having undergone certain diseases, occasioned by particular poisons, in some instances is, and in others is not, again susceptible of the same disease, by the same poison; but the instance before us is the first which has been observed of the constitution being rendered inexcitable to a disease, from a given morbid poison, by having suffered a different disease from another different poison, and yet it remains susceptible of this different disease by this given morbid poison. In the first instance of certain new facts, it is easy to conceive that there may be no analogous fact to the one discovered. When the Small Pox first broke out, on its being discovered that the same constitution could not undergo this disease a second time, no analogous fact was, I think, then known; and on that account it probably was not admitted without much hesitation. But on a subsequent discovery that the same constitution could not be infected more than once with the measles, this, as well as the former fact, readily found acceptance. An evidence for a fact ought not to be rejected because it is incomprehensible or inconsistent with what is already known; but on the present occasion, if the subject be well considered, it does not seem to be difficult to conceive that a change may be effected in the human constitution, by a disease from a morbid poison, so as to render such constitution unsusceptible of a disease from a given different morbid poison, and yet such constitution shall remain susceptible of the former disease, from the former morbid poison. Hence, I apprehend, the only just ground of objection which may be taken, is that of the observations on the authority of which the fact is said to be established. Let us then state the evidence.

Under Case ix., p. 15, Dr. Jenner relates the history of a person who was first affected with the Cow Pox in the year 1780, a second time in 1791, and a third time in 1794. "The disease was equally severe the second and third time as it was the first," which is, in general, otherwise both in the brute and human kind. Inoculation of the variolous poison was twice instituted in this patient, but without producing disease, nor could the patient be infected by associating with persons labouring under the Small Pox.

Another patient (see Jenner, p. 26) suffered the Cow Pox in 1759; in 1797 he was inoculated with the variolous poison, but without exciting the disease. In 1798 the Cow Pox again took place.

With respect to the information which I have gained by my inquiries concerning this fact, some of my correspondents observed, that the Cow Pox occurred so seldom among the human kind, that they had no observations to determine whether a person could undergo the disease more than once; the greater part of my correspondents ventured to say, that it had never been seen more than once in the same person; but some testified that the Cow Pox certainly does take place, repeatedly, in the same constitution.

Mr. Woodman, of *Aylesbury*,* says, "The Cow Pox does not supersede itself on future occasions, for that Cow-boys have it repeatedly."

It may be worth while to notice, that none of the gentlemen of whom I made inquiries, knew an instance of the disease attacking the same Cow more than once; and it was said that it was the current opinion that this was a fact.

The evidence for this fact, to my apprehension, only proves, satisfactorily, that the *local affection* of the Cow Pox may occur in the same person more than once; but whether the *peculiar fever* also occurs more than once in the same person, from the Cow Pox poison, does not appear certain; and must be determined by future observations, to be made with a particular view to this point. Future observations must likewise determine whether, in those cases (if such occur) in which a person, after having gone through the Cow Pox, takes the Small Pox, the Cow Pox was attended with the fever, or was merely a local affection. It seems pretty well ascertained, that the variolous poison may produce the Small Pox only locally, or without any affection of the whole constitution; and in such a case, the constitution is still susceptible of the Small Pox, and yet, in both cases, viz., of the *local affection* only, and of the whole constitution, the matter of the eruptions is capable of infecting others, so as to produce the Small Pox: either locally only, or also in the whole constitution. Hence it seems probable, that similar local and general effects may be produced by the Cow Pox poison, and not only in the human kind, but in Cows. I acknowledge, however, that the Case, p. 26 in *Jenner's* book, militates against this supposition.

V. *A person is susceptible of the Cow Pox, who has antecedently been affected with the Small Pox.*

Dr. Jenner, pp. 15-19, gives some instances of persons taking the Cow Pox who had certainly gone through the Small Pox. But he says, "It is a fact so well known among our dairy farmers, that those who have had the Small Pox either escape the Cow Pox or are disposed to have it slightly; that as soon as the complaint shows itself among the cattle, assistants are procured, if possible, who are thus rendered less susceptible of it, otherwise the business of the farm could scarcely go forward."

I have not got much additional information on this fact. It seems, however, sufficiently authenticated that people may have

* See Mr. Smith's Letter, above cited.

the Cow Pox after they have had the Small Pox, but it will require more nice attention to satisfy the query whether, in such cases, the Cow Pox affects the whole constitution or is only a local affection.

*Mr. Downe,** in particular, speaks of a family who did not take the Cow Pox when much exposed to the infection, because they had all gone through the Small Pox, except one who had been afflicted already with the Cow Pox. I met with a servant at Mr. Rhodes' farm, on the Hampstead Road, who attested that he had suffered the Cow Pox fourteen years ago, but that long before that time he had gone through the Small Pox.

Professor Wall† says: "The answer to the question whether a person is capable of taking the Cow Pox who has gone through the Small Pox, is of some, decidedly, that such a person is not liable to the infection of the Cow Pox. Others of equal experience have answered this question with doubt."

At Mr. Rhodes' farm, at Islington, I found that one of the male servants who had been long employed in taking care of Milch Cows in the environs of London, distinguished the Cow Pox very clearly from common inflammation of the teats with scabs, with which several Cows were at the time that I saw this man affected. He had never contracted the Cow Pox, although he had been repeatedly exposed to the infection, and when others took it. He was deeply pitted with the Small Pox, which he laboured under when a young child.

VI. *The Cow Pox is not communicated in the state of effluvia or gas, nor by adhering to the skin in an imperceptibly small quantity, nor scarce, unless it be applied to divisions of the skin by abrasions, punctures, wounds, etc.*

Some morbific poisons are communicated to animals only in the state of invisible effluvia or gas, *e.g.*, the miasmata which produce intermittent fevers; the contagion which produces the ulcerous sore throat, that which occasions the Hooping Cough, the Measles, etc. Other morbific poisons are communicated both in the state of effluvia and in a palpable or visible quantity, *e.g.*, the variolous poison, the matter which produces in oxen the murrain or lues bovilla, etc. Others again are not propagated in the state of effluvia or gas, but in a palpable or visible quantity only, as the hydrophobic poison, the syphilitic, etc., and to these last must now be added the morbific poison of the Cow Pox.

* Mr. Downe's Letter of August 30th.

† Letter of Professor Wall, above cited.

It does not appear that the disease spreads from any infected Cow among other Cows which are fed in the same stable like a contagious disease. Persons who sleep in the same bed with one who is labouring under the Cow Pox are not in this way liable to be infected. (See Jenner, p. 32). It is not even propagated from the Cows to the milkers for the most part, unless the skin of the part of the hands to which the matter is applied be divided.

This property of the Cow Pox infection not being propagated so as to produce disease, but by contact, and then only when applied in a palpable or visible quantity, and also scarce unless the skin be divided, is the most important one. Yet a few instances I apprehend will suffice to show clearly under what circumstance the Cow Pox infliction produces disease.

A boy who was inoculated for the Cow Pox slept, while he was labouring under the disease, with two other boys, but neither of them by this exposure to the affliction got the Cow Pox. A young woman who had the Cow Pox, with several sores, which maturated to a great extent, slept in the same bed with a fellow dairymaid who never had been infected either with the Cow Pox or Small Pox, but the disease was not communicated. A young woman, on whose hands were several large suppurations from the Cow Pox, was a daily nurse to an infant, but the infant was uninfected. (See Jenner, p. 32).

I am instructed uniformly by my correspondents that the Cow Pox arises only from matter evidently applied most frequently by friction of the diseased teats in milking, but sometimes from the matter lodging accidentally in some soft part, yet even under this circumstance it frequently fails to infect unless there be a cut, scratch, puncture, etc., of the hands.

Mr. Drewe mentions the instance of a woman who lost her eye sight in consequence of the infectious matter being heedlessly applied to the eye, and that the Cow Pox has been observed to take place from handling the milk pail on which the infectious matter has been incautiously allowed to remain.

VII. *The local affection in the Cow Pox produced in the casual way is generally more severe and of longer duration than usually happens in the local affection in the inoculated Small Pox, but in the Cow Pox the fever is in no case attended with symptoms which denote danger, nor has it in any instance been known to prove mortal.*

The Cow Pox in the incidental way, for sufficiently obvious reasons, most commonly affects the palms of the hands. There is a wide difference in the degree of the local affection. I am instructed by my communications that the extreme cases are, 1st. Those in which the patients are inflicted with so much painful inflammation as to be confined to their beds for several days, and have painful phagedenic sores for several months. 2dly. Those cases which are so slight that the patients are not confined at all, but get well in a week or ten days. In the more severe cases, in which the inflamed spots become vesicular with edges of the pustules more elevated than the cuticle, and of a *bluish* or a *purple colour*, there are pains of the axilla, fever, and now and then a little delirium.

These symptoms continue from one to three or four days, leaving ulcerated sores about the hands, which, from the sensibility of the parts, are very troublesome, and commonly heal slowly, frequently becoming phagedenic, like those from which they sprung. The lips, nostrils, eyelids, and other parts of the body are sometimes affected with sores, but these evidently arise from their being heedlessly rubbed or scratched with the patient's infected fingers. Dr. Jenner considers the *bluish* or *livid* tint of the pustules to be characteristic of the Cow Pox (p. 8).

Mr. [illegible]'s information on the fact is, "That the symptoms are similar to the Small Pox, but *less violent.* The pustules are only about the hands, in the parts which have been in contact with the infected teats." But in answer to the question Whether, on the whole, the Cow Pox is a disease of less magnitude than the Small Pox by inoculation, he says: "When I consider what a slight disorder the inoculated Small Pox is, it will not, in my humble opinion, admit of comparison."

Mr. D[illegible]ng says: "There is a swelling under the arm, chilly fits, etc., not different from symptoms of the breeding of the Small Pox. After the usual time of sickening, namely, two or three days, there is a large ulcer, not unlike a carbuncle, which discharges matter."

Dr. P[illegible]ney's account of the symptoms is in these terms: "A soreness and swelling of the axillary glands as under inoculation for the Small Pox, then chilliness, and rigors, and fevers as in the Small Pox. Two or three days afterwards, abscesses, not unlike carbuncles, appear generally on the hands and arms, which ulcerate and discharge much matter."

Mr. D[illegible]n, speaking to this point, says: "The symptoms, as far as could be ascertained in the Cow Pox, were similar to those of the Small Pox, but I never heard of any who had them in any degree alarming." Again, "The symptoms are exactly similar to those of the Small Pox by inoculation, when of the most favourable kind. The disease generally disappears in about the same time that the Small Pox does."

Mr. Giffard tells me that "he never heard of either men or Cows dying of the Cow Pox."

Mr. Woodman (see Mr. Smith's letter) testifies that he never observed symptoms worthy to be called fever; there was merely "feverish heat when the pain was considerable."

Dr. De Salis observes that one of the persons affected with the Cow Pox "was much struck with the resemblance to the symptoms he had lately experienced in the Small Pox."

Professor Wall's information is that "the milkers have the disorder only once, generally with preceding fever, sometimes very violent, sometimes more mild."—"No human creature, or Cow, has been known to be in danger, or to die of the Cow Pox." After a strict inquiry at the milk farms adjoining to London, I could not find that any person had ever died of the Cow Pox.

With respect to the animals from which the human creature derives the disease, it is only known to affect Cows. They have, sometimes, but it is very seldom observed, a disorder of the whole constitution, "the secretion of milk being much lessened."—The local affection appears with irregular pustules on the nipples. "At their first appearance they are commonly of a *palish blue*, or, rather, of a colour somewhat approaching to *livid*, and are surrounded by an erysipelatous inflammation. These pustules, unless a timely remedy be applied, frequently degenerate into phagedenic ulcers, which prove extremely troublesome." See Jenner, p. 8.

Dr. Pulteney acquaints us, that "the disease makes its appearance on the udder of the Cow, and affects the teats principally, which inflame, and then ulcerate, discharging a bloody matter; *but it does not appear that the disease is more than local, as the Cows seem not to be out of health in other respects.*

From *Mr. Drewe's* testimony, however, it appears that the whole constitution of the Cow is affected. There being "loss of appetite and of milk," as well as "ulcerated teats," so as to render the animal, in some cases, totally unfit for the dairy. "It is infectious in the herd, and the infection is probably conveyed by the persons' hands that milk them."

Mr. Downe's information, relating to the present part of our inquiry, is that "the only symptoms were eruptions about the teats of the Cow, exactly similar to the Small Pox, which gradually become sore, and fall off; and the infection was soon communicated to a whole dairy, as was supposed, by the hand of the person who milked. The animals suffered much in the operation of milking."

Professor Wall mentions that the symptoms are "blue or livid blotches on the teats and udder, painful and suppurating. The Cows are seldom ill, so as to refuse their food. Others observe, that Cows being naturally disposed to a lax habit of body, are not so much afflicted with feverish symptoms. Some say Cows suffer no fever at all."

The testimony of several other correspondents has been already stated, that a Cow has never been known to die of the Cow Pox; to which I add in confirmation, that of the milk farmers near London.

VIII. *No consequential disease, which should be attributed to the Cow Pox, has been observed; nor has any disease been excited, to which there previously existed a disposition; nor has it been discovered to produce a predisposition to particular diseases.*

Although a considerable body of evidence might be stated in confirmation of these momentous facts, from the experience of Dr. Jenner, and the uniform testimony of my correspondents; and although we should be inclined to conclude in favour of these facts, from the consideration of the nature of the Cow Pox, as far as yet known; yet it does not appear to my judgment that the observations and arguments warrant more than conclusions on the side of great probability. A number of persons, many hundreds, have gone through the inoculated Small Pox, under the observation of many practitioners, without any disease, or disposition to disease, being produced by the Small Pox; yet no one doubts that, in a certain proportion of instances, disease has been excited, and disposition to disease been produced.

We are led then to think that a greater number and more accurate observations are wanting, to authorize positive conclusions relating to the facts stated under this VIII. head.

IX. *The Cow Pox infection may produce the peculiar local disease belonging to it, but without the disorder of the constitution; in which case, the constitution is liable to be infected by the Small Pox infection.*

This fact is not of small consequence either in respect of general pathology or practice. Dr. Jenner's work, p. 32, furnishes us with an unequivocal example of this fact. A woman was affected with the local disease of the Cow Pox in the ordinary way, but without any pains or swelling of the axillæ, or any disorder of the whole constitution. This person was subsequently infected by the Small Pox; but a fellow-servant who had suffered the Cow Pox (at the same time and from the same source of infectious matter), in which there was fever as well as local disease, could not be infected by inserting the Small Pox poison; even repeated trials for this purpose were successless. Hence, they who offer as evidence, instances of persons taking the Small Pox after they have gone through the Cow Pox, will do well to assure themselves that the whole constitution was affected in the Cow Pox, otherwise such evidence will be inadmissible. Analogous facts have been ascertained, on good authority, in the Small Pox, although the instances are too scarce to afford to scrupulous minds full proof. It has been found that the usual local disease of the inoculated Small Pox may occur, unattended by a disorder of the whole constitution; but yet the matter of such local Small Pox will, in other persons, produce not only the local disease, but general eruption and fever; and that the person who had undergone this local Small Pox only, will be infected at a future time, so as to have both the ordinary local disease and fever of the Small Pox, with eruptions.

It appears from the observations of Dr. Jenner, p. 26, Mr. Drewe, Dr. Pulteney, and others, that during the Cow Pox in the human subject, inflammation and sores are apt to be excited by the matter being lodged upon various parts, especially if the skin be divided; but no mention is made of fresh fever being excited, nor of the peculiar *livid* and *bluish* tint of the Cox Pox pustulous sores. Enough has been said in a preceding part of this paper to direct observers in future to ascertain more accurately the effects of the agency of the Cow Pox infection on the whole constitution, and on part of it only.

It will be necessary also to caution inquirers against the errors of admitting facts to belong to the Cow Pox, as understood in this paper, which, in reality, belong to the Chicken Pox, or Swine Pox, or some other eruptive disease; which it seems, in some provincial situations, are designated by the name of the Cow Pox.

Yet another caution is necessary in investigating the truth, namely, to distinguish from the Cow Pox, "the pustulous sores which appear spontaneously on the nipples of Cows; and instances have occurred, although very rarely, of the hands of the servants employed in milking being affected with sores in consequence, and even of their feeling an indisposition from absorption. These pustules are of a much milder nature than those which arise from that contagion which constitutes the true Cow Pox. They are always free from the bluish or livid tint so conspicuous in the pustules in that disease. No erysipelas attends them, nor do they show any phagedenic disposition, as in the other case; but quickly terminate in a scab, without creating any apparent disorder in the Cow." Like the Cow Pox, "this eruption appears most commonly in the spring, when the Cows are first taken from their winter food, and fed with grass. Jenner, p. 9.

I observed during my visits to the Cow stables near London, in August and September last, that a number of Cows were infected with eruptions, sores and scabs on their breasts, especially on their paps. None of the animals had any constitutional affection, nor could I learn that any of the milkers were infected. The eruptions now spoken of break out, as I was told, especially in new-comers. Fresh Cows, it was said, were apt to be thus affected, on account of the much richer food which is given in London than in the country. The same kind of sores, eruptions, and scabs (which must be distinguished from the Cow Pox), I apprehend are common in the country; of which the following testimonies will be useful:—

Sir Isaac Pennington who could not learn that the Cow Pox was prevalent in Cambridgeshire, says, "I find Cows are liable to inflammations of the udders, but they do not affect the hands of the milkers."

A number of Milch Cows are kept near Twickenham, and *Mr. Beauchamp*,* surgeon, gave himself much trouble to oblige me, by making inquiries according to the direction of my queries. He instructs me, "that all the Cow-keepers agree that warts, and small bladders, or pustules, appear frequently on the teats of the Cow, but never observed the animal, or the milkers, to be affected, and even when these pustules were burst by the hands of milkers who had never suffered the Small Pox.

Dr. Beckwith, of York, who well merits my best thanks, bestowed great pains in making inquiries among the medical practitioners in his neighbourhood, and the farmers. His report is, "I† am well satisfied that no such disease as the Cow Pox has ever appeared here in the memory of man; but soreness and chaps of the paps are observed, from distension by milk in summer, and in winter, without affecting the hands of milkers."

In the *Pestis bovilla*, or murrain, the breasts, and especially the paps, are sometimes affected with pustules, or tubercles;‡ which, however, seem to be in that disease the least of the unfavourable symptoms.

* Mr. Beauchamp's Letter, Twickenham, Sept. 18th, 1798.

† Dr. Beckwith's Letter, York, Sept. 19th, 1798.

‡ Illas duntaxat boves, & quidem admodum raros, mortem effugisse quibus [illegible] ac decubitus in formam tuberculorum, scabiei, depilationis, [illegible], in uberum papillis fieri contegerit.—Lancisi de bovilla peste, [illegible], No. 134.

Dr. Belcombe, of Scarborough, in his obliging letter, observes,* "there is a disease of the paps, which renders them exceedingly sore and difficult to milk, but it is not infectious, and the same Cow has it many times; nor are the hands of the milkers ever sore from it.—It commonly happens in hot and wet summers."

On considering the facts of the preceding history, it appears that some useful conclusions of a practical kind may be drawn from them.

I. The body of evidence is numerous and respectable, declaring that a person who has laboured under the Cow Pox fever and local eruption, is not susceptible of the Small Pox. It does not appear that a single well-authenticated contravening instance has fallen under observation. But I do not apprehend that accurate and able reasoners will consider the fact as compleatly established; although I doubt not they will allow that the testimonies now produced greatly confirm the probability; and that the cautious appropriation of it, in practice, is warrantable.

In the present inquiry, the attestations have been obtained from so many persons, that it seems highly improbable, indeed, that the contrary instances should have been unobserved, or purposely kept out of sight. If the fact had been supported by the testimony of one observer only, the experience of the world would have justified us in demanding the account of the failures; after the example of the keen sceptic of old, who, on being shown the votive tablets of those who had been preserved from shipwreck, instead of yielding his assent, replied, "Where are the tablets of those who have perished?" †

Granting the truth of this fact, its usefulness in practice, in contemplation of it as a substitute of the Small Pox, must depend upon the effects of the Cow Pox, in comparison with the Small Pox, especially in the particulars *of the degree of danger to life; the kind of symptoms and their duration; and the subsequent effects on the constitution.*

1st. The evidences, shewing that no one has ever died, or even

* Dr. Belcombe's Letter, Scarborough, Sept. 22nd, 1798.

† Intellectus humanus in iis quæ semel placuerunt (aut quia recepta funt et credita, aut quia delectant) alia etiam omnia trahit ad suffragationem et consensum cum illis. Et licet major sit instantiarum vis et copia quæ occurrunt in contrarium; tamen eas aut non observat aut contemnit, aut distinguendo summovet et rejicit, non sine magno et pernicioso præjudicio quo prioribus illis syllepsibus authoritas maneat inviolata. Itaque recte respondit, qui, cum suspensa tabula in templo ei monstraretur eorum, qui vota solverant, quod naufragii periculo elapsi sint, atque interrogando premeretur, anne tum quidem eorum numen agnosceret, quæsivit denuo; *At ubi sunt illi depicti qui post vota nuncupata perierunt?*—Verulamii Novum Organum, Aphor. XLVI.

been apparently in danger, are the same as those for the fact itself; that a person is not susceptible of the Small Pox after having suffered the Cow Pox. But the conclusion with respect to the point of danger is far more equivocal. The comparison for this purpose should be made with not fewer than one, or even two thousand instances. For, though in several hundred examples of the Cow Pox, which have been under observation, not one person has fallen a victim, this might, and indeed has been, the fortunate issue of the inoculated Small Pox, of which it will suffice to give two instances.

Dr. William Heberden informs me, that at Hungerford, a few years ago, in the month of October, eight hundred poor persons were inoculated for the Small Pox, without a single case of death. No exclusion was made on account of age, health, or any other circumstance, but pregnancy; one patient was eighty years of age; and many were at the breast, and in the state of toothing.

Dr. Woodville acquaints me, that in the current year, from January to August inclusive, out of upwards of seventeen hundred patients inoculated at the Inoculation Hospital, including the *in* and *out* patients, *only two died*, both of whom were of the latter description.

Such instances of success can only be attributed to a certain favourable epidemic state of the human constitution itself, existing at particular times; for the proportion of deaths is usually much greater; indeed, sometimes it is very considerably greater, owing, probably, to certain unfavourable epidemic states. Of the various different estimates which have been made, the fairest seems to be that which states (under a choice of the most favourable known circumstances which can be commanded) one death out of two hundred inoculated persons. But when it is considered that we are now to make the comparison between the inoculated Small Pox, and what may be called the *natural* Cow Pox; when it is considered that the inoculated Cow Pox, in respect of the local eruption and ulceration, is a much less painful and shorter disease than the natural or casual Cow Pox; when it is considered that the inoculated Small Pox is especially dangerous from the number of eruptions, and that there is only a trifling local eruption of the part poisoned in the inoculated Cow Pox; when it is considered that the Cow Pox infection is not propagated in the state of effluvia;—I say, from such considerations, it seems to be most reasonable to conclude, *that there is great probability of the Cow Pox either not proving fatal at all, or at most being much less frequently* so *than the inoculated Small Pox.*

Further: the comparison of the two diseases should be instituted, with respect to danger, under the particular circumstances of *Pregnancy; Age; Toothing; Peculiar morbid states; Peculiar healthy states, or Idiosyncrasies; and certain Seasons or epidemical States.*

Pregnancy. The inoculated Small Pox is so commonly mortal to the unborn in every period of gestation, and so frequently so likewise to the mother in advanced states of gestation, that no prudent practitioner would choose to inoculate under these circumstances; but to escape the taking the disease by effluvia, in the casual way.* The exposure to infection, being sometimes unavoidable, I confess I feel anxious to ascertain the effects of inoculating the Cow Pox infection in such persons. And on the grounds of the slightness and short duration of the Cow Pox eruptive fever and of the merely local eruption, I apprehend a practitioner would be justifiable in preferring the inoculation of the infection of this distemper to that of the Small Pox.

On another account, the practice of inoculating the Cow Pox seems recommendable in pregnancy, namely, that of preventing the irritable state of the womb, which is produced by abortion, during the Small Pox. From which irritable state, the female will be very liable, in future, to the misfortune of abortions. This is so notorious a fact in brutes, that a cow which has suffered abortion, while labouring under the *Lues bovilla*, or murrain, will seldom, in future, bring forth a live calf; and on this account such Cow becomes greatly degraded in value. Whereas a Cow, which has had the inoculated murrain when a calf, or at least before she was impregnated, is thereby greatly enhanced in value. It was the great *Camper* who recommended to his countrymen in Holland the general inoculation of calves for the murrain. The matter is most advantageously inserted into the ear, tail, or dewlap.

Dr. Layard says, oxen may be inoculated, either with the pus of their eruptions, or with the mucus from the nose; and that few, comparatively with the casual disease, die. Oxen were not infected by eating matter of the pustules with their corn; not by covering their heads with a cloth, which had been impregnated with steam from the breathing of infected oxen.

Whether the unborn animal will take the infection of the Cow Pox from the mother, is a question for future observation to determine.

It has been fully determined (antecedently to the recent contro-

* See my paper "On the Effects of the Variolous Infection on Pregnant Women," *Medical Annals*, vol. ix., Decade 2d, 1795.

versy between two eminent anatomists for the honour of the discovery) by pathological observations, and demonstrated by anatomical* experiments and artifices, that the blood of the mother does not pass to the fœtus, nor return from the fœtus to the mother, for the unborn frequently escapes the disease of the Small Pox, although the mother be affected with it; and when the fœtus is infected, it is uniformly subsequent to the eruption, and even to suppuration of the pustules on the mother.† Further, injections will pass from the umbilical arteries of the fœtus into its body, and return by the umbilical vein, provided the placenta or vicarious lungs of the fœtus be entire. The fœtus then does not receive its blood from the mother, nor does the blood of the fœtus circulate through the mother. Yet the infant, before birth, frequently does receive some kinds of infectious matter from the mother, viz., the syphilitic, variolous, etc., and of consequence it seems possible that it may receive the Cow Pox infection, subsequently to its formation by the mother's constitution. In this case we should expect no local disease, but merely the specific fever.

Age. Whatever doubts may be entertained of very advanced or decrepit age being adverse to the success of the inoculated Small Pox, I am sure that I shall be supported by the opinion and practice of a very decisive majority that *infancy* is the state in which the largest proportion die under inoculation. In medical

---

* Succus nutritius et chylosus matris, ex poris et vasculis uterinis interventu membranæ villosæ tenuissimæ quæ chorio contigua est, non secus ac chylus a tunica intestinorum villosa recipitur, absorbetur, et per umbilicalem venam fertur, ex qua cum sanguine ad hepar infantis deducitur. . . .

Nutritur infans mediante succo temperato, gelatinoso matris, qui per spongiosam uteri substantiam transcolatur et a secundina recipitur, per cujus vasa ad infantem defertur. . . .

Ipsa secundina quatenus utero adhaeret ex ejus substantia porosa succum alibilem, non vero sanguinem matris recipit—Crediderunt veteres, sanguinem matris nutrire infantem et vasa uteri cum vasis secundinæ et foetus invicem connecti: sed notabile est, liquorem siphone umbilicales arterias injectum per venam umbilicalem redire, modo placenta illaesa fuerit; ex quo apparet, nullus dari anostomoses vasorum uteri cum vasis secundinae et foetus, neque sanguinem foetus rursus ad venas matris redire. Placenta uterina ex innumeris capillaribus minimis vasculis est contecta, per quae dum transit sanguis atteritur, comminuitur inque minimas partes ac globulos dividitur, intima unione succi nutritii cum sanguine facta, ut hac ratione per tenues canaliculos embryonis commodius transire et nutritionem praestare possit; unde revera secundina in foetibus vice fungitur pulmonum, qui in foetu a munere fuo vacant, quod identidem in intima sanguinis partium comminutione earumque unione cum chyloso succo consistit: qua de causa etiam vena umbilicalis id habet peculiare cum vena pulmonali ut sanguinem fluxilem floridum, et arterioso similem vehat quod omnibus aliis venis negatum est.—F. Hoffmann, t. 1 lib. 1 sect. 11 cap. XIII.

† See the paper above cited on the effects of variolous matter on pregnant women.

families, and in large towns, where, to the reproach of our police, persons labouring under the Small Pox are suffered to appear in the streets and public walks, even the most cautious practitioners deem inoculation of infants warrantable, but not even then otherwise than to avoid the casual disease. Of the effects of inoculation of infants with the Cow Pox infection, we have but one or two examples; however, these are in favour of the practice.

Toothing. Though the tender, irritable state of a new-born child may be a more dangerous one with the Small Pox, than even the state of actual great irritation during the cutting of teeth with this disease, yet the evidence in point of safety is against inoculating the Small Pox in the latter cases. This being the fact, we shall feel inclined, under the circumstances of dentition, to inoculate for the Cow Pox, if exposure to the Small Pox infection be unavoidable.

Peculiar morbid states. Certain diseases have been found to have no influence in occasioning the inoculated Small Pox to take place in a severe manner. On the contrary, it appears that some of these diseased states render the Small Pox milder. But of the influence of such morbid conditions on the Cow Pox, we possess no experience to authorize an opinion. There are some states induced by particular diseases, namely, by the Measles, Hooping Cough, etc., which are considered to be the occasion of a severe disease in the inoculated Small Pox; and from this consideration, under the circumstance of unavoidable exposure to the Small Pox infection, it seems warrantable to prefer the inoculation of the Cow Pox.

Peculiar states of health, Idiosyncrasies. The cases of certain families in which the Small Pox is uncommonly severe, and of other families in which it is very mild, are so frequent as to have fallen under the notice of every physician of experience. Some families have been so unfortunate that all their children have died in the Small Pox, either in the casual way, or by inoculation. It is not a very great rarity to find a family in which several children have fallen victims to the Small Pox, and in which a single surviving child remains; in such a case, the parents, and perhaps the child, are under constant apprehensions of the casual Small Pox, for they are deterred from inoculation by what has happened. Surely, in such circumstances, one would be inclined to recommend inoculation for the Cow Pox.

During certain seasons, or epidemical states.* At certain times,

* A very mild and innocent endemial Small Pox occurred in the practice of Dr. Hicks, of which a history is expected by the professional public.

when the Small Pox is epidemical, it is mostly violent and very fatal, and at other times it is mostly neither violent nor very fatal.

Such different sorts of Small Pox seem to depend upon prevalent peculiar states of health of people, rather than on the properties of the atmosphere. When an unfavourable epidemical state is discovered, the judicious practitioner will find the question worthy of his contemplation, whether it will not be justifiable to introduce the inoculation of the Cow Pox to supersede the Small Pox.

2. *The kind of symptoms and the duration* of the two diseases must be compared together.—If an inoculator could, at his will, command an inoculation of the Small Pox, a slight local affection, a trifling eruptive fever, and a very small number of eruptions, there would be no temptation held out on the score of symptoms to inoculate for the Cow Pox, because, in this disease, it appears that we are liable, even by inoculation, to produce a painful phlegmonic inflammation, extensive and very irritating inflammation of the skin around the part poisoned, and ulceration of the phagedenic kind. A sufficient number of cases of the inoculated Cow Pox have not been attested to enable us to form an accurate judgment of the degree of the symptoms in comparison with those of the inoculated Small Pox. It does not appear that there is nearly so great a difference between the constitutional disorder, or fever, of the inoculated Cow Pox and of the casual Cow Pox, as between the disorder of the constitution of the inoculated Small Pox and the casual Small Pox; nor, of course, are the advantages of the inoculated Cow Pox so eminently great, comparatively with those of the casual disease, as the advantages of the inoculated Small Pox are superior to those of this disease in the casual way. On comparison of the symptoms of the inoculated Chicken Pox, the inoculated murrain, and the inoculated Measles, with these diseases, in the casual way, by effluvia, the difference is not so great as to raise considerably our expectation of advantages from the practice of inoculation. Although Camper and Layard are advocates for inoculation for the murrain, *Mons. de Berg* gives a contrary opinion, declaring,* "Que l'inoculation n'offre aucuns avantages reels; sur-tout dans les cas où l'epizootie est très-meurtrière, circonstance qui d'ailleurs est la seule dans laquelle elle puisse être de quelque utilité."

3. *The subsequent effects on the constitution*, from the Cow Pox,

* Lettre à Mons. Linguet, p. 28, Appendix.

must be compared with those from the inoculated Small Pox. A disposition to certain diseases, and even diseases themselves, are not rarely brought on by the Small Pox; but sometimes also dispositions to diseases, and diseases themselves of the most inveterate kind, are removed by the Small Pox. In families wherever certain dispositions to diseases are hereditary, and which diseases are known to have been excited by the Small Pox; inoculation for the Cow Pox on this account may be a considerable benefit; but that is on the supposition that no diseases, or morbid dispositions, are induced by it. As far as my inquiries have extended, I have found that no such morbid effects have ensued from the Cow Pox; but I apprehend that many more observations than have hitherto been made are requisite to ascertain this point satisfactorily.

Although pits from the Small Pox are not a disease, they are at least a deformity, which it is of the greatest moment for many persons to prevent; but which, however, no one can certainly guard against, even by inoculation; and as in the Cow Pox no such consequences take place, an inducement is afforded to inoculate for this disease.

II. As the Small Pox infection is propagated in the state of effluvia, and by adhering, in an unseen and even invisibly small quantity, to cloths, furniture, etc.; but as the Cow Pox infection is only propagated in a visible quantity, and for the most part, only when applied to the divided cuticle; the means of avoiding the Cow Pox are easy and obviously simple. On account of the extremely contagious nature of the variolous poison, the extensive dissemination of it by inoculation, and the practice of inoculating for the Small Pox being only partial, it appears that the mortality by the Small Pox, has been in a greater proportion since, than before the introduction of inoculation. And no sagacity is required to predict, that should the practice of inoculating for the Cow Pox ever become very general amongst young persons, the variolous infection must be extinguished; and, of consequence, that loathsome and destructive disease, the Small Pox, be known only by name. And this benefit will accrue, without even the alloy of the introduction of a new disease, it being plain from the nature of the Cow Pox poison that it will be easy to avoid and prevent its dissemination.

III. The Cow Pox poison appears to alter the human constitution, so as to render it unsusceptible of the agency of a different morbific poison, namely, of the variolous, in producing the Small Pox. This fact is, I believe, quite a novelty in physiology and pathology; it indicates a new principle in the mode of prophylactic practice. And we now see upon what principle diseases from various other morbific poisons may possibly be prevented from taking place, such as the measles, ulcerous sore throat, hooping cough, syphilis, etc., viz., in consequence of destroying the excitability of the constitution to such poisons by the agency of different and perhaps less hurtful ones. Whether the Cow Pox preserves the constitution from other morbific poisons, besides the variolous, is an undecided question. This fact also suggests the idea that the œconomy of live beings may be liable to undergo permanent changes in the state of excitability of each, in respect of certain stimuli, both morbific and innocent ones, which observation has not hitherto discovered. And on account of the unobserved agency of such stimuli, some constitutions are utterly incapable, either permanently or for a limited time, of taking the Small Pox, and perhaps other diseases. But if there are in nature means of rendering the human constitution unsusceptible, it must be allowed that it is probable there are also means of rendering it particularly disposed to certain diseases. And it is possible that the same constitution may, in the course of life, undergo repeatedly a temporary state of inexcitability to certain stimuli; but there is no reason to suppose that a state of inexcitability, which would otherwise be permanent, may be removed by certain morbific stimuli.

In the veterinary branch of physic it is a matter of still greater importance to possess the means of rendering the constitution unsusceptible of the agency of the morbific poison which produces the murrain; because,

(1) This malady is more destructive when it is epizootic than the Small Pox is among human creatures; (2) because inoculation for it is not nearly so beneficial, a great proportion dying under inoculation.

It seems of small consequence in practice, but it is very important on account of physiology to determine, whether the human œconomy is rendered unsusceptible of the Cow Pox by having undergone the Small Pox. In the instances related, of people taking the Cow Pox who had gone through the Small Pox, the observation was not directed with a view to determine, satisfactorily, whether the local affection was certainly attended or preceded by a constitutional affection.

IV. If it be true that the same constitution is liable to undergo repeatedly the Cow Pox, to which distemper no one has fallen a victim, practitioners may avail themselves of this means of exciting an innocent fever as a remedy of various disorders, it being a truth, admitted by men of experience, that fevers are occasionally efficacious remedies, especially for inveterate Chronic maladies, such as Epilepsy, Hysteria, Insanity, St. Vitus' Dance, Tetanus, Skin deformities and diseases, etc.

V. Concerning the *Ætiology* of the disease which is the subject of our inquiry. The Cow Pox in the human animal has, in every *casual instance* of the disease, been so clearly traced immediately to the Cow's breasts, affected with the Cow Pox, that it would be misspending time to relate particularly the history of cases, to prove what is asserted. The inoculation with matter from the Cow produces the same disease as the casual Cow Pox. It appears also that the Cow Pox matter of the human animal excites the same disease as the matter from the Cow. It has not been determined by experiment, nor by any observation of incidental agency of Cow Pox matter, that this matter generated in the human animal will excite the same disease in the Cow; but from the facts just spoken of, probably few persons will doubt that this must be the case. The Cow Pox of the brute is either excited by the matter conveyed from a beast labouring under the disease (in an obvious way by the hands of milkers) to uninfected cows; in which manner one diseased beast may infect an unlimited number of beasts, or the disease is excited by aboriginal Cow Pox matter, that is, by matter compounded in the animal œconomy of the Cow, without any matter of the same kind having been applied. The means by the agency of which the animal œconomy is put into such a state as to compound this peculiar matter are not yet found out. A connection is, however, observed between the disease and the spring season, the autumn, and change from less nutritious to more nutritious food.

It has been concluded by Dr. Jenner that the aboriginal matter is from the matter of the grease of horses, which gains admission through the milkers who handle such greased horses; but this conclusion has no better support than the coincidence in some instances of the prevalence of the two diseases in the same farm, and in which the same servants are employed among the horses and Cows. This assertion stands in need of support from other observations. The *experimentum crucis* seems to have been already instituted, but without success, namely, the inoculation, with the grease matter, of the Cow's breast by Dr. Jenner. It is to excite farther research that I shall mention how successful my inquiries have been to find the origin of the Cow Pox to be in the grease.

1. I have found that in many farms the Cow Pox breaks out,

although no new-comer has been introduced into the herd; although the milkers do not come in contact with horses; although there are no greased horses; and even although there are no horses kept on the farm.

2. It appears that the Cow Pox does not break out under the most favourable circumstances for its production if it be occasioned by *the grease*. Through the application of my inestimable colleague, Dr. Wm. Heberden, I have got much instruction relating to this head from *Sir Isaac Pennington*. "I * have had," says Sir Isaac, "Dr. Jenner's book some weeks, and the particulars stated in it are really astonishing. I have made inquiries upon the subject at Cottenham and Willingham; in which two parishes 3,000 Milch Cows are kept, also a great many horses of the rough-legged cart kind (much liable to the scratches or grease), half the parishes being under the plough, and the men being much employed in milking. But I cannot find that any pustulous eruptions on the teats of the Cow, or on the hands of the milkers, have ever been heard of, and, what seems to prove the negative in this case, I understand inoculation succeeds just as well in these parishes as anywhere else. I cannot find from those concerned in inoculation that shoeing-smiths are less liable to the infection of the Small Pox than other people."

Dr. Parr is one of the few men of learning, and acknowledged ability, who has imbibed an unfavourable opinion of the whole of the facts and reasoning of Dr. Jenner. But as my Exeter friend merely opposes reasoning and gratuitous suppositions to at least some well-attested facts, I do not think anything will be gained by stating, particularly, his sentiments on the subject, yet I acquiesce to his judgment, "that the assertion that the Cow Pox proceeds from the heels of horses is gratuitous." He reprobates the conclusions on this part of the subject in somewhat opprobrious terms, in which, however, the doctor himself argues more on gratuitous suppositions than admitted truths.

"Limpid † fluid is always more active than pus, for a wound no longer spreads when the matter becomes purulent. If a disease does proceed from the matter of the heel of the horse, it is no other than such as occurs in the human subject, namely, topical ulcers, from a putrid fomes; since it is probable (p. 25, Jenner) on Dr. Jenner's own foundation, the eruptions must precede its influence. Men servants seldom milk Cows in this country, and when they do, such insufferable dirtiness as to milk

* Sir Isaac Pennington's Letter, Cambridge, Sept. 14th, 1798.
† Dr. Parr's, M.D., Letter, Exeter, July 22nd, 1798.

with hands streaming with the running of a sore heel would not be tolerated in any milking court in this country. Indeed, I think this publication (Dr. Jenner's) is a libel on his own neighbourhood."

At the close of these adverse observations, it is but fair to represent that this opinion respecting the origin of the Cow Pox is not merely that of Dr. Jenner, for Mr. Smith (letter above cited) says, "Mr. Woodman had a notion of the Cow Pox originating from the sore heels of horses." And several male servants at the milk farms near London said, "There was such a notion entertained in several parts in the country, whatever might be its foundation."

The Cow Pox poison, and the hydrophobic poison, are the only specific morbific matter to the human animal œconomy which are clearly proved to be derived from brute animals; for there is only small probability on the side of the opinion that the syphilitic poison is from the *bull,** the Small Pox from the *camel,*† and the itch from the *dog.* The œconomy then of the human kind, and of Cows, resemble, in the particular of being excitable to a disease, the Cow Pox, by a certain specific poison. Whether other animals, especially males of the bovine kind, can take the Cow Pox has not been determined by experiment or accidental observation. Morbific poisons, which produce specific diseases, act in this way only on one species of animal, except in a few instances, such as the hydrophobic and Cow Pox poisons. Camper, Ingenhousz, and Woodville in vain attempted to produce the Small Pox by inoculation in a number of different brute animals.‡ J. Hunter failed in attempting to excite the syphilis in a dog by inoculating him with the poison of the gonorrhœa and of a syphilitic ulcer. Camper attests that in the most malignant epizootic murrain, which spread most rapidly among oxen, yet other animals, such as sheep, horses, asses, dogs, etc., were not infected by associating with the distempered oxen, nor even by feeding with them in the same compartments of a stable.

In the eruptive contagious disease among sheep in France

---

* Bulls so diseased are said to be *stung.*—Sir Isaac Pennington's Letter.

† See Bruce's *Travels* and Dr. Woodville's *History of Inoculation.*

‡ Berrier, of Chartres, asserts that monkeys, dogs, sheep, rabbits, oxen, and other brute animals, are susceptible of the Small Pox; but his evidence has not the weight of a feather against the contrary authorities.

Swediaur asserts that monkeys are never affected with the syphilis, although in England they are subject to the scrofula, and that other animals are equally unsusceptible of the syphilis, although *Pauw* affirms that in Peru dogs are affected with this disease.

forty years ago, other species of animals which associated with them were not infected.

The newly-observed disease, which prevailed among domestic cats in 1796, throughout great part of Europe, and even America, did not appear to affect other animals.

These observations may serve to remove the fears of those who apprehend, that in consequence of domesticating brute creatures, we are liable to render their diseases *endemial.*

VI. As it appears that the Cow Pox poison, after its admission into the human constitution, takes effect, or sensibly exerts its agency upon the whole economy, in seven or eight days, it seems probable that it will anticipate, in many instances, the agency of the Small Pox poison, if the two poisons be introduced at the same time, or nearly so; in which case the patients should be in future incapable of the Small Pox.

If the morbific poison of the varicella, or Chicken Pox, were to be inserted at the same time with the Cow Pox poison, it is probable also that the Cow Pox would suspend the Chicken Pox, and perhaps render the constitution unsusceptible of its action in future. But if it be a truth that the rubeolous poison can be inserted by inoculation, and that it affects the constitution in six days, when this poison and that of the Cow Pox are introduced at the same time, it is most likely the Measles will suspend the Cow Pox.

So long as the constitution is under the agency of the Cow Pox poison, it is not probable that it will be infected by those morbific poisons whose existence is only known by their effects (for they operate in too minute a quantity to fall under the notice of our senses), namely, the poison which occasions the Influenza, Hooping Cough, ulcerous Angina, that which occasions the Typhus fever, the miasmata and the contagion of intermittent fevers, etc.

To give an instance of the application of facts to practice. If a woman be far advanced in pregnancy, and exposure to Small Pox infection has been or is unavoidable, in that case it will be of vast importance to avert the present impending danger from the female. Under such a circumstance the temptation to inoculate for the Cow Pox will be felt by the practitioner. And provided the inoculation be instituted in not more than six or seven days after exposure to the variolous infection, it should, according to principle, pretty certainly preserve the patient from Small Pox; or if it be done within ten or twelve days, it should frequently answer the purpose. For the variolous poison lies within the human body, most frequently fifteen days, and often four or five days later, before its general agency is perceived; whereas the Cow Pox poison acts upon the whole constitution in seven or eight days after its admission.

VII. The Cow Pox poison is, according to the present facts, totally different in its nature and effects from every other morbific poison, both of cattle and human creatures. It is not necessary to enter minutely into the distinguishing characters of it as it appears in Cows, as these will be collected from the history of the disease. I think it right just to mention that care should be taken not to confound the Cow Pox with the common warty-eruptions and inflammations ending in scabs, which affect the paps only, or at most the paps and the udders. It must also be recollected that the Cow Pox is quite different from the diseases of cattle which are attended with eruptions of the skin in general, such as take place in the murrain, or *pestis bovilla*, already spoken of, on which eruptive diseases more has been written by the Italian, French, and Dutch physicians than by the English.*

On account of the notion which, by some, is entertained, that the Cow Pox infection is of the same nature as the variolous, it may be useful to point out the great differences between them.

1. The Cow Pox poison, introduced by inoculation, affects the whole constitution at the same time in the same degree and manner as when admitted in the casual way; and if the local affection be more severe in the casual than in the inoculated way, it seems to be owing to the structure of the part, namely, the thick cuticle in the palms of the hands.

2. The Cow Pox poison only affects the constitution through the intervention of the part poisoned.

---

* Gli assistenzi a'bovi ammalati e molt' altri uomini degni di fede m'attestarono d'aver osservati, in alcuni tumori crudi in diverse parti del corpo con lingue aride, nere e tagliate, in altri aver veduti tumori maturate.—*P. A. Michelloti*, p. 12, 1711.

La terza osservazione fu circa alcuni buovi, che dimorarano in ima stalla come alle pecore: due di essi cacciarono d' alla cute certi tubercolletti.—*Padre Boromeo*, p. 48.

Annis 1713, 1714, in nostro Ferrariensi Ducatu, lues contagiosa boum, etc. Correpti enim boves cibum respuebant; aures subito collapsæ procidebant: pili erigebantur; tremor pené universalis aderat: oculi lacrymabant: per nares multa lymphæ copia exibat; alvus solvebatur et in aliquibus pustulæ sub cute prodibant, ita ut crederent aliqui Variolis boves ipsos assici; tandemque brevi septem dierum spatio moriebantur.—*J. Lanzoni*, t. 20, b. 202.

Maculis denique et pustulis infecta cutis, adeo ut quibusdam, in mentem venerit cogitare boves non lue, ut nunc res est, sed ipsis pustulis quas Variolas vocant interire.—*J. M. Lancisi* de bovilla peste.

Schreiben an die Generalstaaten betreffend die Einimpfung der Viehseuche geschrieben den 16 Febr. 1770. CAMPER Von Einimpfung der Kindviehseuche. ihren Vortheilen und Bedingungen.—CAMPERS Berliner Gesellschaft.

3. This morbific poison produces no eruption or inflammation but of and near the part to which the poison is applied.

4. The Cow Pox poison from the human subject will, in all probability, infect the cow with the Cow Pox, which the variolous poison will not.

5. It is asserted that a person may have the Cox Pox who has had the Small Pox.

6. The local pustulous eruptions in the Cow Pox are rather of the nature of vesicles, or phlyctenæ, than purulent eruptions, and the ulceration is apt to be of the phagedenic kind.

7. The Cow Pox infection is not propagated in the state of effluvia or gas.

8. Cow Pox matter applied to the eyes, lips, and various other soft parts, or to any parts which are punctured or wounded, in persons who already have had the Cow Pox, or are then ill of the disease, will excite the peculiar local affection from this poison, and perhaps fever.

VIII. There are some who are not certain whether or not they have gone through the Small Pox, yet they have such a dread of the disease as not to submit even to inoculation for it. To such persons the inoculation for the Cow Pox as a substitute for the Small Pox must prove a happy discovery.

Some who have never gone through the Small Pox have been repeatedly inoculated for the Small Pox, and also been exposed much to the infection of it in the casual way, yet could not be infected. Persons so circumstanced, to be more secure, may be inoculated for the Cow Pox.

Such is the representation which I shall venture to lay before the public of the benefits likely to accrue to human society from inoculation for the Cow Pox. I shall be no better contented with those who will consider the facts to be already completely demonstrated, than with the opposite extreme opinion, that the whole of the prospects displayed are merely *Utopian*. The fortunes of the new proposed practice cannot, with certainty, be told at present by the most discerning minds. More instances are required to establish practical and pathological truths. Without assuming pretensions which I think unwarrantable, the number of instances farther requisite cannot be stated; but one may safely assert that well-directed observation in a thousand cases of inoculated Cow Pox would not fail to produce such a valuable body of evidence as will enable us to apply our knowledge with much usefulness in practice, and establish, or at least bring us nearer the establishment of, some truths.

They who take a part in the present inquiry must not expect to escape detraction. But such a prospect will not divert him from his path who labours in the culture of physic for the satisfaction of his own mind, well knowing that it argues egregious ignorance of what is passing in the world to do so from any other motive.

COMMUNICATIONS RECEIVED AFTER THE PRECEDING SHEETS WERE PRINTED; AND ADDITIONAL OBSERVATIONS.

Mr. Rolph, Surgeon in *Peckham*, practised physic nine years at Thornbury in Gloucestershire. During two of these years he was the colleague of the late *Mr. Grove*, who had been a medical practitioner at Thornbury for near forty years. The greater part of the facts above stated, relating to the Cow Pox, are familiarly known to Mr. Rolph from his own observation, and from the experience of Mr. Grove.

Mr. Rolph tells me, that in Gloucestershire the Cow Pox is very frequently epizootic in the dairy farms in the spring season. It especially breaks out in Cows newly introduced into the herds. When a number of Cows in a farm are at the same time affected, the infection seems generally to have originated in the constitution of some one Cow, and before the milker is aware of the existence of the disease the infectious matter is probably conveyed by the hands to the teats and udders of other Cows; hence they are infected. For if the disease in the Cow first affected be perceived in a certain state, and obvious precautions be taken, the infection does not spread, but is confined to a single beast. Whether the morbific poison is generated in the Cow first diseased in a given farm, *de novo*, from time to time, and disseminated among the rest of the herd, or, like the Small Pox poison, is only communicated from animals of the same species to one another, is not ascertained. No Cow has been known to die or be in danger from this disorder.

A great number of instances of the Cow Pox in milkers had fallen under Mr. Rolph's observation, and many hundreds more under that of his late partner, Mr. Grove; but not a single mortal, or even dangerous, case had occurred. The patients were ordinarily ill of a slight fever for two or three days, and the local affection was so slight that the assistance of medical practitioners was rarely required. He had no doubt that the inoculated Cow

Pox was attended with as little pain and uneasiness as the ordinary cases of inoculated Small Pox.

Mr. Rolph says, there is not a medical practitioner of even little experience in Gloucestershire, or scarce a dairy farmer, who does not know from his own experience, or that of others, that persons who have suffered the Cow Pox are exempted from the agency of the variolous poison.

The late Mr. Grove was a very extensive Small Pox inoculator, frequently having two or three hundred patients at one time, and the fact of exemption now asserted had been long before his death abundantly established by his experience of many scores of subjects who had previously laboured under the Cow Pox being found unsusceptible to the Small Pox, either by inoculation or by effluvia.

While Mr. Rolph practised at Thornbury, he thinks not fewer than threescore instances of failure in attempting to produce the Small Pox by inoculation occurred in his own practice, all of which were persons who had been previously affected with the Cow Pox. In almost all of these cases the uninfected persons associated with those who took the Small Pox, and many were repeatedly inoculated. Although Mr. Rolph has not, in his recollection, any instances of people taking the Small Pox who gave admissible evidence of their having laboured under the Cow Pox, he thinks such cases may, and have indeed occurred to others, where the Cow Pox had been *only* local, it being requisite that the whole constitution should be affected in order to destroy the excitability to the variolous poison.

Mr. Rolph declared that his confidence in the efficacy and safety of inoculation for the Cow Pox was such that he regretted he could not, at present, procure Cow Pox matter to inoculate two of his own children who had not yet had the Small Pox. This measure is, however, determined upon.

As a particular instance, Mr. Rolph related the following:—A soldier's wife, while in the Small Pox, was accidentally in the company of several farmers at an ale-house in Thornbury. Two of the company who had gone through the Cow Pox, but not the Small Pox, were not infected by the variolous infection; but three others, who had not laboured under the Cow Pox, took the Small Pox.

Mr. Rolph's mind was not satisfied that a person could be constitutionally affected by the Cox Pox poison more than once, but he had no doubt that the local affection might be produced repeatedly. Neither did he certainly know that a person was unsusceptible of the Small Pox who had been constitutionally affected by the Cow Pox.

Mr. Rolph, in a letter to Dr. Beddoes, dated June 10th, 1795, communicated the following observations. Speaking of a man who could not be infected, although he was repeatedly inoculated for the Small Pox, and although he lived in the same room with another man who died of the Small Pox, Mr. Rolph says, "It is worthy * of remark that this man had some years before a complaint incident to Cows, and commonly called the Cow Pox, a malady more unpleasant than dangerous. It is generally received by contact in milking. In the human species the complaint is sometimes local; at other times absorption takes place, and the glands in the course of the absorbents become indurated and painful. When this is the case, *I have learned from my own observation, and the testimony of some old practitioners, that susceptibility to the Small Pox is destroyed.* Some advantage may probably, in time, be derived from this fact."

LETTER FROM DR. JENNER TO DR. PEARSON.

CHELTENHAM, *27th September*, 1798.

MY DEAR SIR,—The perusal of your proof sheets has afforded me great pleasure, both from the handsome manner in which you mention my name, and from the mass of evidence which has poured in upon you from different countries in support of the fact which I so ardently wish to see established on a steady and durable basis.

Your first query respecting the Fœtus in Utero I cannot resolve.

With respect to your second, you may be assured that a person may be repeatedly affected, both locally and generally, by the Cow Pox, two instances of which I have adduced, and have many more in my recollection. But, nevertheless, on this important point, I have some reason to suspect that my discriminations have not been, till lately, sufficiently nice. I must observe to you, that what the constitution feels from the absorption of the Virus † is of a mild and transient nature, but the sores (which sores, when casual, are

---

* See the queries of Dr. Beddoes concerning inoculation, subjoined to his translation of Gimbernat's *Method of Operating for the Femoral Hernia.* London: Johnson, 1795.

† I use this expression as the common language of the day, without consenting to the truth of it.

Pox was
cases
Mr.
exper
not
with
the

free
and

the system.
effects
feel
determine.
the Small Pox
disturb the
of the
the Cow Pox
spreads
not unlike

not an atom of the
the experiments.
not take matter
efficacy,—for after it
I fear its specific
necessary in the pro-
that the discovery
conducting
example, a person
when, in
scratches
subjected
will
at once
however,
appearance

ER.

bury,

length the cause of the failure was discovered from the case of a farmer who was inoculated several times ineffectually, yet he assured us he had never suffered the Small Pox, but, says he, "*I have had the Cow Pox lately to a violent degree, if that's any odds.*" We took the hint, and, on inquiry, found that all those who were uninfectable had undergone the Cow Pox. I communicated this fact to a medical society of which I was then a member, and ever afterwards paid particular attention to determine the fact. I can now, with truth, affirm *that I have not been able to produce the Small Pox, in a single instance, among the persons who have had the true Cow Pox,* except a doubtful case which you are acquainted with. I have, since that, inoculated near two thousand for the Small Pox, amongst whom there were a great number who had gone through the Cow Pox; the exact numbers of these I cannot tell, but I know that they all resisted the infection of variolous matter.

With regard to your questions:

1. As to danger from Cow Pox. In the course of thirty years I have known numberless instances of the disease, but never knew one mortal, or even dangerous, case.

2. Is a person susceptible of the Cow Pox more than once? I cannot answer this question.

3. Is the Cow Pox, in the natural way, a more or less severe disease than the inoculated Small Pox? I think it is a much more severe disease in general than the inoculated Small Pox. I do not see any great advantage from the inoculation for the Cow Pox. Inoculation for the Small Pox seems to be so well understood, that there is very little need of a substitute. It is curious, however, and may lead to other improvements.*

4. Have you ever known any pregnant woman labour under the Cow Pox? Yes, many, but it *never produced abortion.* The state of the fœtus I cannot speak of.

5. Are Cows affected at certain times more than at others? They are especially affected from February to May, when there is the greatest number of greased horses.

I cannot procure any Cow Pox matter this season.

From Mr. Bird *to* Dr. Pearson, *October 16th,* 1798.

Mr. G. G. Bird, of *Hereford,* who is now attending medical lectures in London, tells Dr. P. that he has very often seen the

* I have stated the writer's opinion of inoculation for the Cow Pox, in obedience to a law imposed on myself, of not suppressing any part of the evidence communicated, however differently I might reason on the facts.—Note *by the author of this inquiry.*

Cow Pox in Cows and human creatures near *Gloucester;* that it attacks the same person repeatedly, and once the third attack was observed to be more severe than the preceding ones, but ordinarily the reverse is the fact. It appears with red spots on the hands, which enlarge, become roundish and suppurate—tumours take place in the armpit—the pulse grows quick—the head aches—pains are felt in the back and limbs, with sometimes vomiting and delirium. It is most common in a wet spring. No one dies of the disease.

Dr. Currie, of *Chester*, informs Mr. Thomas that the disease called Cow Pox is unknown to the medical practitioners and farmers in Cheshire.

Dr. Richard Pearson, of *Birmingham*, in his obliging letter of the 26th September last, says, "From this united evidence (that of medical persons and farmers), I think that it may be inferred that the disease, which Dr. Jenner calls *Variolæ vaccinæ*, is not epizootic in the counties of Warwick, Worcester, and Stafford."

Dr. Woodville acquaints me, "that not being able to procure Cow Pox matter he is making trials with *grease matter*, from which no doubt some useful information will be obtained."

Extracts of a Letter from Mr. Thomas Wales, Surgeon at Downham, Norfolk, dated October 18th, 1798, to Dr. Pearson.

I shall endeavour to give you satisfactory answers to your queries.

Previous to my conversation with Dr. Redfearn, I had no knowledge of the disease called Cow Pox, nor was it known to any medical practitioner in this district. But on inquiring at the dairy-farms, I have got much information concerning the disease. I this day saw two persons who have had the Cow Pox. One of them, a man above sixty years of age, who has been a milker all his life, knows the disease very well by the name of *Pap-pox*, having himself experienced the disorder a great many years ago. He remembers that on that occasion he was sick at the stomach and otherwise ill for two or three days. The eruption on his hands was considerable, and the fingers were swollen; probably owing to improper applications the places healed slowly, and left scars, which are evident at this day; and when the hands are very cold these scars are of a *livid cast*. He had not gone through the Small Pox before he had the Cow Pox, nor has he had the Small Pox since this disease, although he has been repeatedly inoculated.

The other case above mentioned is that of a young woman, who had the Cow Pox some time ago, but never suffered the Small Pox, although she had been several times inoculated.

There are, I find, many other instances of persons who have gone through the Cow Pox, and who have not been able to take the Small Pox, either naturally or by inoculation.

As the public in this part are not at all aware of the advantages of inoculation for the Cow Pox, there are no instances of this disease by this mode of producing it.

I do not find that any person has had the Cow Pox more than once, that is, a fever with the local affection more than once; but the local affection without the fever has occurred in the same person repeatedly. I have met with two cases in which the matter of the Cow Pox, by being applied to the eyes, destroyed the power of vision, from the opacity of the cornea so produced.

No person has been known to die, or even to be in danger, with the Cow Pox, although the axillary glands have been much affected, and the sores on the hands have healed with difficulty. I have not met with a case of a woman who has gone through the disease during pregnancy.

No instance has fallen under my observation of a person who has gone through the Cow Pox after having had the Small Pox.

With regard to Cows, they are subject to the Cow Pox more than once. It comes on in the spring, when they first begin to taste luxuriant food, but not uniformly every year. One farmer informed me that he thought it broke out especially when the cows were fed with turnips in autumn; but I do not depend much upon this observation.

Remarks on the term VARIOLÆ VACCINÆ.

For the sake of precision in language, and of consequence justness in thinking, and considering that there is no way of disabusing ourselves from many of the errors in physic but by the use of just terms, it is not unworthy of our attention to guard against the admission of newly appropriated names which will mislead by their former accepted import.

Variola is an assumed Latin word, and its meaning will be popularly understood in the English tongue by saying that it is a name of a disease, better known by another name—the Small Pox. Granting that the word "Variola" is a derivative from *Varius* and *Varus*, used by Pliny and Celsus to denote a disease with spots on the skin, the etymological import of Variola is any cutaneous spotted distemper; but one of the most formidable and distinct of the cutaneous order is what is called the *Small Pox*, and therefore, as I apprehend the name, *Variola* has been used technically (κατ' ἐξοχην) to signify this kind of spotted malady, and no other.

Now as the Cow Pox is a specifically different distemper from the Small Pox in essential particulars, namely, in the nature of its morbific poison, and in its symptoms,—although the Cow Pox may render the constitution not susceptible of the Small Pox,—it is a palpable *catachresis* to designate what is called the Cow Pox by the denomination *Variolæ vaccinæ;* for that is to say, in English, *Cow-Small Pox*, and yet the Cow is unsusceptible of infection by the variolous poison.

To the name Cow Pox, or better, perhaps, *Cow Pocken*,* in our language, I think no reasonable objection can be urged. According to the more distinct and lucid arrangement of cutaneous distempers, by Dr. Willan,† the Cow Pox belongs to the *order* entitled *pustules;* the word *pock* is known to signify *pustule*, and the prefix *Cow* denotes the only animal in which the morbific poison of the disease has its γενεσις. Further, if hereafter, by the practice of universal inoculation, the human animal should be much more abundant and better known source of this morbific matter, than the brute animal, it is fit that the latter, to which obligations will be owing for an inestimable benefit, should live in the grateful memory of mankind, as ought also the name of JENNER, who will be so great a PUBLIC BENEFACTOR.

QUERIES.

It may save some persons the trouble of thinking and time, if a set of questions be stated, which will serve to guide observation in the acquisition of facts belonging to the subject of inquiry. For this purpose the following queries are proposed.

With Respect to Brutes.

1. If a distemper of Cows has been noticed, called the Cow Pox, or by any other name, in which the breasts, especially the paps, are affected with pustulous, and generally purple, or livid eruptions and sores, by which the hands of milkers are infected, what are the symptoms?

* Instead of the modern orthography Small PoX, etc., in which *cs* and *cks* are denoted by *x*, it will be, perhaps, thought preferable to follow the original orthography *pock* with its plural *pocken*, as the Germans still do; from whose language we have received the words.

† *Description and Treatment of Cutaneous Disorders* (Order 1: Pustulous Eruptions on the Skin), by Robert Willan, F.A.S. 4to, with plates, Johnson, 1798.

2. Can any connection be traced betwixt this disease and the grease of horses' heels? between the disease and particular kinds of food and water? between it and any particular states of the atmosphere? between it and any particular season?

3. Is the same Cow liable to the disease more than once?

4. Has any Cow ever appeared to die of this disease?

5. Is the Cow susceptible of the Cow Pox by the inoculation of the breasts with grease matter of horses?

6. Are males of the Ox kind; or other different kinds of brutes, susceptible of the disease by inoculation with Cow Pox matter of Cows?

7. Have Cows in a state of pregnancy been observed to be affected with this distemper?

8. Is the Cow susceptible of the disease by inoculation of other parts beside the breasts?

9. Is the Cow Pox matter of human creatures capable of producing Cow Pox in Cows?

With Respect to Human Creatures.

1. What parts are affected, and what are the symptoms of the distemper when contracted in the casual way?

2. Has any person been supposed to be in danger or to have died of the disease?

3. Is the whole constitution disordered previously, or *only at the same time* the pustules break out? Does the disorder of the constitution disappear on the appearance of the pustules? Does the same or a different disorder of the constitution again appear; and under what circumstances in the course of the disease?

4. If in the course of the disease, when there is no disorder of the whole constitution, the infectious matter of the Cow or of the human patient already labouring under the Cow Pox be applied to fresh parts, does a disorder of the whole constitution arise, as well as a local affection; and of the same kind as those which have already taken place?

5. Is the same person susceptible of the Cow Pox local affection, and fever, or disorder of the whole constitution more than once, or only of the local affection more than once? In the instances in which the disorder of the whole constitution was said to have occurred more than once, is it not probable that in one case only the specific fever of the infection occurred, and in the others a different disorder of the whole constitution, such as was merely from the irritation of the local affection?

6. Is the local affection of the same nature on a second or on further attacks in the same person as on the first?

7. In the instances of Cow Pox in persons who had gone through the Small Pox, were the local affection and disorder of the constitution of the same nature as in persons who had not laboured under the Small Pox?

8. Has it been observed that a person has ever taken the Small Pox after having gone through the Cow Pox? In the instances in which the Small Pox was said to have taken place, was it certain that the preceding Cow Pox was attendant with its specific fever, or was there only a local affection, or at most was there only disorder symptomatic of the local affection?

9. Does the Cow Pox render the human constitution unsusceptible of any other disease besides the Small Pox; or, on the contrary, increase its susceptibility to any particular diseases?

10. What are the effects of the Cow Pox on pregnant women?

11. In the inoculated Cow Pox is the fever less considerable than in the casual way?

12. In the inoculated Cow Pox is the local affection slighter and of shorter duration than in the casual Cow Pox?

13. How long after the insertion of the matter is it before the constitution is affected?

14. If a person were to be inoculated at the same time with the Cow Pox and variolous matter, which disorder would appear first, or what other effects would be produced?

15. If the Cow Pox morbific matter be applied to a secreting membrane, *e.g.*, to the urethra, will it produce a gonorrhœa or pustulous sores?

16. Does the disease appear to injure the constitution, by producing or exciting other diseases?

17. Does the disease appear to eradicate any other disease already present?

18. Does the mildness or severity of the inoculated Cow Pox depend upon the quantity of the matter inserted, or on the wounds inflicted for inoculation?

19. Does the Cow Pox matter produce the disease as certainly in its dried as in its fluid state; and when old as when recent; and with equal mildness?

20. Are there any particular states of the constitution in which the Cow Pox is particularly mild; or, on the contrary, severe; as after the Measles, Hooping Cough, etc.?

21. Are there particular idiosyncrasies in families or individuals which influence the Cow Pox, as is the case in the Small Pox?

22. Is the inoculation of the Cow Pox equally successful in infancy, manhood, and decrepit age?

23. Do certain epidemic states appear to prevail which influence this disease?

Answers to the preceding questions will be principally obtained by inoculation for the Cow Pox, of which there are many opportunities in provincial situations; which practice it is one of the chief objects of this publication to encourage.

P.S.—Extract of a letter from Dr. FOWLER *to Dr.* PEARSON, *dated Sarum, October 24th,* 1798.

MY DEAR SIR,—The disease called Cow Pox is known in this neighbourhood only to a few farmers, but they understand that it is a preservative from the Small Pox. This morning, *Anne Francis*, a servant girl, aged twenty-six years, was brought to me; she informs me, that some years ago bluish pustules arose on her hands, from milking Cows diseased by the Cow Pox. These pustules soon became scabs, which, falling off, discovered ulcerating and very painful [sores?—E.M.C.], which were treated by a Cow doctor, and were long in healing. Some milk from one of the diseased Cows having spurted on the cheek of her sister, and on the breast of her mistress, produced on these parts of both persons pustules and sores, similar to her own on her hands. None of these three had suffered the Small Pox, nor have they gone through it since that time, although they have been much exposed to the infection; and the sister above mentioned has been inoculated three times for the Small Pox. The Cow doctor who attended these three women said he would forfeit his life if any of them should afterwards have the Small Pox.

With sincerest good wishes for the success of this and all your undertakings,

I am, etc., etc.,

R. FOWLER.

NOTE.—*Mr. Hughes'* Letter, dated Stroud-Water, Gloucestershire, October 27th, 1798, to *Mr. Bliss*, Surgeon, Hampstead, has been just sent to the Author, in answer to his Queries. Unfortunately this valuable letter cannot now be published. It especially confirms, by a number of instances, the facts of the safety of the Cow Pox, and of its producing unsusceptibility of the Small Pox.

FINIS.

REPORTS

OF

A SERIES OF INOCULATIONS

FOR THE

VARIOLÆ VACCINÆ,

OR COW-POX;

WITH REMARKS AND OBSERVATIONS ON THIS DISEASE, CONSIDERED AS A SUBSTITUTE FOR

THE SMALL-POX.

By WILLIAM WOODVILLE, M.D.,

PHYSICIAN TO THE SMALL POX AND INOCULATION HOSPITALS.

LONDON:

PRINTED AND SOLD BY

JAMES PHILLIPS AND SON,

George Yard, Lombard Street.

TO

THE RIGHT HONORABLE

SIR JOSEPH BANKS, Bart.,

Knight of the Bath,

President of the Royal Society, etc., etc., etc.

Sir,

The great attention with which you honoured some of the first cases described in the following sheets has induced me to hope that an account of the whole, though not affording the satisfactory evidence upon the subject that I expected, may still not be entirely unacceptable to you.

I have the honour to be,

With the utmost regard,

Your obedient servant,

W. WOODVILLE.

Ely Place,

May 16th, 1799.

REPORTS, ETC.

LAST summer Dr. Jenner presented to the public* several curious and interesting facts, respecting a disease known to dairy farmers by the name of Cow-Pox. The most important of these is, that persons who have been affected with this distemper are thereby rendered as secure from the effects of the variolous infection as if they had actually undergone the Small-Pox.

However extraordinary this circumstance may appear, it is supported by numerous experiments made under Dr. Jenner's inspection, and also by concurrent testimonies since collected by Dr. Pearson,† who with much laudable zeal and industry instituted a farther inquiry into the subject.

Dr. Jenner, who, from his situation in Gloucestershire, had many opportunities of seeing the Cow Pox, supposes it to originate from the matter of the grease in horses, and to take place in the following manner:

"In this dairy country a great number of cows are kept, and the office of milking is performed indiscriminately by men and maid servants. One of the former having been appointed to apply dressings to the heels of a horse affected with the grease, and not paying due attention to cleanliness, incautiously bears his part in milking the cows with some particles of the infectious matter adhering to his fingers. When this is the case, it commonly happens that a disease is communicated to the cows, and from the cows to the dairy-maids, which spreads through the farm, until most of the cattle and domestics feel its unpleasant consequences. The disease has obtained the name of the Cow Pox. It appears on the nipples of the cows, in the form of irregular pustules. At their first appearance they are commonly of a palish blue, or rather of a colour somewhat approaching to livid, and are surrounded by an erysipelatous inflammation. These pustules, unless a timely remedy

* See "*An Inquiry into the Causes and Effects of the Variolæ Vaccinæ*, a Disease discovered in some of the Western Counties of England, particularly Gloucestershire, and known by the name of the Cow Pox."

† See *An Inquiry concerning the History of the Cow Pox.*

conceiving that the distemper might be produced by inoculating the nipples of cows with the matter of the grease of horses, in conformity with the opinion above stated I proceeded to try whether the Cow Pox could be actually excited in this manner.

Numerous experiments were accordingly made upon different cows, with the matter of grease, taken in the various stages of that disease, but without producing the desired effect. My friend, Mr. Coleman, the ingenious professor at the Veterinary College, likewise made similar trials, which proved equally unsuccessful.* Neither were inoculations with this matter, nor with several other morbid secretions in the horse, productive of any effects upon the human subject.

I am aware that the experiments I allude to may, by some, not be deemed wholly conclusive, from the supposition that the peculiar predisposition of the cows, necessary to render the inoculations efficient, might not exist at the time the matter was applied to their nipples.

But I have also other reasons for believing that the Cow Pox does not originate from any disease of the horse. In the first place, the affirmative opinion is confessedly gratuitous. A horse, at a certain season of the year, becomes affected with the grease, and the cows at the same time are affected with Cow Pox; and from this coincidence the two diseases have been considered as cause and effect. Yet is it not equally probable that the same temporary causes which produce a certain disorder in one animal may so operate upon another animal of a different genus as to excite another disorder? Therefore, though the Cow Pox may break out among the cows at the time that the grease affects the horses kept on the same farm, yet the consecutive appearance of these diseases affords no proof of their connection; while, on the other hand, I can adduce instances in which the former disease has broken out under such circumstances as render it highly improbable, if not impossible, that it should have been caused by the latter.†

But, though Dr. Jenner seems to have been misled with respect to the origin of the Cow Pox, still his facts and observations concerning its effects upon mankind are not the less valid and important; nor did I feel the less desirous to try how far they

* Mr. Coleman caused one of his cows to be inoculated in its teats with Cow Pox matter and that taken from a variolous pustule, without effect; but the former matter, after being regenerated by the human subject, produced the disease in the cow.

† Those who wish for further information on this subject may consult Mr. Simmons' *Experiments* and Dr. Pearson's *Inquiry*, pp. 75-76.

would be invalidated or confirmed by a more enlarged experience than he had the opportunity of acquiring.

Towards the latter end of January last I was informed that the Cow Pox had appeared among several of the milch cows kept in Gray's Inn Lane, and upon examination of these, three or four were discovered to be affected with pustulous sores upon their teats and udder. These pustules corresponded in their appearance with the representation and description of the genuine Cow Pox, as given by Dr. Jenner. I should not, however, call the surrounding inflammation erysipelatous; it was evidently an indurated tumefaction of the skin. The number of cows kept at this place was at the time about two hundred, and about four-fifths of them were eventually infected.*

The hands of three or four persons became sore in consequence of milking the cows thus affected; and one of them, Sarah Rice, exhibited so perfect a specimen of the disease that I could entertain no doubt of its being the true, and not the spurious, Cow Pox. Several gentlemen, who I knew would be highly gratified by seeing the disease as it appeared upon this girl's arm, were invited to meet me at the cow-house on the following day, when Lord Somerville, Sir Joseph Banks, Sir Wm. Watson, Drs. Simmons, Pearson, Willan, and others, attended. This was on the 24th of January last, and Sarah Rice had then been affected five days. The appearance of the disease upon this girl's hand and arm very much resembled the representation of it given in the first plate of Dr. Jenner's pamphlet. At first a small tumour or circular vesicle appeared between her fingers; next day she discovered [illegible] the first, namely, one upon her finger, another at [illegible] upon the middle of her forearm. The two [illegible] larger, and exactly resembled the vesicle upon [illegible] the plate alluded to; that at the wrist was now [illegible] third of an inch in diameter, and the other upon her [illegible] larger; they were both of a circular form, not [illegible] the centre, and had a simple inflammatory border; [illegible] of both these tumours, but more especially of the [illegible] acquired a blue colour, which was deepest [illegible] The blueness had come on during the last [illegible] for I had seen the tumours the preceding day, [illegible] could scarcely be perceived, and that too [illegible] at that time also it contained a colourless fluid, [illegible] appeared brownish. The girl now perceived

* [illegible] not in milk escaped the disease.

an uneasiness at the axilla; and I afterwards learned that this symptom was followed by a slight headache. None of the tumours were painful, and they all gradually went off without producing ulceration.

Sarah Rice had undergone the Small Pox when a child; and the only reason why she was more affected by milking the diseased cows than the other milkers were, was that her hands and arms were more red, swollen, and disposed to chap than theirs; though it does not appear that there were any abrasions of the cuticle of those parts of the skin which were infected by the Cow Pox.

Before relating the cases of inoculation with the matter of Cow Pox, I have judged it proper in the first place briefly to state what are the local effects produced by inoculating variolous matter, so that the progress of the infection in both cases may be compared, and the subject of inoculation at large be better understood.

In cases wherein inoculation of the Small Pox proves effectual, a small particle of variolous matter being applied by a superficial puncture of the skin usually produces, in the course of three or four days, or sooner, a little elevation of the punctured part, discoverable by the touch, and a red speck distinguishable by the eye. From this time the redness advances in a circular form, more or less rapidly, according to the constitutional circumstances of the patient; and the first effect of this superficial inflammation is the formation of a vesicle upon its centre, which usually appears between the fourth and seventh day after the inoculation. The extent of the vesicle is generally found to bear some proportion to the intensity of the inflammation; and contains a limpid fluid, by the absorption of which the Small Pox is produced. The vesicle soon bursts, and the central part of the puncture becomes depressed, and often of a dark hue; which appearances, together with the marginal inflammation, continue to increase till the eruptive symptoms subside, when the edges of the depressed part begin to swell with a purulent fluid, and the inflammation gradually recedes.

Thus it appears that the variolous matter, first inserted by the puncture, like that of other morbid poisons, is not capable of being immediately absorbed, but lodges in the skin, and there excites an inflammatory process, by which a new matter producing the disease is generated.* It would seem also that this

* In the second volume of the *History of Inoculation*, (now nearly ready for the press,) I have endeavoured to show that the general greater mildness of the inoculated than the casual Small Pox depends upon this circumstance.

process is carried to a greater or less extent in different persons before the matter enters the absorbents, owing probably to the greater or less aptitude in these vessels to receive it; hence we find the local inflammation, in some cases, considerably advanced before the system becomes affected, while in others the eruptive symptoms supervene when it appears to have made but very little progress; and, therefore, though the eighth day after the inoculation proves the usual period at which the patient feels indisposed, yet this frequently happens much sooner or later, and the progress of the Cow Pox infection will be found to take the same latitude.

Monday, January 21st, 1799, I took the matter of Cow Pox in a purulent state upon the teats of a cow, with which I immediately inoculated seven persons by a single puncture in the arm of each, or rather by scratching the skin with the point of a lancet till the instrument became tinged with blood.

First Case.

Mary Payne, a child two years and a-half old, of a strong, robust constitution. *Third Day.*—The inoculated part was evidently elevated and slightly inflamed. *Sixth Day.*—The local tumour extended to about one-third of an inch in diameter, and was nearly of a circular form, with its edges more elevated than the centre, and, with the surrounding inflammation not greater than is usual in cases of inoculated Small Pox. The vesicle, upon the middle of the tumour, was now very large, and distended with a limpid fluid, some of which I took upon a lancet and with it inoculated another person, John Talley. She appeared dull and drowsy, and her pulse was quicker than usual. She had no appetite for food, and had been very thirsty since yesterday. *Eighth Day.*—The redness surrounding the tumour seems returning; and the thirst and other febrile symptoms are much abated; but she still appears listless and somewhat indisposed. *Eleventh Day.*—She is perfectly free from complaint; the inoculated part s scabbing, but surrounded with a hard tumefaction of a bright red colour. She was this day inoculated with variolous matter. *Fifteenth Day.*—She has no ailment. The variolous inoculation produced considerable inflammation, which gradually disappeared after the fifth day.

Second Case.

Elizabeth Payne, aged four months, in appearance weak and somewhat emaciated. The progress of the infection on this child's arm was very much like that of her sister's, just mentioned; but the vesication seemed rather more extensive, and the surrounding inflammation less. The sixth day after inoculation her mother informed me that the child had been very unwell the preceding night with what were called inward convulsions, and had vomited two or three times. On examination, the heat of her skin, and the frequency of her pulse, indicated the presence of some degree of fever. *Eighth Day.*—I learned that the febrile state had continued, more or less, till this morning; nor was it then wholly gone off. The inoculated part, I judged from its appearance, had not entirely ceased from disordering the constitution. *Eleventh Day.*—The redness of the tumour is subsiding, and its general appearance resembles the effects of inoculation with variolous matter when the eruption is completed, and the maturation proceeding favourably. The patient's mother now thinks her as well as usual. She was this day inoculated with variolous matter. *Thirteenth Day.*—She manifests no signs of indisposition. The redness about the tumour is gone off, and the matter is forming a scab. The second inoculation produces no effect. *Fifteenth Day.*—She is now very well; but her mother says she was seized with inward convulsions yesterday, and was extremely ill afterward for two hours; this, however, cannot be justly ascribed to inoculation, as the part in which the Cow Pox matter was inserted is now covered with a dry scab, not attended with inflammation; and the variolous matter produced no redness whatever. She was this day brought to a man labouring under the casual Small Pox, and kissed by him, in order more fully to try if she was secure from the infection of the Small Pox. Her sister, Mary Payne, was also subjected to the same test, but neither of them have since taken the disease.

Third Case.

Thomas Buckland, a strong child, four months old. The progress of the infection on this boy's arms was even more regular, and produced appearances more analogous to those of the inoculated Small Pox than in the case of Mary Payne. The vesicle on the inoculated part formed on the third day, and the surrounding inflammation never became phlegmonous, nor was it attended with any hardness of the integuments. *Seventh Day.* —In the evening he was discovered to be feverish and restless, when two pustules exactly resembling those of the Small Pox appeared near to the inoculated part. The following day he still continued indisposed, and the cutaneous inflammation had that peculiar irritable or angry aspect which is observed on the accession of the eruptive 'symptoms in cases of inoculation with variolous matter. *Tenth Day.*—The suppuration was more extended, and the efflorescence immediately encompassing it had nearly disappeared, leaving its outer border more strongly marked than the inner; a circumstance of the most favourable import in inoculation. The two pustules upon his arm were more advanced, and several others were now visible upon different parts of his body; his ankles and feet were beset with a rash like scarlatina. He is still feverish, and his mother reports that last night he vomited. *Eleventh Day.*—The soreness of his arm and the fever had ceased. Nine distinct pustules were now discovered upon his body and limbs, somewhat smaller than variolous pustules; from one of these I obtained an ichorous matter, and with it inoculated Sarah Price. *Thirteenth Day.*—The febrile symptoms returned yesterday, nor is he wholly free from them to-day. Nine additional pustules have appeared; no inflammation remains at the inoculated part, and the matter it contains begins to dry. *Fifteenth Day.*—He is free from disorder; six pustules more have appeared, making in the whole twenty-four; some of them maturate at the apex, but they mostly die away without proceeding to suppuration. He was this day exposed to the effluvia of the casual Small Pox, in the same manner as the two Paynes.

Fourth Case.

Richard Payne, a healthy boy, ten years old. The inoculated part was not sensibly elevated nor inflamed till the fourth day. *Seventh Day.*—The tumour had spread considerably; and the vesication upon it was very evident. He felt a sensation of itching in the part; and the next day complained of a pain in the axilla, which continued two days. *Tenth Day.*—The centre of the tumour became depressed, its edges elevated, and surrounded by a deep-coloured inflammatory border. The central part of the tumour was now assuming externally a brown colour, and in a few days afterwards it formed a dark scab. Though considerable tumefaction, with hardness and redness, remained at the inoculated part several days, yet no ulceration ensued. *Fifteenth Day.* —Five pustules appeared resembling those in Buckland. This boy was twice inoculated with variolous matter during the progress of the Cow Pox infection, and exposed to patients under the Small Pox the whole time, without being infected by it; and the only complaint arising from the Cow Pox was the pain in his arm-pit.

Fifth Case.

Matthew Redding, sixteen years old. *Third Day.*—The insertion of the matter did not appear to have produced any inflammation or hardness in the part; he was therefore inoculated with variolous matter, at the distance of two inches from the part in which the Cow Pox matter was inserted. Next day a little redness could be discovered at the first puncture, and from this time both inoculations proceeded very regularly, but slowly, so that on the seventh day they appeared to be inflamed in an equal degree, the extent of the inflammation not exceeding the tenth of an inch in diameter. *Eighth Day.**—He has pain in the axilla. *Tenth Day.*—Both tumours are approaching to suppuration. They are of the same form, and attended with an equal degree of efflorescence. *Eleventh Day.*—He complains of headache; the red tinge now extends in a circular form, and includes both tumours. *Thirteenth Day.*—There appears more tension and pain at the variolous tumour than at the other, but the latter tumour is more prominent. *Fifteenth Day.*—Both tumours began to dry, and no inconvenience followed. This boy made no other complaint, during the process of infection, than of uneasiness in the axilla, followed by a slight headach, of very short duration; however, on the seventeenth day, four small pustules appeared, viz., one upon his nose, one upon his thigh, and two on his head; none of which suppurated. This case strikingly resembles that of Richard Payne, on which the pustules did not appear till the arm scabbed.

Sixth Case.

Jane Collingridge, a healthy, active girl, seventeen years of age. *Third Day.*—The inoculated part began to be elevated and inflamed. *Fifth Day.*—It was vesicated, and attended with itching. She was inoculated with variolous matter in the right arm, the former inoculation having been in the left. *Eighth Day.*—The whole tumour is much increased in all dimensions; its form is perfectly circular, and it appears of a lemon-coloured tint. She now complains of a stiffness across her arms, and of a pain in the

* Here, as well as in the subsequent cases, where the patient was twice inoculated on different days, I date the time from the first inoculation.

left axilla; the puncture in the right arm begins to be elevated and inflamed. *Eleventh Day.*—She complains of headach and pains about the loins; the tumour produced by the Cow Pox matter is now more inflamed at the margin, which is beset with minute confluent pustules; the variolous tumour is also advanced to a state of vesication; and she reports that last night both axillæ were painful. *Twelfth Day.*—She continues indisposed; the tumour is surrounded by an extensive efflorescence; the variolous tumour is of a deeper red colour. *Thirteenth Day.*—The Cow Pox tumour is subsiding and forming a scab; that of the Small Pox is efflorescent; her headach continues; pain in the right axilla; several pustules appear. *Fifteenth Day.*—There are small pustules round the edges of the variolous tumour; more pustules appear scattered over the face, body, and limbs. *Seventeenth Day.*—The scab over the Cow Pox tumour is completely formed; at its edges however, a fluid is still visible: the variolous tumour is in a state of suppuration; she complains of a sore throat; the number of pustules is now from one to two hundred, in no respect differing from variolous pustules of the mild sort. From this time both the tumours gradually healed, and the pustules dried at the usual time.

SEVENTH CASE.

Ann Pink, a tall girl, of a brown sallow complexion, aged fifteen years. This girl was inoculated with variolous matter, on the fifth day, in the same manner as Collingridge, and both tumours proceeded to maturation, though more slowly than in that case. Neither of the tumours began to scab till the *seventeenth day*, when they resembled each other so perfectly that the one could not easily be distinguished from the other. She had no pain in either axilla, nor made any complaint during the whole progress of the infection, neither did one pustule appear upon her.

The only other persons whom I first inoculated with the matter of Cow Pox, and on the *fifth day* afterwards with variolous matter, were William Harris, William Bunker, and James Crouch.

EIGHTH CASE.

William Harris, twenty-one years of age, of a tall and slender make, and of a delicate constitution, was inoculated January 24th with the matter of Cow Pox, taken from the arm of Sarah Rice, who received the disease by milking the cows. *Third Day.*—The inoculated part was evidently elevated and inflamed. *Fifth Day.*—It advanced to vesication, and a sensation of itching was perceived in the part; he was this day inoculated with variolous matter. *Ninth Day.*—The tumour of the first inoculation presents prominent callous edges with but very little redness; its centre is depressed and contains a lymphatic fluid; he perceives a tenderness in the axilla; the variolous tumour is considerably inflamed and vesicated, and itches more than the other. Next day a pain was perceived in the axilla of the arm in which the variolous matter was inserted, as well as in the other. *Twelfth Day.*—Redness of the Cow Pox tumour is going off; but that of the variolous still spreads with an irregular margin. *Fourteenth Day.*—Several pustules appear. The Cow Pox tumour is now dry at the centre, but its surrounding edges appear of a bluish tinge, and still abound with ichorous matter. The variolous tumour is much inflamed, and beset with confluent pustules at its edges; its centre is depressed and of a dark hue. *Nineteenth Day.*—The Cow Pox tumour has formed into a dry scab, with a finely polished surface, and of a mahogany brown colour; the variolous tumour is in a purulent state, with an extensive inflammation at the margin; the pustules are about three hundred in number, very large, and all in a state of maturation. From this time all the effects of inoculation went off gradually; he never complained of headach nor of any febrile symptom during the whole progress of the disease.

Ninth Case.

William Bunker, a strong, healthy boy, fifteen years of age, was inoculated in his left arm, on the same day and with matter from the same person as Harris. *Third Day.*—The inoculated part was elevated and reddened. *Fifth Day.*—The inflammation was much increased; he was now inoculated in his right arm with variolous matter. *Eighth Day.*—The tumour upon his left arm is much elevated, and the vesication considerable since the *sixth day;* he now complains of pain in the axilla and of headach. The pustule on the right arm advances very slowly. *Tenth Day.*—The pain in the axilla and the headach continue. The tumour of the left arm begins to scab in the centre, and is surrounded with a red tinge of considerable extent. The tumour on the right arm now also presents a red tinge of a similar appearance, but not of half the extent; its centre is in a state of vesication, and its edges studded with small pustules; his headach is not entirely gone off. *Twelfth Day.*—The red tinge surrounding the tumour on the left arm has disappeared, except a narrow ring at its outer ambit, the tumour on the right arm is depressed at the centre, where it is also of a livid colour; its edges are hard and inflamed; he now discovers two or three pustules upon his body. *Seventeenth Day.*—The matter of both tumours is almost wholly formed into a dry incrustation; no more pustules have appeared; one upon his hip has maturated. *Twentieth Day.*—Both tumours are perfectly scabbed: that upon his left arm appears browner and smoother than the other.

Tenth Case.

James Crouch, seven years old, inoculated on the same day as the last patient with matter taken from the same girl, and with variolous matter five days afterward. *Fifth Day.*—The inoculated part was considerably elevated and inflamed. *Ninth Day.*—The Cow Pox tumour is much advanced; the pellicle filled with ichor; the marginal inflammation not considerable; the variolous puncture now displays a small red speck, which begins to spread. *Eleventh Day.*—The Cow Pox tumour exhibits an extensive efflorescence, or red stain upon the surrounding skin, and its centre begins to dry; the variolous tumour is spreading a little, and in a state of vesication. *Fourteenth Day.*—Pain in the axilla is now produced by the Cow Pox tumour, which is drying at the centre; the variolous tumour is now efflorescent, but not to half the extent of the other. From this time the tumours quickly healed, no eruption took place, and no farther inconvenience was experienced.

Eleventh and Twelfth Case.

Thomas Fox, aged twenty-five, and John Dennis, twenty-three years of age, both strong men, and accustomed to hard labour, were inoculated on the 22nd of January with variolous matter, and on the following day with Cow Pox matter, taken from the arm of Sarah Rice. In both these cases the first inoculation was performed by two punctures at the distance of two inches from each other, and the latter by one puncture at the same distance from the two former. The local effects and appearances of the inoculation were very similar in both these men; the Cow Pox tumours seemed to advance equally with those of the variolous, and bore a strong resemblance to them; the former, however, were more elevated and circumscribed; for about the *ninth day* the variolous tumours became angulated or ragged at the margin, which was not so conspicuous as the others, though both had small confluent pustules at their margins. Those of the Cow Pox also sooner healed, and formed a smoother scab. The eruptive fever came on about the *eighth day* with Dennis, but not till the *tenth* with Fox; the former had more than three hundred pustules, and the latter about one hundred; all of which were in every respect similar to variolous pustules.

THIRTEENTH AND FOURTEENTH CASE.

John Talley, fourteen, and Thomas Brown, fifteen years old, were, January 25th, inoculated with variolous matter in the left arm, and the following day they were both inoculated in the right arm with the matter of Cow Pox, taken from the arms of Mary and Elizabeth Payne (see cases first and second). The progress of both the infections on the arms of these boys was perfectly regular and equal throughout. On the *seventh day* all the tumours were considerably inflamed and in a state of vesication, attended with itching. Brown also at this time complained of a pain in each axilla; but with Talley the pain was confined to the left till the next day, when both arm-pits were affected. *Tenth Day.*—They both complained of headach and of pains about the loins; these, however, were very slight, and no further indisposition ensued. On the evening of the *twelfth day* some pustules appeared upon Brown, but upon Talley they did not appear till the *fourteenth day;* the former had in all about thirty, and the latter only six, all of which were apparently variolous. The Cow Pox tumours were more elevated at the edges and less depressed at the centre after the *ninth day* than those of the variolous; and they eventually formed a smoother and browner scab, as in the case of Fox and Dennis.

January 30th.—William Mundy, Elizabeth George, and Sarah Butcher were inoculated by two punctures with the matter of Cow Pox, taken from the arm of Collingridge (case six).

FIFTEENTH CASE.

William Mundy, a strong labouring man, aged twenty-five years, was inoculated as above described by two punctures in his left arm. The local infection of both punctures advanced, and the inflammation and its effects proceeded rapidly, so that on the *eighth day* he complained of uneasiness in his axilla, and of pain in the head and loins, which continued about two days; the tumours were then considerably elevated, and their margins much inflamed. *Thirteenth Day.*—They were surrounded with an extensive redness, in the form of a halo, and beginning to scab at the centre; the edges continued circular, well defined, and elevated. *Fourteenth Day.*—Several pustules appeared upon his neck and back, but disappeared in two or three days without suppurating. He was this day inoculated with variolous matter, but it produced no other effect than a little redness of two or three days' duration.

Sixteenth Case.

Elizabeth George, a strong woman, twenty-five years old, was inoculated in the same manner, and on the same day above mentioned, with Cow Pox matter taken from the same person. The punctures quickly rose, but the inflammation was inconsiderable till the *sixth day*, when vesication and itching commenced. *Ninth Day*.—Has no pain in the axilla, but complains of headache and pain in the loins. *Eleventh Day*.—Her pains continue; pulse quick; the central pellicle of the tumours is extending, and replete with a watery humour; the margins swollen and red. *Thirteenth Day*.—The same appearances continue. *Fifteenth Day*.—The symptoms are abated; says she has no other complaint than a giddiness of the head; the inflammation at the margins of the tumours is greatly abated; the matter in the centre is beginning to dry; some pustules appear on her face. *Sixteenth Day*.—She makes no complaint; more pustules show themselves; the tumours appear circular, with the centre equally elevated as the edges, and exhibiting an uniform, smooth surface, which is becoming hard. *Eighteenth Day*.—More pustules have appeared; the tumours are scabbing, and the surrounding redness is almost wholly gone. *Twentieth Day*.—Her face is swelled; the pustules are very sore, and in a purulent state; their number is five hundred and thirty, and two in the throat are a little troublesome. *Twenty-fifth Day*.—The pustules in a state of desquamation. She was now inoculated with variolous matter, which produced no effect. The scabs at the inoculated parts were of that brown, smooth kind peculiar to the Cow Pox.

Seventeenth Case.

Sarah Butcher, a healthy little girl, thirteen years old, was inoculated with the matter of Cow Pox at the same time and in the same manner as above mentioned. *Sixth Day*.—The tumours were much [illegible]ted, the inflammation inconsiderable; the vesication fully [illegible]ed, and attended with itching. *Ninth Day*.—There was a [illegible]ht efflorescence around the tumours, uneasiness in the axilla, [illegible]ach, pain in the loins. *Eleventh Day*.—Suppuration at the inner edges of the tumours, redness at the outer edge very extensive. *Sixteenth Day*.—Tumours scabbing; no eruption; complains of pain in her bowels and diarrhœa. *Sixteenth Day.*—No complaint, central part of the tumours scabbed ; inflammation still surrounding the edges. She was inoculated this day with variolous matter. *Eighteenth Day.*—The redness gone off, leaving a red tinge at its outer margin. The variolous inoculation produced a little redness, which disappeared in two days.

January 31st.—Thomas Wise, aged fourteen, and Sarah Price, aged thirteen years, were inoculated with the matter of Cow Pox, taken from Matthew Redding, and at the same time with variolous matter, but the effects of the latter inoculations were the following day prevented by applying the concentrated acid of vitriol to the punctures.

Eighteenth Case.

Thomas Wise, above mentioned. *Fifth Day.*—The inoculated part was considerably inflamed and vesicated. *Eighth Day.*—The tumour advances with much marginal redness, and a pain in the axilla is perceived. *Twelfth Day.*—Pain in the axilla continued two days. He has had no other complaint. The centre of the tumour is forming a scab, but is surrounded with an appearance like the areola papillæ. Two pustules were discovered upon his body this day, and two more appeared on the *fifteenth day*, but none of them became purulent. The tumour upon his arm had at that time formed a hard, smooth scab.

Nineteenth Case.

Sarah Price, inoculated, as above stated, in her left arm ; on the same day was inserted in her right arm Cow Pox matter, taken from a pustule from Buckland. *Fifth Day.*—There was a redness and elevation at the two punctures, each arm, but in consequence of the caustic effects of the vitriolic acid none at the variolous puncture. *Eighth Day.*—Both tumours were advanced ; vesication and a considerable degree of inflammation, especially in that on the left arm. She now complains of *rigor* and of a pain in the left axilla. These symptoms, together with a headach, continued two days. *Thirteenth Day.*—No complaint, both tumours subsiding ; three small pustules have appeared upon her face and neck, and two days afterwards three others, none of which suppurated. This girl, as well as Thomas Wise, was constantly exposed to the Small Pox during the progress of their inoculation.

Twentieth Case.

Thomas Dorset, inoculated February 1st, with the matter of Cow Pox, taken from the arm of Jane Collingridge (see case six).

Seventh Day.—The inoculated part was much elevated and in a state of vesication, attended with the usual degree of redness. *Eleventh Day.*—Last night he perceived an uneasiness in his axilla, and he now complains of pain about his loins; the tumour encircled by an extensive efflorescence. *Thirteenth Day.*—The tumour scabbing at the centre. He was inoculated this day with variolous matter. The variolous inoculation produced no effect. About the *twelfth day* this man had four or five pustular appearances which he called pocks, but they seemed to me more like common pimples than variolous pustules.

Twenty-First Case.

John Keys, twenty-five years old, inoculated February 4th, with matter of Cow Pox taken from the arm of James Crouch. On the *fourth day* the inoculated part was considerably inflamed, and affected with a sensation of itching; but from this time the redness gradually disappeared, and was entirely gone on the *ninth day*, when he was inoculated with variolous matter in both arms, but without effect. On the *tenth day*, however, he complained of pain in his head and loins, with which he was affected three days, but no eruption ensued.

Twenty-Second Case.

Edward Turner, a strong man, twenty-four years of age, inoculated by two punctures with the matter of Cow Pox taken from the arm of James Crouch (case ten) February 5th. *Seventh Day.*—The tumours were much advanced, in a state of open vesication, and attended with itching. *Twelfth Day.*—They began to dry in the centre, but the margins were of a dark red colour, and studded with minute vesiculæ; he now complains of pain in the axilla, stiffness of his neck, and pain in the loins. *Fourteenth Day.*—Headach and pain in the loins continue; the inner edges of the tumours are distended with an ichorous fluid. *Sixteenth Day.*—Complaint of headach and sore throat; next day about one hundred pustules appeared, many of which were very small. *Nineteenth Day.*—He has no complaint; the number of the pustules now amounts to about two hundred and twenty; all of them afterwards suppurated. On the *twenty-second day* he was inoculated with the variolous matter, which produced no effect.

Twenty-Third Case.

Hannah Morgan, a strong child, one year old, was inoculated with the matter of Cow Pox taken from the arm of James Crouch,

February 5th. *Fifth Day.*—The inoculated part is much elevated and inflamed. *Seventh Day.*—The tumour contains ichor, and the redness and elevation are greatly increased; yesterday she became feverish, and last night was sick and vomited; her skin at this time is hotter than usual. *Fourteenth Day.*—The febrile symptoms continued, and at times were very severe, till the *eleventh day*, since which time they have not returned: no pustules have appeared, and the tumour is now scabbing. She was afterwards inoculated with variolous matter, but it only produced a transient redness in the part.

Twenty-Fourth Case.

Jane West, twenty-one years of age, was inoculated February 6th with the matter of Cow Pox, taken from the arm of Sarah Butcher. *Seventh Day.*—The inoculated part was considerably elevated and inflamed; the vesication was also extensive and attended with itching. *Ninth Day.*—She complained of headache, and next day of a pain in the axilla and upon her shoulder, attended with rigors and shivering; the border of the tumours appeared of a deep red, and its inner edges contained an ichorous matter. *Thirteenth Day.*—Yesterday an efflorescence appeared round the tumour. She complains of a sore throat, and says she has a pain across her chest. *Fifteenth Day.*—Two pustules have appeared upon her side; the tumour begins to dry. She makes no complaint. *Seventeenth Day.*—Twenty pustules appeared, all of which suppurated. *Twenty-third Day.*—The variolous inoculation produced no inflammation.

Twenty-Fifth Case.

Ann Bumpus, aged twenty years, was inoculated February 6th with the matter of Cow Pox, taken from the arm of Sarah Butcher. The appearances of the inoculated part in this girl's arm corresponded in every respect with those stated in West's case. *Eighth Day.*—She complained of headache. *Tenth Day.*—Pain of the head and loins; shivering. *Eleventh Day.*—Two or three pustules appear upon her face. *Thirteenth Day.*—Pains continue; more pustules appear. *Fifteenth Day.*—No complaint; the pustules were counted and found to be three hundred and ten, resembling those of the Small Pox. *Seventeenth Day.*—Complains of sore throat. *Nineteenth Day.*—Pustules drying. *Twenty-second Day.*—Inoculated with the matter of Small Pox, but no inflammation was produced by it.

Twenty-Sixth Case.

Thomas Slade, twenty years of age, was inoculated with the

matter of Cow Pox taken from the arm of William Mundy, February 6th. On the *eighth day* the inoculated part was much elevated and in an advanced state of vesication. He complained of headach and pain in the axilla; and on the next day of a pain in the loins. *Eleventh Day.*—Pains abated; three or four pustules appear; the tumour is bordered with small confluent vesicles. *Fourteenth Day.*—No complaints; tumour beginning to scab. *Nineteenth Day.*—The centre of the tumour formed a brown, hard scab. The pustules do not suppurate and are receding. *Twenty-second Day.*—He was inoculated with the matter of Small Pox, which produced a redness for two or three days and afterwards gradually disappeared.

Twenty-Seventh Case.

Frances Jewel, a healthy young woman, twenty years of age, who had undergone the Small Pox by inoculation when a child, was inoculated with the matter of Cow Pox taken from the arm of Sarah Butcher, February 5th. The inoculated part advanced into a tumour equal in extent and duration to that in the case last mentioned; on the *ninth day* headach and pain of the loins came on, and continued two or three days. The tumour began to scab on the *thirteenth day*, but no pustules appeared. She was afterwards inoculated with variolous matter, and also with that of the Cow Pox, neither of which produced any inflammation.

Twenty-Eighth Case.

Charlotte Fisk, four months old, was, on February 13th, inoculated with the matter of Cow Pox, taken from the arm of Frances Jewel. In this child the local disease proceeded very regularly. She became indisposed on the *eighth day*, and continued feverish for three or four days, when about forty pustules appeared; but the greatest part of these pustules did not proceed to suppuration. The mother of this child laboured under the natural Small Pox, and was covered with pustules in a purulent state at the time her child was inoculated; yet the infant was suckled by her during the whole course of the disease, and was frequently seen besmeared with variolous pus. Whence it would appear that the vaccine infection not only prevents but actually supersedes the casual Small Pox.

Twenty-Ninth Case.

James Tarrent, nineteen years old, was on the 16th of February inoculated with the matter of Cow Pox, taken from a pustule upon Elizabeth George. In this case the inflammation at the inoculated part proceeded very rapidly, and was more extensive than usual on the *sixth day;* but from this time it began to recede, and was entirely gone on the *tenth day*, only a small dry scab at the puncture being left. He was now inoculated with variolous matter, which did not produce any inflammation whatever. I consider this man as one of the few whose constitutions cannot be affected either by the virus of the Cow Pox or the Small Pox. It is true he complained of headach about the *ninth day*, but I should not be disposed to attribute this symptom to the inoculation.

Thirtieth Case.

William Hull, aged eleven years, was, on the 8th of February, inoculated with the matter of Cow Pox taken from the arm of Sarah Butcher. *Seventh Day.*—The tumour at the inoculated part is advanced in the usual manner, and he this day complains of headach. *Tenth Day.*—His headach and pain in the loins continue, and several pustules now appear upon him. *Twelfth Day.*—The pains are gone off and more pustules have appeared. *Fifteenth Day.*—The pustules amount to about two hundred. They vary much in size, and are proceeding to maturation. *Eighteenth Day.*—He was inoculated with variolous matter, which produced no effect.

Thirty-First and Thirty-Second Case.

February 8th, Hannah Hull, aged thirteen years, and Sarah Hull, eight years old, were inoculated with the matter of Cow Pox taken from Sarah Butcher. These two sisters had the disease rather more favourably than their brother, William Hull, for the inoculated part was in both surrounded by an efflorescence on the *eleventh day*, and the number of pustules upon the two was not equal to that of their brother's, nor were the eruptive symptoms of half the duration of his. On the *twentieth day* they were inoculated for the Small Pox, but no disease ensued.

Thirty-Third Case.

George Reed, aged fifteen years, was inoculated with the matter of Cow Pox taken from the arm of F. Jewel, February 14th. The inoculated part tumified in the usual manner; he complained of headach on the *eighth day*, and this symptom continued with occasional intermissions till the *thirteenth day*. Some pustules began to appear about the *eleventh*, and the eruption was completed on the *fourteenth day*. They were in number about seventy, some of which were very small, but they all maturated in a favourable manner. He was afterwards inoculated with variolous matter, which formed a pustular appearance; but no disorder was produced. Frances Pedder, Amelia Hoole, George Hickland, and Elizabeth Morton were inoculated on February 13th and 14th with Cow Pox matter taken from the arm of Sarah Price, who was inoculated from a pustule on Buckland (see case three).

Thirty-Fourth Case.

Frances Pedder, a child eleven months old. The inoculated part was gradually elevated and inflamed. *Eighth Day.*—The eruptive symptoms supervened and she continued feverish till the *thirteenth day*, when several pustules appeared. *Sixteenth day.*—The tumour began to scab, and the number of pustules then upon her was forty, all of which maturated without becoming purulent. She was afterwards inoculated for the Small Pox without effect.

Thirty-Fifth Case.

Amelia Hoole, five months old, was inoculated as above described. The local tumour advanced in the usual manner. *Seventh Day.*—She became feverish, and several small pustules appeared at the border of the tumour. *Tenth Day.*—She has continued slightly indisposed since the last report, and nine pustules are now visible upon her body and extremities. *Fourteenth Day.*—The pustules amount to one hundred and two in number, and form yellowish scabs. *Eighteenth Day.*—The inoculated part was perfectly healed; the pustules appeared in a state of desquamation. She was at this time inoculated with variolous matter, but without effect.

Thirty-Sixth Case.

George Hickland, six months old, was inoculated from the person above-mentioned. The eruptive symptoms in this child were less severe, and of shorter duration, than in the last case. However, the number of pustules which appeared amounted to three hundred, but only about one-third of them suppurated. This patient also resisted the infection of the Small Pox by inoculation.

Thirty-Seventh Case.

Elizabeth Morton, nine months old, was more severely disordered than any of the four children inoculated with the matter taken from Sarah Price. The fever continued with some degree of violence from the *seventh* to the *fifteenth day*, and the number of pustules amounted to two hundred. On the *twentieth day* she was inoculated with variolous matter without effect.

Thirty-Eighth Case.

L. Davy, aged eleven weeks, was on February 19th inoculated with the matter of Cow Pox taken from the arm of Charlotte Fisk. This child had the disease very favourably. On the *tenth day* the tumour was surrounded by an efflorescence, and her skin was a little hotter than usual during that day only. On the *thirteenth day* one pustule appeared near to the inoculated part, and two upon her forehead, which were all she had. She was afterwards inoculated for the Small Pox without effect.

Thirty-Ninth Case.

Maria Murrell, aged four months, was inoculated with matter taken from the same person and on the same day as Davy. *Fifth Day.*—The inoculated part was much elevated and inflamed. On the evening of the *eighth day* she vomited. *Tenth Day.*—The tumour was surrounded by a very extensive efflorescence, and she became hot and restless. *Twelfth Day.*—She seemed free from fever, and about twenty pustules appeared upon her. *Fourteenth Day.*—The inflammation upon the arm was gone off, and the pustule seemed to be scabbing. The subsequent inoculation of the Small Pox, as upon the others, produced no effect upon this patient.

A cow kept by Professor Coleman, at the Veterinary College, was inoculated on its teat with the matter of Cow Pox taken from the arm of James Crouch, which produced the disease in the cow (see case ten). A man-servant, by milking this cow, was also affected with an extensive tumour upon his thumb; this soon acquired a livid blue colour, and was attended with a considerable degree of fever for several days, and with a rash upon his ankles and feet.

With the matter produced in the nipple of this cow were inoculated Martha Streeton, James Smith, and George Meacock.

Fortieth Case.

Martha Streeton, aged twenty-two years, was on the 18th of February inoculated with the matter above mentioned. The inoculated part tumefied in the usual manner, and on the *ninth day* she complained of headach, and afterwards of a pain in the axilla. The headach and pain in the loins continued, but not with severity, for five or six days. Pustules began to appear on the *twelfth day*, and the eruption was completed on the *sixteenth day*, when the number was about three hundred. During the maturation of the pustules, which in no respect differed from those of the Small Pox, she complained of her throat being sore. On the *nineteenth day* this patient was perfectly well. She was afterwards inoculated for the Small Pox without effect.

Forty-First and Forty-Second Case.

James Smith, sixteen, and George Meacock, thirty years of age, were, on the 19th of February, inoculated with the same matter as that mentioned in the preceding case. The latter of these patients had the disease nearly in the same manner as Streeton; but in a greater degree, for Meacock's pustules were more numerous, and the inoculated part did not exhibit a tumour so well defined and elevated as Streeton's did. Smith's case differed widely from both; his arm tumified rapidly, and an erythema or blush extended from the puncture several inches up his arm, and down to his elbow. The eruptive symptoms began on the *seventh* and continued in a slight degree till the *eleventh day*. He had four or five pustules upon his face, and nearly a hundred upon his body and limbs, all of which matured favourably, and the erysipelatous appearance of the inoculated part soon went off, though no application was employed for that purpose. Both the above patients were inoculated with variolous matter, which produced no effect upon Meacock, but in Smith it was followed by a cutaneous inflammation of several days' continuance.

Samuel Fairbrother, fifteen years old, Richard Calloway, aged nineteen years, James Camplin, aged seventeen years, John Turner, eight months old, Joanna Buckley, five months old, and Mary Welch, three months old, were all, on the 21st and 23rd of February, inoculated with the matter of Cow Pox taken from the arm of Edward Turner (see case twenty-two).

Forty-Third Case.

Samuel Fairbrother began to be indisposed on the *ninth day*, [illegible] had repeatedly slight feverish paroxysms with pain in the [illegible] the *fourteenth day*, when four small pustules appeared, [illegible] no farther complaint ensued.

FORTY-FOURTH CASE.

In Richard Calloway the inoculated part tumefied in the usual manner, and on the *ninth day* he first complained of a pain in the axilla, and headach, which continued till the *twelfth day;* an extensive bright red blush then surrounded the tumour, and no farther complaint ensued. At this time also some pustules appeared, but their number never exceeded twenty. He had been inoculated in the hand as well as in the arm, in order to discover if the appearance of the tumour in a part constantly exposed to the air would be the same as in the arm kept covered by his dress. The difference was very evident, for the tumour upon his hand was much more extensive, of a more livid colour, and attended with more inflammation than the other.

FORTY-FIFTH CASE.

James Camplin suffered rather more from the eruptive complaints than Calloway, and they continued with him a day longer. However, the disease gave him very little uneasiness, and he had only thirty pustules.

FORTY-SIXTH CASE.

John Turner's arm was inflamed very extensively, and he became feverish on the *eighth day*. The following day many pustules appeared, and on the *eleventh day* he was almost covered with pustules, having about one thousand. These, however, were perfectly distinct, and they all maturated favourably, so that about the *seventeenth day* he was completely well.

FORTY-SEVENTH AND FORTY-EIGHTH CASE.

Joanna Buckley and Mary Welch had the disease in its mildest form. On the *eighth day* an efflorescence surrounded the inoculated part in both these children, and during this day only appeared a little indisposed. No pustules appeared upon either of them.

All the six patients thus infected with vaccine disease from E. Turner were subsequently inoculated with variolous matter, which did not produce any disorder.

February 18th, William Walker, eleven months old; February 24th, Sarah Dixon, nineteen years old; Thomas Ellistone, aged fifteen months; Maria Dunn, aged twenty months; and James Cummins, aged fourteen weeks, were all inoculated with the matter of Cow Pox taken from the arm of Hannah Bumpus.

Forty-Ninth Case.

*William Walker's arm tumified in the usual manner, but he did not manifest the least indisposition during the course of the infection; neither did any pustules appear, except one or two at the inoculated part.

Fiftieth Case.

Sarah Dixon's arm tumified in the usual manner, and on the *tenth day* she began to complain of a pain in her head and loins: this was followed by shiverings and a pain in the axilla and across her shoulders. *Thirteenth Day.*—The pains were much abated, and some pustules appeared. *Sixteenth Day.*—She makes no complaint but of a soreness of her throat; the eruption is now completed, and the number of pustules is found to be one hundred and seventy-four; all of these afterwards maturated.

Fifty-First Case.

Thomas Ellistone was feverish from the *sixth* to the *eighth day,* when the tumour was surrounded with an extensive efflorescence. After this time he had no ailment. No pustules appeared.

Fifty-Second Case.

Maria Dunn was hot and restless from the *sixth* till the *ninth day.* She had no eruption.

Fifty-Third Case.

James Cummins did not seem the least disordered from the inoculation, although the inoculated part tumified very considerably, and several pustules appeared at the margin of the tumour on the *eleventh day.*

All the above-mentioned persons, inoculated with the matter of Cow Pox, taken from the arm of Bumpus, have been since inoculated with variolous matter, but without effect.

John Giles, twenty years of age; Wm. Bigg, eighteen years old: William Briaris, fifteen years old; Sophia Dobinson, five years old; Sarah Dobinson, three years old; and Hannah Dobinson, one

* The father of this child is an ingenious engraver in Rosamond Street, Clerkenwell, who having lost a child under the effects of the inoculated Small Pox was induced to inoculate his only son for the Cow Pox. The particulars of the case are related by Mr. Walker himself, in the *Medical and Physical Journal* for March, 1799. [There is an interesting coloured plate facing p. 217 of this journal, illustrating the progress of the vesicle.—E.M.C.]

year old, were inoculated with the matter of Cox Pox, taken from the arm of Jane West, February 21st.

FIFTY-FOURTH CASE.

John Giles complained of head-ach from the *ninth* till the *eleventh day*. A slight soreness of the throat came on, and continued several days. He had about thirty pustules.

FIFTY-FIFTH CASE.

William Bigg also complained of head-ach and sore throat several days, and had about twelve pustules.

FIFTY-SIXTH CASE.

Wm. Briaris first complained of indisposition on the *seventh* and continued somewhat disordered till the *eleventh day*. Only two pustules appeared.

FIFTY-SEVENTH CASE.

Sophia Dobinson's arm tumified extensively, but she made no complaint during the whole progress of the infection, and had no eruptions.

FIFTY-EIGHTH CASE.

Sarah Dobinson's case was in every respect similar to that of her sister Sophia.

FIFTY-NINTH CASE.

Hannah Dobinson suffered as little from the disease as either of her sisters till the *fourteenth day*, when, according to her mother's report, she was seized with convulsive fits for two or three hours. She had no eruption.

The above six patients have since been inoculated for the Small Pox without effect.

Mary Greenville, twenty years old; Edward Honeywood, two years old; Thomas Rood, one and a half year old; Charlotte Mile, fifteen months old; John Jenkins, one month old; Henry Barber, eleven months old; Thomas Dix, eleven months old; Ann Walker, ten months old; Samuel Francis Brough, ten months old; Alexander Towser, eight months old; Wm. Knighton, eight months old; Sarah Price, eight months old; Elizabeth Spilsbury, four months old; Elizabeth May, four months old; Mary Ann Sully, three months old; Francis Terry, two months old; Wm. Scott, two months old; Wm. Johnstone, two months old; and

Mary Stewart, two months old, were inoculated with the matter of Cow Pox, taken from the arm of Martha Streeton, on February 25th.

SIXTIETH CASE.

Mary Greenville, on the *ninth day*, began to complain of head-ach, which continued till the *twelfth day*, when a sore throat came on, and gave her a little uneasiness for about two days. She had thirty-five pustules.

SIXTY-FIRST CASE.

Edward Honeywood was not perceptibly disordered from the inoculation, although his arm was much tumified; and on the *eleventh day* it exhibited an efflorescence. No eruption appeared.

SIXTY-SECOND CASE.

Thomas Rood was feverish from the *seventh* till the *tenth day*, and at the commencement of the fever he had two or three short convulsive paroxysms; but no eruption took place.

SIXTY-THIRD CASE.

Charlotte Mile. A little redness was observed at the inoculated part on this child's arm for two or three days; but this had wholly disappeared on the *seventh day*, when she was inoculated with variolous matter, which produced the disease in a favourable manner.

SIXTY-FOURTH CASE.

John Jenkins became indisposed on the *twelfth day*, and was very restless for three days. He had about three hundred pustules.

SIXTY-FIFTH CASE.

Henry Barber had a slight fever on the *eighth day*, when symptoms of dentition supervened, but the fever was of short duration. He had but one pustule, and that was upon his upper lip.

SIXTY-SIXTH CASE.

Thomas Dix's arm exhibited an extensive efflorescence on the *eleventh day*, and some evanescent pustules appeared; but he never manifested any indisposition during the progress of the infection.

Sixty-Seventh Case.

Ann Walker became indisposed on the *ninth day*, and continued fretful about twenty-four or thirty hours; the fever then ceased, and she has since been wholly free from disorder. No eruption appeared.

Sixty-Eighth Case.

Samuel Francis Brough was taken ill on the *ninth day* with spasmodic paroxysms, succeeded by fever; the former were of short duration, but the latter, with occasional intermissions, continued for three days. *Eleventh Day.*—Some pustules appeared; their number, however, when the eruption was completed, did not exceed twenty.

Sixty-Ninth Case.

Alexander Towser was restless and feverish about two days. Ten pustules appeared.

Seventieth Case.

William Knighton had no eruption. He was a little indisposed between the *seventh* and *tenth days*.

Seventy-First Case.

Sarah Price had some indisposition on the *ninth day*, which terminated in a diarrhœa. On the *thirteenth day* she was perfectly well; two pustules were now discovered upon her right foot, which were all she had.

Seventy-Second Case.

Elizabeth Spilsbury was somewhat indisposed on the *tenth*, and on the *fifteenth day;* but the latter indisposition was the effect of teething. She had no eruption.

Seventy-Third Case.

Elizabeth May was a little feverish on the *eighth day*, and continued somewhat restless till the *thirteenth day;* five pustules appeared.

Seventy-Fourth Case.

Mary Ann Sully was feverish on the *ninth day*, and passed a restless night, but on the next morning she was better; she made no farther complaint, and no pustules appeared.

Seventy-Fifth Case.

Francis Terry became feverish on the *ninth day;* the next morning a rash appeared, when he seemed to be as well as usual. He had only one pustule.

Seventy-Sixth Case.

William Scott was a little feverish on the *eighth day* only; no eruption ensued.

Seventy-Seventh Case.

William Johnstone's arm tumified in the usual manner. He had no pustules, nor did he appear feverish during the course of the disease; but on the evening of the *thirteenth day* he was thought to be a little restless.

Seventy-Eighth Case.

Mary Stewart, like Johnstone, was not perceptibly indisposed during the whole progress of the infection, neither had she any pustules.

The above patients inoculated with the matter taken from Streeton were subsequently inoculated for the Small Pox, without affecting any but Charlotte Mile, in whom the inoculation for Cow Pox took no effect.

February 27th, Joseph Wrench, twenty-four years old; Stephen Peters, nineteen years old; Peter Peters, eighteen years old; Elizabeth Brown, five years old; Mary Shipley, three years old; Margaret Crosby, ten months old; and John Evans, seven months old, were inoculated with the matter of Cow Pox, taken from the arm of James Smith.

Seventy-Ninth Case.

Joseph Wrench continued indisposed from the *tenth* till the *thirteenth day*. An efflorescence appeared at the inoculated part on the *eleventh day*. *Fifteenth Day.*—Several pustules appeared, and he now complained of a sore throat, which continued three days. The number of pustules was thirty.

Eightieth Case.

Stephen Peters began to complain on the *eighth day*, and continued to be affected with the usual febrile symptoms till the *thirteenth day*. He had only one pustule.

Eighty-First Case.

Peter Peters' complaints were similar to those in the preceding case. The efflorescence did not appear till the *eleventh day.* He had twenty-four pustules, all of which were very small.

Eighty-Second Case.

Elizabeth Brown's tumour on the *eighth day* was surrounded by an efflorescence. She made no complaint, nor had she any eruption.

Eighty-Third Case.

Mary Shipley's arm exhibited an efflorescence on the *eighth day;* but she was not perceptibly indisposed, and had only one pustule.

Eighty-Fourth Case.

Margaret Crosby had no eruption, nor was she perceptibly ill during the progress of her inoculation. Her arm, however, tumified in the usual manner, and displayed an efflorescence.

Eighty-Fifth Case.

On John Evans' arm there was an efflorescence on the *sixth day,* and the following day a slight fever commenced with a spasmodic paroxysm, but he was perfectly well on the *ninth,* and no eruption took place.

The above five persons have been since inoculated with variolous matter without effect.

Sarah Hat, twenty years old, and Elizabeth Platford, seventeen years old, were inoculated with matter of the Cow Pox taken from the arm of Maria Murrell.

Eighty-Sixth Case.

Sarah Hat began to complain on the *sixth day,* and she continued much indisposed till the *eleventh day,* when the tumour was surrounded by an efflorescence, and she made no farther complaint. The number of the pustules which appeared was about forty.

Eighty-Seventh Case.

Elizabeth Platford was taken ill on the *ninth day,* when she complained of pain in the head and loins, with chilliness, etc.; the inoculated part at this time was considerably inflamed; the tumour was circular, but flat, and not surrounded by any efflorescence. *Eleventh Day.*—The pains and shiverings continue; pulse very frequent and weak; tongue white. *Thirteenth Day.*—The symptoms still continue; she also complains of pain across her shoulders; some pustules appear. *Fifteenth Day.*—She complains of pain in the loins and of giddiness; the number of the pustules is much increased. *Seventeenth Day.*—The pains continue; she is very weak and faint; her eyes and throat are inflamed and painful; the edges of the tumour are beset with confluent pustules; the pustules upon her face are about two hundred or three hundred, and approach to confluency. *Nineteenth Day.*—Her face is considerably swelled, and the pustules are now maturating rapidly; she makes no complaint but of the soreness occasioned by the eruption. *Twenty-first Day.*—Swelling of the face much subsided; the pustules in a state of desiccation. *Twenty-third Day.*—She continues recovering. *Twenty-sixth Day.*—She complains of a sore throat, and a cough is troublesome to her. *Twenty-eighth Day.*—The sore throat is almost gone, but the cough continues; pulse 100. *Thirtieth Day.*—The cough is still violent. *Thirty-second Day.* The cough is abated, and her appetite improves; from this time she gradually recovered.

Both the above patients were afterwards inoculated with variolous matter, which produced no effect.

Isaac Cowling, twenty-three years old; Mary Webb, twelve years old; Sophia Mason, two years and a half old; and Elizabeth Goodluck, three months old, were, on the 2nd of March, inoculated for the Cow Pox with matter from the arm of G. Reed.

Eighty-Eighth Case.

Isaac Cowling sickened on the *ninth*, and the eruptive complaints did not wholly go off till the *fourteenth day*. He had about fifty pustules.

Eighty-Ninth Case.

Mary Webb began to complain on the *seventh day*, and continued feverish for a week. On the *tenth day* a redness was diffused over the greatest part of her arm, between the elbow and shoulder, and did not wholly disappear till the fourteenth day. She had about twelve pustules.

Ninetieth Case.

Sophia Mason's arm inflamed in the usual way, and exhibited an efflorescence on the *ninth day*. She had four or five small [illegible] vesicles, but did not seem indisposed during the course of the infection.

Ninety-First Case.

Elizabeth Goodluck was taken ill on the *eighth day*, when she had a slight spasmodic fit; the tumour at this time exhibited an efflorescence. *Eleventh Day.*—Has had no indisposition since yesterday. No eruption took place.

None of the above three patients took the Small Pox in consequence of inoculation with variolous matter.

Ninety-Second and Ninety-Third Cases.

March 3rd.—C. S. Cooke, four years old, and A. T. Cooke, two years old, were inoculated with the matter of Cow Pox, taken from the arm of George Meacock.

An efflorescence at the inoculated part took place in both these children on the *tenth day*, but neither of them seemed indisposed from the inoculation, nor did any pustules appear upon them. They were also put to the test of inoculation with variolous matter, but no disease ensued.

March 3rd.—A. K. Gunter, one year old; Matthew Sears, nine months old; and Eliz. Giles, nine months old, were inoculated with the matter of Cow Pox, taken from the arm of H. Dobinson.

Ninety-Fourth Case.

A. K. Gunter was a little feverish for two days. On the *tenth day* the tumour was surrounded by an efflorescence, which became very extensive. Only two or three imperfect pustules appeared.

Ninety-Fifth Case.

Matthew Sears was indisposed for about four or five days. The tumour was small and angular, nor was it ever surrounded with an efflorescence. He had about two hundred pustules.

Ninety-Sixth Case.

Elizabeth Giles became indisposed on the *tenth day*. The tumour had a dark red-coloured border without any efflorescence. She had from seventy to one hundred pustules.

The above patients have been inoculated with variolous matter without effect.

Richard Scott, two years and a half old; Sarah Bennett, one year old; Maria Black, one year old; Mary Jenkins, nine months old; John Lawyer, eight months old; Eliz. King, six months old; William Jones, six months old; Esther Phipps, six months old; Thomas Newman, six months old; and Ann Harper, five months old, were inoculated with the matter of Cow Pox, taken from the arm of Elizabeth Brown.

NINETY-SEVENTH CASE.

... became feverish for a short time on the *tenth day*. ... fourteen pustules.

NINETY-EIGHTH CASE.

... King's tumour, on the *ninth day*, was surrounded ... She did not manifest any indisposition, ... any eruption.

NINETY-NINTH, ONE HUNDREDTH, AND ONE HUNDRED AND FIRST CASES.

... of John Lawyer, William Jones, and Sarah Bennett ... similar to that of King.

ONE HUNDRED AND SECOND CASE.

... Phipps was a little restless and feverish from the ... till the *thirteenth day*, but had no eruption.

ONE HUNDRED AND THIRD CASE.

... Black became feverish on the *ninth day*, and was ... for two or three days, during which time she had ... convulsions. Some pustules appeared, but did not ...

ONE HUNDRED AND FOURTH CASE.

... was a little indisposed on the *tenth day*. She ... eruption.

ONE HUNDRED AND FIFTH CASE.

... a little restless during the *seventh* and *eighth* ... eruption took place.

ONE HUNDRED AND SIXTH CASE.

... was feverish from the *seventh* till the *twelfth* ... appeared.

... Paul, three years old; Ann Paul, one year ... months old; Martha Hat, one year old; ... old; Samuel Lampart, two years ... a half old; Jane Carter, five weeks ... months old; Susan Sermon, six ... years old; Harriet Marshall, ... Henley, five years old, were ... Cow Pox, taken from the arm of

One Hundred and Seventh Case.

George Paul was not perceptibly indisposed from the inoculation. He had two pustules.

One Hundred and Eighth Case.

Ann Paul was feverish for about three days, and had forty pustules, all of which were much smaller than those of the Small Pox.

One Hundred and Ninth Case.

Martha Chandler's inoculation produced a very extensive efflorescence; but neither fever nor eruption ensued.

One Hundred and Tenth Case.

Martha Hat did not become indisposed till the *thirteenth day*, when a few small pustules appeared.

One Hundred and Eleventh Case.

Elizabeth Boardore's arm tumified considerably; but neither efflorescence, fever, nor eruption took place.

One Hundred and Twelfth Case.

Samuel Lampart was somewhat disordered from the *ninth* till the *twelfth day*, and had three small imperfect pustules.

One Hundred and Thirteenth Case.

Ann Page was not sensibly indisposed from the inoculation, neither had she any eruption. The tumour was surrounded with an efflorescence on the *twelfth day*.

One Hundred and Fourteenth Case.

Jane Carter was slightly indisposed from the *seventh* till the *tenth day*, and had two or three pustules.

One Hundred and Fifteenth Case.

William New was ill four days, and had about one hundred pustules.

One Hundred and Sixteenth Case.

Susan Sermon was taken ill on the *ninth day*, when she vomited. She continued feverish till the *twelfth day*. Only five pustules appeared.

One Hundred and Seventeenth, One Hundred and Eighteenth, and One Hundred and Nineteenth Cases.

Alice Marshall, Frances Henley, and Harriet Marshall had no eruption, nor appeared to have any disorder from the inoculation. The local disease, however, was considerable in all these patients, and was attended with an efflorescence.

All the above patients, who received the infection from Brown and May, have since been inoculated for the Small Pox without effect.

One Hundred and Twentieth Case.

Mary Crouch, aged three years, was inoculated with matter taken from one of the pustules upon John Turner (see case forty-six). A tumour formed at the inoculated part in the usual manner, which was surrounded with an efflorescence; but neither fever nor eruption took place.

One Hundred and Twenty-First and One Hundred and Twenty-Second Cases.

Elizabeth Wood, aged three years, and Wm. Clifford, two years and a half old, were inoculated with Cow Pox matter, taken from the arm of Mary Stewart, March 4th. Both these children were slightly indisposed about the *tenth day*, but neither of them had any pustules.

March 6th.—The following persons were inoculated with the matter of Cow Pox, taken from the arm of Ann Walker :—

Amelia Restieux, four months old; John Bates, six weeks old; Martha Thompson, two years old; William London, six months old; James London, six months old; Frances Wallace, three years old; Joseph Rogers, forty-two years old; Thomas Thoroughgood, fourteen years old; and Ann Thoroughgood, seventeen years old.

One Hundred and Twenty-Third and One Hundred and Twenty-Fourth Cases.

Amelia Restieux and John Bates neither experienced any disorder from the inoculation nor had any eruption; but both their arms tumified in the usual manner.

One Hundred and Twenty-Fifth Case.

Martha Thompson was feverish from the *eighth* till the *tenth day*. She had only one pustule.

One Hundred and Twenty-Sixth Case.

William London was taken ill on the *tenth day*, and vomited; but the following day was as well as usual. He had no eruption.

One Hundred and Twenty-Seventh Case.

James London had no perceptible disorder; and no pustules appeared. On the *tenth day* the tumour was surrounded with an efflorescence.

One Hundred and Twenty-Eighth Case.

Frances Wallace was feverish for two or three days, but no eruption ensued.

One Hundred and Twenty-Ninth Case.

Joseph Rogers on the *eighth day* complained of pain in the axilla, and was affected with head-ach for two or three days; but he had no eruption.

One Hundred and Thirtieth Case.

Thomas Thoroughgood made the same complaints as Rogers. He had thirty-three pustules.

One Hundred and Thirty-First Case.

Ann Thoroughgood was indisposed for six or seven days, but she had only ten pustules.

The preceding twelve patients have had variolous matter inserted in their arms without effect.

The following persons were inoculated with the matter taken from the pustules of Martha Streeton, viz.:

Susan Reeve, eighteen months old; Ann Reeve, five weeks old; Susan Richardson, thirteen years old; and Mary Adams, six months old.

One Hundred and Thirty-Second and One Hundred and Thirty-Third Cases.

Susan Reeve and Ann Reeve were very little disordered by the inoculation; the former, however, had twenty and the latter twelve pustules.

One Hundred and Thirty-Fourth Case.

Susan Richardson continued indisposed from the *tenth* till the *fourteenth day*, but she had only twelve pustules.

One Hundred and Thirty-Fifth Case.

Mary Adams had about two hundred pustules; but the eruptive symptoms were not severe. The tumour in this case spread, and formed an irregular margin, which was studded with confluent pustules.

March 7th.—The disease was transferred from the pustules upon Sarah Dixon to the following children, viz.:

Caroline Harriskind, four years old; William Harriskind, two years old; Daniel Harding, fourteen weeks old; Elizabeth Harding, three years old; James Waters, twelve years old; and Joseph Harding, seventeen years old.

One Hundred and Thirty-Sixth and One Hundred and Thirty-Seventh Cases.

Caroline and William Harriskind were feverish for two or three days. The former had one hundred and the latter had twelve pustules.

One Hundred and Thirty-Eighth and One Hundred and Thirty-Ninth Cases.

Daniel and Elizabeth Harding were but very slightly indisposed from the inoculation. Daniel had fifteen very small pustules; Elizabeth had only two.

One Hundred and Fortieth Case.

James Waters complained of headach, pains of his limbs, and sore throat, from the *eighth* till the *fourteenth day*. The tumour at the inoculated part was never much elevated above the skin, and had an angulated border. He had a hundred and twenty pustules.

One Hundred and Forty-First Case.

Joseph Harding was very slightly disordered, and had no pustules.

March 8th.—William Shipton, four years old; George Staits, two years old; Elizabeth Youngman, three months old; Mary Dudley, two years old; William Cade, ten months old; and William Piper, four months old, were inoculated with the matter of Cow Pox taken from the arm of Esther Phipps.

One Hundred and Forty-Second, One Hundred and Forty-Third, One Hundred and Forty-Fourth, and One Hundred and Forty-Fifth Cases.

William Shipton, Elizabeth Youngman, William Cade, and William Piper had no pustules; and none of them appeared to be disordered from the inoculation, except Piper, who was a little feverish on the *eighth day.* An efflorescence took place around the tumour in all of them.

One Hundred and Forty-Sixth Case.

George Staits was indisposed for two days, and had three or four small pustular eruptions.

One Hundred and Forty-Seventh Case.

Mary Dudley was a little feverish on the *ninth day*, when a rash appeared, which receded the following day, and about fifty small pustules were discovered; these, however, disappeared in the course of twenty-four hours.

March 11th.—Hannah Timms, nineteen years old; Susan Timms, seventeen years old; Jane Franklin, twelve years old; and Henry Lee, fifteen years old, were inoculated with the matter of Cow Pox, taken from the arm of Mary Webb.

One Hundred and Forty-Eighth Case.

Hannah Timms was affected with the febrile symptoms from the *eighth* till the *sixteenth day*, and had one hundred and sixty-five pustules, all of which suppurated.

One Hundred and Forty-Ninth Case.

Sarah Timms was ill from the *ninth* till the *fourteenth day.* She had no eruption.

One Hundred and Fiftieth Case.

Jane Franklin was very little indisposed from the inoculation, and had no eruption.

One Hundred and Fifty-First Case.

Henry Lee complained for two or three days, and had only one pustule.

March 13th.—The following persons were inoculated with the matter of Cow Pox, taken from the arm of Sarah Hat, viz.: Ann Spooner, twenty-one years old; Matthew Wall, fourteen years old; John Wall, ten years old; William Ockendon, twelve years old; Joseph Ockendon, ten years old; William Jennings, seven years old; George Jennings, six years old; John Pluckrose, seven years old; Charlotte Webb, fourteen weeks old; Charles Dibden, three months old; Elizabeth Eaton, two years old; Charlotte Eaton, ten months old; and Joseph Pigg, eleven years old.

One Hundred and Fifty-Second Case.

Ann Spooner was indisposed for three or four days, and had a hundred and fifty pustules.

One Hundred and Fifty-Third Case.

Matthew Wall was a little indisposed for three days. He had ten pustules.

One Hundred and Fifty-Fourth Case.

John Wall made no complaint, and had no eruption.

One Hundred and Fifty-Fifth Case.

William Ockendon was indisposed from the eighth till the tenth day. He had only one pustule.

One Hundred and Fifty-Sixth Case.

Joseph Ockendon was ill for three days. He had no eruption.

One Hundred and Fifty-Seventh Case.

William Jennings complained of headach two days. He had only one pustule.

One Hundred and Fifty-Eighth Case.

George Jennings was disordered in the same manner as his brother William, but he had no eruption.

[illegible] Hundred and Fifty-Ninth Case.

[illegible] made no complaint and had no eruption.

[illegible] and One Hundred and Sixty-[illegible] Cases.

[illegible] and Charles Dibden.—The former was percep-[illegible] the inoculation, and had no pustules. The [illegible] on the *ninth day* and vomited. He had [illegible]

One Hundred and Sixty-Second and One Hundred and Sixty-Third Cases.

Elizabeth Eaton and Charles Eaton were both slightly indisposed on the *eleventh* and *twelfth day*, and each had about twenty pustules.

One Hundred and Sixty-Fourth Case.

Joseph Pigg complained of a pain in the axilla, and of a slight headach for four days. He had fourteen pustules only.

March 13.—The following were inoculated with the matter of Cow Pox, taken from the arm of Samuel Lampart, viz.: Mary Ockendon, sixteen years old; Sarah Ockendon, seven years old; Sarah Stacey, twelve years old; Ann Stacey, seven years old; Mary Fuller, eleven years old; Isabella Barrett, eleven years old; Mary Perry, three years old; Susan Vinicum, five months old; Elizabeth Brensden, eighteen months old; Mary Ward, ten months old; William Terry, two months old; Caroline Poorey, three years old; Ann Poorey, eleven months old; John Langstaff, four years and a half old; Emma Lightfoot, thirteen months old; Daniel Sinclair, seven months old; M. H. Hills, eighteen weeks old; and Catharine Donaldson, nineteen months old.

One Hundred and Sixty-Fifth Case.

Mary Ockendon was indisposed from the *ninth* till the *fourteenth day*. She had only six pustules.

One Hundred and Sixty-Sixth Case.

Sarah Ockendon complained of headach, pain of her limbs, etc., from the *tenth* till the *fourteenth day*, but only four pustules appeared.

One Hundred and Sixty-Seventh Case.

Sarah Stacey was indisposed from the *tenth* till the *fifteenth day*. No pustules appeared.

One Hundred and Sixty-Eighth Case.

Ann Stacey's case was similar to that of her sister Sarah.

One Hundred and Sixty-Ninth and One Hundred and Seventieth Cases.

Mary Fuller and Isabella Barrett both complained of the febrile symptoms from the *ninth* till the *fourteenth day*. The former had six and the latter twenty pustules.

One Hundred and Seventy-First, One Hundred and Seventy-Second, and One Hundred and Seventy-Third Cases.

Mary Perry, Susan Vinicum, and Elizabeth Rensden did not appear to be indisposed from the inoculation, and had no eruption; but the tumours in all were considerable, and surrounded by an efflorescence.

One Hundred and Seventy-Fourth Case.

Mary Ward was a little feverish for two days, and a few small pustules appeared for one day only.

One Hundred and Seventy-Fifth, One Hundred and Seventy-Sixth, One Hundred and Seventy-Seventh, and One Hundred and Seventy-Eighth Cases.

William Terry, Ann Poorey, Caroline Poorey, and John Langstaff had no pustules, neither did any of them appear to be indisposed, except Ann Poorey, who was feverish for two days.

One Hundred and Seventy-Ninth and One Hundred and Eightieth Cases.

Emma Lightfoot and Daniel Sinclair were both a little disordered for two or three days, and the former had four or five small pustules, but the latter had no eruption.

One Hundred and Eighty-First and One Hundred and Eighty-Second Cases.

Ann Hills and Catharine Donaldson had neither fever nor eruption.

One Hundred and Eighty-Third Case.

Ann Clarke was inoculated with the matter of Cow Pox, taken from the arm of Peter Peters, which produced two or three small evanescent pustules; but no fever took place.

March 15.—John Buckthorpe, twenty-two years old; John Cater, fourteen years old; Susan Tomlins, nineteen years old; Maria Burgess, four years old; and Sophia Burgess, three years old, were inoculated for the Cow Pox, with matter taken from the arm of Joseph Wrench.

One Hundred and Eighty-Fourth Case.

John Buckthorpe was indisposed from the *ninth* till the *fourteenth day*. He had nearly one hundred pustules.

One Hundred and Eighty-Fifth Case.

John Cater complained of headach, etc., from the *eighth* till the *eleventh day*. He had forty pustules.

One Hundred and Eighty-Sixth Case.

Susan Tomlins continued ill for three days. She had twenty-four pustules.

One Hundred and Eighty-Seventh and One Hundred and Eighty-Eighth Cases.

Maria and Sophia Burgess were neither indisposed from the inoculation. Sophia had no pustules and Maria only three.

March 18th.—The following persons were inoculated with the matter of Cow Pox, taken from the arm of Elizabeth Platford: John Williams, seven months old; James Runtsman, three months old; Robert Lear, seventeen months old; John Selby, five months old; Samuel Ariell, two years old; James Ariell, five years old; Henry Servy, two years and a half old; Sarah Lovell, four years old; Henry Lovell, two years old; Rebecca Salmon, nine months old; John Corwell, eight months old, and Francis Cundell, six months old.

One Hundred and Eighty-Ninth Case.

John Williams had no indisposition nor pustules. The tumour was surrounded with an efflorescence on the *eleventh day*.

One Hundred and Ninetieth Case.

James Runtsman was a little feverish on the evening of the *tenth day*. He had no eruption.

One Hundred and Ninety-First Case.

Robert Lear's case was similar to that of Runtsman.

One Hundred and Ninety-Second Case.

John Selby was feverish two days, and had forty pustules.

ONE HUNDRED AND NINETY-THIRD AND ONE HUNDRED AND NINETY-FOURTH CASES.

Samuel Ariell and James Ariell were both feverish on the *tenth* and *eleventh days*, but neither had any eruption.

ONE HUNDRED AND NINETY-FIFTH AND ONE HUNDRED AND NINETY-SIXTH CASES.

Henry Servy and Sarah Lovell were disordered two days. The former had no pustules, the latter forty.

ONE HUNDRED AND NINETY-SEVENTH CASE.

Henry Lovell was ill three days, and had one hundred and seventy pustules.

ONE HUNDRED AND NINETY-EIGHTH CASE.

Rebecca Salmon was very slightly indisposed, but had about two hundred pustules, which were very small.

ONE HUNDRED AND NINETY-NINTH AND TWO HUNDREDTH CASES.

John Corwell and Francis Cundell were both feverish for two or three days; the former had thirty-six and the latter twelve pustules.

All the above patients, inoculated since the 6th of March, have subsequently had variolous matter inserted in their arms, except the two Ariells, but it produced no disorder.

In order that the progressive descent of the Cow Pox infection from patient to patient, as well as the magnitude of the disease which was excited by the inoculation, may be comprehended at one view, I have subjoined the following tabular statement.

It may be observed that the matter used for the preceding inoculations was not only derived immediately from the pustular eruptions upon the teats of the cow, but also from Sarah Rice, who contracted the disease by milking the infected cows. I begin with the former. In the first and second divisions opposite to the names the age in years or months is recorded; in the third the number of days during which the febrile symptoms continued; and in the last, the number of pustules produced :

TABLE.

	Years of Age.	Months.	Days of Illness.	No. of Pustules.
From the cow to—				
M. Payne	2	6	3	0
E. Payne	...	4	5	0
Buckland	...	4	4	24
R. Payne	10	...	0	5
Redding	16	...	1	4
Collingridge	17	...	4	170
Pink	15	...	0	0
From M. and E. Payne to—				
Talley	14	...	...	...
Brown	15	...	...	...
From Collingridge to—				
Mundy	25	...	2	15
George	25	...	6	530
Butcher	13	...	2	0
Dorset	19	...	1	0
From Buckland's pustules to—				
S. Price	13	...	2	6
From Redding to—				
Wife	14	...	0	4
From Mundy to—				
Slade	21	...	5	4
From George to—				
Tarrant	19	...	1	0
From Butcher to—				
Jewel	20	...	2	0
Bumpus	20	...	6	310
West	21	...	5	20
W. Hull	11	...	4	200
H. Hull	13	...	1	8
S. Hull	8	...	2	120
From Jewel to—				
Fisk	...	4	4	40
Reed	15	...	5	70
From S. Price to—				
Pedder	...	11	5	40
Hoole	...	5	5	102
Hickland	...	6	3	300
Morton	...	9	7	200
From Fisk to—				
Davy	...	3	1	3
Murrell	...	7	4	20
From Bumpus to—				
Dixon	19	...	4	174
W. Walker	...	11	0	0
Cummins	...	3	0	0
Ellistone	...	3	2	0
Dunn	...	8	3	0
From West to—				
So. Dobinson	5	...	0	0
Sarah Dobinson	3	...	0	0
H. Dobinson	1	...	1	0
Giles	20	...	3	30

	Years of Age.	Months.	Days of Illness.	No. of Pustules.
From West to—				
Bigg	18	...	5	12
Briaris	16	...	4	2
From Reed to—				
Cowling	23	...	4	50
Webb	12	...	0	12
Mason	2	6	0	4
Goodluck	...	3	2	0
From Murrell to—				
Hat	20	...	4	40
Platford	17	...	8	1000
From H. Dobinson to—				
Gunter	1	...	2	3
Sears	...	9	5	200
E. Giles	...	9	3	90
From Dixon's pustules to—				
C. Harriskind	4	...	4	100
W. Harriskind	2	...	3	12
D. Harding	...	3	1	15
E. Harding	3	...	1	2
Waters	12	...	6	120
J. Harding	17	...	1	10
From Webb to—				
H. Timms	19	...	7	165
S. Timms	17	...	5	0
Franklin	12	...	1	0
Lee	15	...	2	3
From Hat to—				
Spooner	21	...	4	150
M. Wall	14	...	3	10
J. Wall	10	...	0	0
J. Ockendon	10	...	3	0
W. Ockendon	12	...	3	1
W. Jennings	7	...	2	1
G. Jennings	6	...	2	0
Pluckrose	7	...	0	0
C. Webb	...	3	0	0
Dibden	...	3	1	0
E. Eaton	2	...	2	2
C. Eaton	...	10	2	2
Pigg	11	...	4	14
From Platford to—				
Williams	...	7	0	0
Runtsman	...	3	1	0
Lear	1	5	1	0
Selby	...	5	2	40
S. Ariell	2	...	2	0
J. Ariell	5	...	2	0
Servy	2	6	2	0
S. Lovell	4	...	2	40
H. Lovell	2	...	3	170
Salmon	...	9	1	200
Corwell	...	8	3	36
Cundell	...	6	2	12
From S. Rice to—				
Harris	21	...	0	300
Bunker	15	...	3	3

	Years of Age.	Months.	Days of Illness.	No. of Pustules.
From S. Rice to—				
Crouch	7	...	0	0
Fox	25	...	...	...
Dennis	23	...	...	...
From Crouch to—				
Keys	25	...	1	0
Turner	24	...	6	220
Morgan	1	...	5	0
Mr. Coleman's cow.				
From the cow to—				
Streeton	22	...	6	300
Smith	16	...	4	105
Meacock	30	...	5	350
From Turner to—				
Fairbrother	15	...	4	4
Calloway	19	...	3	20
Camplin	17	...	4	30
J. Turner	...	8	2	1000
Buckley	...	5	1	0
Welch	...	3	1	0
From Streeton to—				
Greenville	20	...	3	35
Honeywood	2	...	0	0
Rood	1	6	2	0
Mile	1	3	0	0
Jenkins	1	...	3	300
Barber	...	11	2	1
Dix	...	11	0	6
A. Walker	...	10	2	0
Brough	...	10	3	20
Towser	...	8	2	10
Knighton	...	8	2	0
Price	...	8	1	0
Spilsbury	...	4	2	0
May	...	4	4	5
Sully	...	3	1	0
Terry	...	2	1	1
Scott	...	2	1	0
Johnston	...	2	0	0
Stewart	...	2	0	0
From Smith to—				
Wrench	24	...	3	30
S. Peters	19	...	4	1
P. Peters	18	...	4	24
Brown	5	...	0	0
Shipley	3	...	0	1
Crosby	...	10	0	0
Evans	...	7	2	0
From Meacock to—				
C. Cooke	4	...	0	0
A. Cooke	2	...	0	0
From Brown to—				
R. Scott	2	6	1	14
Bennett	1	...	0	0
Black	1	...	3	7
M. Jenkins	...	9	1	0
Lawyer	...	8	0	0

	Years of Age.	Months.	Days of Illness.	No. of Pustules.
From Brown to—				
King	...	6	0	0
Jones	...	6	0	0
Phipps	...	6	3	0
Newman	...	6	4	0
Harper	...	5	2	0
From May to—				
G. Paul	3	...	0	2
A. Paul	1	...	3	40
Chandler	...	5	0	0
M. Hat	1	...	1	5
Boardore	...	7	0	0
Lampart	2	...	2	3
Page	1	6	0	0
Carter	...	1	2	3
Sermon	...	6	3	5
A. Marshall	2	...	0	0
H. Marshall	...	4	0	0
Henley	5	...	0	0
New	1	6	4	100
From Turner's pustules to—				
M. Crouch	3	...	0	0
From Stewart to—				
Wood	3	...	1	0
Clifford	2	6	1	0
From A. Walker to—				
Restieux	...	4	0	0
Bates	0	1½	0	0
Thompson	2	...	2	1
W. London	3	6	1	0
J. London	...	6	0	0
Wallace	3	...	2	0
Rogers	42	...	3	0
T. Thoroughgood	14	...	3	33
A. Thoroughgood	17	...	6	10
From Streeton's pustules to—				
S. Reeve	1	6	1	20
A. Reeve	...	1	1	12
Richardson	13	...	3	12
Adams	...	6	3	200
From Phipps to—				
Shipton	4	...	0	0
Staits	2	...	2	3
Youngman	...	3	0	0
Dudley	2	...	1	50
Cade	...	10	0	0
Piper	...	4	1	0
From Lampart to—				
M. Ockendon	16	...	4	6
S. Ockendon	17	...	3	4
S. Stacey	12	...	4	0
A. Stacey	7	...	4	0
Fuller	11	...	4	6
Barrett	11	...	4	20
Perry	3	...	0	0
Vinicum	...	5	0	0
Bensden	1	6	0	0

	Years of Age.	Months.	Days of Illness.	No. of Pustules.
From Lampart to—				
Ward	...	10	2	7
Terry	...	2	0	0
C. Poorey	3	...	0	0
A. Poorey	...	11	2	0
Langstaff	4	6	0	0
Lightfoot	1	1	2	5
Sinclair	...	7	2	0
Hills	...	4	0	0
Donaldson	1	7	0	0
From Wrench to—				
Buckthorpe	22	...	4	100
Cater	14	...	3	40
Tomlin	19	...	3	24
M. Burgess	4	...	0	3
S. Burgess	3	...	0	0
From P. Peters to—				
Clarke	5	...	0	3

The preceding table comprehends all the cases originally intended to have been given in this work, the publication of which, from a concurrence of circumstances, has been delayed much longer than the author expected, and has thereby afforded him an opportunity of making the following additions:—

	Years of Age.	Months.	Days of Illness.	No. of Pustules.
From Platford's pustules to—				
Prince	1	...	0	30
Chandler	1	9	0	40
Jervoise	...	6	1	0
Palmer	...	3	3	100
Henderson	...	10	4	300
Crawford	1	10	3	250
From Dudley to—				
A. Valentine	3	...	2	0
J. Valentine	2	...	3	0
From S. Timms to—				
S. Harris	21	...	7	6
S. Clarke	...	9	2	0
M. Harris	23	...	6	60
Ludgrove	...	11	2	0
Stringer	20	...	4	2
From Greenville to—				
B. Crane	2	...	3	200
T. Crane	4	...	2	12
Garrett	14	...	4	62
M. Crane	8	...	4	30
From A. Stacey to—				
M. Stacey	38	...	3	5
R. Stacey	...	7	0	12
J. Stacey	3	6	0	5
Harriott	...	8	1	6

	Years of Age.	Months.	Days of Illness.	No. of Pustules.
From A. Stacey to—				
M. Waite	...	10	2	50
J. Waite	3	...	2	20
From M. Ockendon to—				
H. Pigley	22	...	4	100
Dach	...	4½	2	0
G. Pigley	...	5	0	0
Morgon	...	2½	0	0
Bradley	19	...	6	156
Harrison	...	2	1	0
Morton	...	5	0	0
Cooper	4	11	0	0
E. Cooper	...	4	1	0
Ellikins	3	3	0	0
M. Hide	4	11	0	0
D. Hide	1	5	0	0
Phillips	...	8	0	0
From Tomlin to—				
C. Hopes	3	...	1	0
S. Hopes	1	...	0	0
Oliphant	3	...	1	0
Castin	...	6	3	0
Hamm	2	...	0	0
A. Smith	4	...	0	0
Reynolds	...	4	0	0
From J. Wall to—				
Galliway	...	3	1	0
Barnaby	1	6	0	0
Dick	2	8	0	3
Dalkins	...	5½	1	0
Bromley	1	2	2	3
Ford	...	6	2	0
From J. Valentine to—				
Merrin	...	3	0	0
Loathis	4	...	3	5
Gedge	...	4½	0	0
Beasley	...	3	0	4
Goodman	1	10	2	40
From Spooner to—				
Stainer	16	...	3	34
M. Pepler	4	...	0	0
Swannell	10	...	3	6
F. Pepler	2	...	0	0
Brown	19	...	4	35
P. Roberts	6	...	4	12
M. Roberts	4	...	0	6
C. Roberts	1	8	3	6
Freeman	11	...	4	40
A. Palmer	...	9	2	40
Wade	16	...	4	3
From Cooper to—				
Munden	...	7	1	50
From H. Timms' pustules to—				
Stiles	...	6	3	500
Burrows	...	5	1	12
From M. Bartlett to—				
J. Mundy	...	6	3	100

	Years of Age.	Months.	Days of Illness.	No. of Pustules.
From Cowley to—				
Nash	15	...	1	0
From Spooner's pustules to—				
Serjeant	16	...	4	35
Cook	15	...	2	11
From Stringer's pustules to—				
Argant	17	...	7	19
From H. Timms' pustules to—				
E. Gilbert	17	...	3	4
Brewster	11	...	4	6
Truluck	...	6	2	250
Wiggins	...	5	0	7
Th. Turner	...	6	0	50
Gilbert	...	6	3	500
Downes	...	4	2	30
King	...	2	2	4
Talbot	...	4	3	500
From Corwell to—				
Graham	...	4	0	0
Sellers	15	...	0	0
From Barrett to—				
T. Barrett	32	...	3	200
M. Barrett	5	...	0	0
J. Barrett	2	3	1	0
H. Barrett	...	7	2	30
E. Wybrow	5	...	3	200
T. Wybrow	9	...	3	150
J. Wybrow	1	...	1	6
Harwood	2	3	1	6
M. Harwood	4	...	0	12
J. Harwood	5	...	2	6
P. Harwood	...	5	4	200
Higgins	...	3	0	0
M. Higgins	2	6	0	5
From Henderson to—				
Upstone	19	...	5	12
I. Bumpus	16	...	5	20
From S. Harris to—				
Tyler	13	...	0	0
W. Meacock	18	...	5	400
R. Meacock	29	...	5	20
M. Meacock	1	...	3	6
Porch	3	6	0	2
E. Porch	2	...	0	0
J. Porch	...	4	3	350
Fermoy	...	11	0	60
Gurney	...	11	0	0
Downs	1	6	2	300
From Wade to—				
Mays	1	1	2	500
From J. Mundy to—				
Matthews	...	4	2	0
From Brewster to—				
M. Brewster	...	11	0	0
From Lee's pustules to—				
Baker	29	...	3	140
Caterer	15	...	5	8

	Years of Age.	Months.	Days of Illness.	No. of Pustules.
From Lee's pustules to—				
R. Featherstone	12	...	3	40
C. Featherstone	9	...	3	120
Porter	5	...	0	9
J. Porter	1	6	1	12
J. Jennings	5	...	1	30
C. Jennings	3	...	1	30
W. Jennings	1	1	0	9
Mansfield	1	6	2	12
S. Wybrow	6	...	2	300
S. Baker	1	1	3	25
J. Goss	2	8	1	0
W. Goss	...	8	2	30
Odell	...	9	3	90
Murphield	...	6	2	0
From Dalkins to—				
Sharp	...	4	2	0
From Waite to—				
T. Jennings	1	6	0	0
Kitchen	5	...	1	0
S. Pluckrose	4	...	2	0
T. Pluckrose	...	10	2	0
Rout	...	6	1	20
W. Houghton	2	6	1	0
From Swannell to—				
Mickland	...	2	0	3
Ferguson	...	7	1	7
Goddard	1	...	2	0
Roberts	...	9	1	0
Gran	...	6	1	0
Benson	...	8	2	0
Floaks	...	2	1	2
From M. Gilbert to—				
Welch	15	...	3	100
Rowley	...	3	2	25
A. Waite	17	...	4	10
Tarbotts	1	1	2	600
S. Tarbotts	3	3	4	300
Bell	...	3	3	250
From S. Hopes to—				
Snell	17	...	2	200
I. Houghton	32	...	2	200
Stedman	...	5	3	60
M. Broadwood	...	6	2	150
W. Broadwood	...	6	2	200
Sorrell	4	11	4	500
S. Sorrell	6	...	1	1
Underwood	...	9	2	105
From Ellikin to—				
G. Cooke	2	2	3	20
Costin	...	5	2	0
From Reynolds to—				
Walford	...	6	2	600
From Wade to—				
Wenworth	1	8	3	500
Gibson	...	8	0	0
Lister	...	5	0	0

	Years of Age.	Months.	Days of Illness.	No. of Pustules.
From Wade to—				
Wooden	1	4	4	0
Smart	6	...	2	0
Taylor	1	...	1	200
Arnold	...	5	3	0
Turvey	...	3	2	12
Guilder	2	3	2	0
Gallap	...	2	2	0
Stanny	2	2	4	2
Moore	...	4	0	0
M. Moore	2	6	1	0
From Oliphant to—				
Absalom	...	7	1	0
From M. Ford to—				
Clark	2	4	3	0
Cox	1	7	2	0
Sandaw	...	2	0	0
From J. Roberts to—				
T. Roberts	3	...	3	0
From Kitchen to—				
T. Foster	5	...	2	5
J. Foster	1	...	1	2
M. Foster	1	...	1	24
S. Gobby	27	...	2	20
W. Gobby	5	...	0	2
J. Gobby	...	6	3	0
Putney	...	7	2	0
Bush	1	7	1	0
E. Franklin	3	...	2	0
S. Franklin	...	8	0	0
Neat	2	...	2	9
Hicks	3	...	2	0
More	...	5	0	0
Barker	6	...	2	6
North	2	...	3	0
Cowland	1	3	3	12
Harrison	...	8	1	5
R. Lawyer	36	...	1	1
E. Lawyer	3	6	1	7
F. Lawyer	4	6	0	0
M. Lawyer	1	...	0	0
E. Dunn	5	...	0	0
F. Dunn	2	6	0	0
T. Dunn	...	3	2	6
N. Collop	9	...	1	0
J. Collop	7	...	1	0
A. Collop	3	...	1	0
E. Collop	...	5	0	0
T. Wiggins	7	...	0	0
W. Wiggins	4	...	0	0
P. Wiggins	1	6	0	0
Ruffles	19	...	2	6
Bridges	...	1	0	0
From J. Barrett to—				
I. Mitchell	6	...	2	200
P. Mitchell	4	...	2	50
T. Mitchell	2	...	2	26

	Years of Age.	Months.	Days of Illness.	No. of Pustules.
From Cook to—				
E. Chapman	12	...	2	27
M. Chapman	9	...	3	67
Good	13	...	4	400
From Styles to—				
Edwards	18	...	3	0
From Talbot to—				
Brandrom	12	...	0	0
From Caterer to—				
Stapler	22	...	4	300
Marsham	17	...	4	43
Waller	18	...	3	15
Wall	8	...	3	200
R. Johnston	...	3	2	0
Fletcher	...	6	3	500
From Bradley's pustules to—				
Vaughan	...	5	2	12
Vethall	...	4	3	200
Hope	...	6	4	100
Masterson	...	5	2	20
Green	2	4	3	30
Lutman	1	...	2	20
Roberts	...	4	3	450
Starbuck	...	5	2	20
M. Phillips	2	2	3	500
S. Phillips	3	11	3	5
Wicks	...	4	2	36
Terry	...	3	2	8
Sheriff	7	...	3	34
Steers	13	...	3	40
From I. Houghton to—				
S. Houghton	19	...	0	0
W. Houghton	58	...	0	0
Jolly	1	8	0	0
From T. Pluckrose to—				
Lineau	12	...	3	3
Woodlard	2	...	0	0
From Kitchen to—				
Kettridge	16	...	1	3
Raymond	1	...	1	3
From I. Harwood to—				
A. Harris	26	...	4	100
M. Harris	...	1	4	500
S. Harris	4	6	5	50
W. Harris	5	6	2	25
G. Harris	2	6	1	5
S. Boyton	8	...	4	700
E. Boyton	6	...	3	600
J. Boyton	3	...	3	350
From Talbot to—				
Lemare	...	6	3	60
Williams	...	9	4	650
English	1	3	2	100
Churchman	...	3	4	30
Hunt	1	2	4	700
Whitburn	...	9	4	430
Chartau	...	10	4	17

	Years of Age.	Months.	Days of Illness.	No. of Pustules.
From Talbot to—				
Callen	...	8	3	75
Russel	...	5	4	15
E. Russel	3	6	3	12
Knight	...	8	3	500
Richardson	...	6	2	200
Johnston	1	7	3	150
From J. Goss to—				
Blinkinhorn	...	2	0	0
Millward	...	7	0	5
Haywood	1	8	4	46
A. Godden	1	...	2	300
W. Godden	3	...	3	650
Jones	...	6	0	0
Paradise	3	...	3	50
Kelly	2	...	0	100
Hales	...	6	4	500
I. Mountain	4	6	2	300
M. Mountain	2	...	2	150
A. Mountain	1	...	1	75
From Brewster to—				
Barnett	1	1	0	0
Balling	...	9	2	6
Upton	1	9	3	0
Finn	1	1	2	0
Hilliard	...	6	0	0
White	1	4	1	0
From W. Meacock to—				
Westbrook	...	3	0	0
From E. Chapman to—				
Hider	...	2	1	0
Hughes	1	8	3	12
C. Hughes	...	5	2	4
From M. Chapman to—				
Sharp	18	0	3	30
Calburn	16	...	3	12
Ledger	...	4	2	50
Vautin	1	...	1	2
McKennish	4	3	2	150
Wright	...	7	3	10
Rance	...	2	0	0
From Ruffles to—				
Thornton	17	...	1	0
Boreham	16	...	2	3
Hill	...	5	1	0
Towler	1	3	1	0
French	...	11	0	0
Brestley	...	8	0	0
Thomas	...	4	1	0
Richardson	...	9	0	0
Morgan	...	5	0	0
From A. Waite to—				
Wood	22	...	4	6
Young	16	...	2	0
Norman	12	...	2	0
M. Bartlett	...	11	1	20
Askew	...	3	0	15
Clark	...	9	0	0

Those who are acquainted with the history of the Cow Pox will, no doubt, be surprised to find from the preceding cases that pustules have frequently been the consequence of the inoculation of this disease. Indeed, when I first observed a pustular eruption upon Buckland (case three), the occurrence being wholly unexpected, I was not without apprehension that the lancet which was employed in its inoculation might have had some particles of variolous matter adhering to it. But this suspicion was soon removed, for, upon enquiry, I found that all the lancets which I had used on the 21st of January were then made use of for the first time since they had been ground by the cutler.

Among the patients inoculated for the Cow Pox during the first week in which I obtained the matter of this disease, several were so circumstanced as to be afterwards constantly exposed to the infection of the Small Pox. Having then had no proof that the progress of the infection of the former would supersede that of the latter, I used the precaution to inoculate the patients with variolous matter on the fifth day after that taken from the cow had been inserted. This led some medical gentlemen to suppose that the matter locally formed in the arm from the first inoculation might be variolated by the progress of the second inoculation in the other arm, and that consequently the matter generated in the Cow Pox tumour with which others were inoculated would produce a hybrid disease and not the genuine Cow Pox. But as the matter employed in the Cow Pox inoculations was always taken before the constitution could be affected by the variolous matter, and during the time that both inoculations were merely local diseases, I apprehend its effects would be the same as if the variolous inoculation had not taken place. Nay, had this not been the case, but had several patients been inoculated with matter taken from the Cow Pox tumour on the arm of Jane Collingridge, after both the inoculations were supposed to have affected the constitution for several days, neither facts nor analogy lead us to believe that the matter thus obtained would produce any other disease than that of its own species, or that its specific morbid quality would be changed by entering into combination with the virus of the Small Pox. The general character of the tumour formed by the inoculation of the Small Pox is very different from that of the Cow Pox; and though on the same day a person be inoculated in one arm with the matter of the Cow Pox, and in the other with that of the Small Pox, yet both tumours preserve their respective characteristic appearances throughout the whole course of the disease.

This is certainly a strong proof that the two diseases, in respect to their local action, continue separate and distinct.

Twenty-eight patients were on the same day inoculated with the matter of Cow Pox and that of the Small Pox, mixed together in equal quantities, in order to try which would prevail, or, if it were probable, to produce a hybrid disease by a union of both. The result was that in more than one-half of the patients thus inoculated the local affection distinctly assumed the characters of the Cow Pox; in the others it more resembled the Small Pox, but in none of them was there much indisposition or many pustules.

At the request of Dr. Jenner, I transmitted to him, in Gloucestershire, some of the Cow Pox matter from the patients then under my care, which he used for the purpose of inoculation; after a trial of it he informed me that "the rise, progress, and termination of the pustule created by this virus on the arm was exactly that of the true uncontaminated Cow Pox." The matter sent was taken from the arm of Ann Bumpus, who had three hundred and ten pustules, all of which suppurated; yet with the matter of this stock Dr. Jenner inoculated twenty, and another gentleman in the same county a hundred and forty persons, without producing any pustules which maturated.

This fact would appear to confirm an opinion entertained by Dr. Jenner. In his second publication on the variolæ vaccinæ he seems disposed to attribute the pustules which so often attended this disease in London and its vicinity to some peculiar influence of the town air. But, of the cases which I have stated, several were those of patients who were inoculated eight miles' distance from London; yet these patients, in the proportion of about one in five, had an eruption. And at a small village, still farther from London, eighteen persons were inoculated with similar matter, in all of whom it produced pustules.

The twenty-seventh case also affords decisive evidence that the matter employed in it was that of the Cow Pox, for Jewel had undergone the Small Pox when a child; yet the inoculation excited febrile symptoms of two or three days' duration, and the tumour which was produced upon her arm did not begin to scab till the thirteenth day.

Having now, I presume, given sufficient reasons for establishing the point for which they have been adduced, I shall proceed to enquire how far the effects of the Cow Pox upon the human subject seem to differ from or correspond with those of the Small Pox when communicated by inoculation.

The vaccine disease, as it has lately been called, affords a striking example, and perhaps the only one yet discovered, of a disorder which can be transferred from brute animals to man, and carried back again from him to the brute. A remarkable instance of this is related at p. 115, which shows that the matter of the Cow Pox, as reproduced by inoculation in the human animal and inserted into the teat of a cow, produced the disease. Similar attempts were also made with variolous matter, which had no effect; hence in this respect these two morbid poisons appear to differ. The Cow Pox also differs from the Small Pox in acting upon the constitutions of those who have undergone the latter disease, as was fully exemplified in the case of Frances Jewel. However, I am disposed to think that the matter of the Cow Pox is not so capable of affecting persons who have had the Small Pox as has been represented. I made several trials to inoculate this disease in patients at the hospital who were recovering from a full eruption of the natural Small Pox, but in no instance did any tumour appear on the arm; neither does the insertion of the variolous matter, in such cases, excite the least inflammation in the skin. It is probable, therefore, that the matter of the Cow Pox, like that of the Small Pox, does not manifest any local action upon persons who have lately undergone the variolous disease. If a person has casually received the infection of the Small Pox, and be inoculated with variolous matter three or four days before the eruptive symptoms supervene, the inoculated part does not tumify, as in other cases, but becomes a simple pustule; on the contrary, if a person has been inoculated, and the progress of the inoculation be so far advanced that the patient is within one day of the approach of the eruptive fever, and be then inoculated a second time, the tumour produced from the second inoculation will become nearly as extensive as the first, and be in a state of suppuration a few hours after the fever commences. Hence it appears that the process of variolation in the natural and in the inoculated Small Pox is different. The Cow Pox, in every case with which we are acquainted, has been introduced into the human constitution through the medium of external local inflammation, and is therefore to be considered as an inoculated disease; the virus of it seems also to effect a similar mode of action, and to be governed by the same laws as that of the Small Pox. Thus if a person be alternately inoculated with variolous matter and with that of the Cow Pox every day till fever is excited, all the inoculations make a progress; and as soon as the whole system becomes disordered, they appear to be all equally advanced in maturation. However, the local tumour excited from the inoculation of the Cow Pox is commonly of a different appearance from that which is the consequence of inoculation with variolous matter; for if the inoculation be performed by a simple puncture, the consequent tumour, in the proportion of three times out of four, or more, assumes a form completely circular, and it continues circumscribed, with its edges elevated and well defined, and its surface flat, throughout every stage of the disease; while that which is produced from variolous matter either preserves a pustular form or spreads along the skin, and becomes angulated and irregular, or disfigured by numerous vesiculæ.

Another distinction, still more general and decisive, is to be drawn from the contents of the Cow Pox tumour; for the fluid it forms, unless from some accidental circumstance, very rarely becomes puriform, and the scab which succeeds is of a harder texture, exhibits a smoother surface, and differs in its colour from that which is formed by the concretion of pus. All the appearances here described, however, do not constantly attend the disease, but are sometimes so much changed they can in no respect be distinguished from those which arise from the inoculation of the Small Pox. When the disease thus deviates from its usual appearance at the inoculated part, its effects upon the constitution have commonly, though not always, been felt more severely than where the tumour was distinctly characterised.

As I have now pointed out the principal circumstances in which the two diseases usually differ in their local effects, I shall proceed to examine them in a more important point of view, and to compare their general effect upon the constitution, in order, if possible, to ascertain, from the facts already adduced, whether or not the inoculation of the vaccine disease produces a milder distemper, and of less dangerous consequences to the patient, than that of the Small Pox. For if it be an established fact, as I presume it is, that those who have undergone the former disease are thereby rendered secure against the effects of the latter, it only remains to be proved, in order to make the former be generally adopted, that the disorder which attends the Cow Pox is also less severe and less fatal than the other. The number of cases of Cow Pox inoculated under my direction have amounted to about six hundred, but all these could not be included in the table, as at the time it was printed the disease, in many patients, was not far enough advanced to give the result; and to these may be added others who did not give proper attendance, and also some whose names I am not permitted to make public.

The table, however, contains a sufficient number of cases to enable the medical reader to form a tolerably correct judgment respecting the disease; and from considering what would have probably been the effects of an equal number of cases of variolous inoculation, he may draw his own conclusions. But before this is done, I have to observe that, since the table was composed, an infant at the breast died on the eleventh day after the Cow Pox matter had been inserted in its arm. In this solitary fatal case, the local tumour was very inconsiderable, and the eruptive symptoms took place on the seventh day, when the child was attacked with fits of the spasmodic kind, which recurred at short intervals with increased violence, and carried it off at the time above mentioned, after an eruption of eighty or one hundred pustules.

It appears, therefore, that out of about five hundred cases of the inoculated Cow Pox, one proved fatal, and the preceding table shows that in some others the disease, from the number of the pustules, was of formidable severity; while, on the other hand, a very large proportion of the patients were scarcely disordered from the inoculation, and had no pustules.

Were I enabled to state a number of cases of variolous inoculation, equal to those given above, and reduced to a similar tabular form, the comparative magnitude of the two diseases might be estimated with tolerable precision. It is evident, however, that the matter of the vaccine disease has generally produced much fewer pustules, and less indisposition, than that of the Small Pox; for it appears from the preceding statement that about two-fifths of all the persons inoculated for the variolæ vaccinæ had no pustules, and that in not more than a fourth part of them was there experienced any perceptible disorder of the constitution. But it must be acknowledged, that in several instances, the Cow Pox has proved a very severe disease. In three or four cases, out of five hundred, the patient has been in considerable danger, and one child, as I have already observed, actually died under the effects of the disease. Now, if it be admitted that, at an average, one of five hundred will die of the inoculated Cow Pox, I confess I should not be disposed to introduce this disease into the Inoculation Hospital, because out of the last five thousand cases of variolous inoculation the number of deaths has not exceeded the proportion of one in six hundred. But I am inclined to think, that if the matter of the Cow Pox, used for the purpose of inoculation, were only taken from those in whom the disease appeared in a very mild form, the result would be more favourable than in the statement here given. For though it has occasionally happened that the matter taken from the arm of a patient, in whom the disorder neither produced fever nor eruption, has in others produced both; yet still it has much more commonly had the effect of exciting a milder disease than the matter of the pustules, or than that which was obtained from a patient who had the disease in a severe manner, as may be seen by an examination of the table.

Thus we find that out of sixty-two persons, who were inoculated with the pustule matter, fifty-seven had an eruption; and those who received the disease from any of these fifty-seven patients, appear also to have had pustules in nearly the same proportion. I may also remark that the disease, before noticed as proving fatal to a patient, was excited from matter of this description, and taken from Talbot. Whence it appears, that the Cow Pox, from certain circumstances, is not only liable to lose the characters which distinguish it from the Small Pox, but also to continue to propagate itself under this new and casual modification. The vaccine variolæ, the human variolæ, ought, therefore, to be considered as only varieties of the same disease, rather than as distinct species.

One important advantage which the Cow Pox is supposed to have over the Small Pox is that the former is not a contagious disease, and not to be propagated by the effluvia of persons infected with it. This is certainly true when the disorder is confined to the inoculated part, but where it produces numerous pustules upon the body the exhalations they send forth are capable of infecting others in the same manner as the Small Pox. Two instances of casual infection in this way have lately fallen under my observation; in one the disease was severe, and the eruption confluent; in the other the disease was mild, and the pustules few.

It has been asserted, that persons have had the Small Pox after having been affected with the Cow Pox; and some facts have been published with a view to show that instances of this kind have actually happened. But all these, as far as I have seen, have been very defective in not affording sufficient proof that the affection, supposed to have been the Cow Pox, was in reality that disease. On the other hand, the instances which have been brought forward to prove that those who had undergone the genuine Cow Pox resisted the infection of the Small Pox are unquestionably decisive, and sufficiently numerous to establish the fact in the most satisfactory manner. This circumstance then appears to be as much a general law of the system, as that a person having had the Small Pox is thereby rendered unsusceptible of receiving the disease a second time. For of all the patients whom I inoculated with variolous matter, after they had passed through the Cow Pox, amounting to upwards of four hundred, none were affected with the Small Pox; and it may be remarked, that nearly a fourth part of this number was so slightly affected with the Cow Pox, that it neither produced any perceptible indisposition nor pustules.

We have been told that the Cow Pox tumour has frequently produced erysipelatous inflammation and phagedenic ulceration; but the inoculated part has not ulcerated in any of the cases which have been under my care, nor have I observed inflammation to occasion any inconvenience, except in one instance, where it was soon subdued by the application of aqua lithargyri acetati. It should seem, then, that the advantages to be derived from substituting the Cow Pox for the Small Pox must be directly in proportion to the greater mildness of the former than the latter disease.

FURTHER

OBSERVATIONS

ON THE

VARIOLÆ VACCINÆ

OR

COW POX.

By EDWARD JENNER, M.D., F.R.S., F.L.S., &c.

London:

PRINTED, FOR THE AUTHOR,

By SAMPSON LOW, No. 7, BERWICK STREET, SOHO:

AND SOLD BY LAW, AVE MARIA LANE, AND MURRAY AND HIGHLEY, FLEET STREET.

1799.

TO

C. H. PARRY, M.D.,

AT BATH.

My Dear Friend,

THE same motives which impelled me to dedicate to you my first Essay on the Variolæ Vaccinæ, induce me to offer you my further Observations on the same subject.

I am pleased at seeing the investigation so generally entered into, and I hope that the spirit with which this important inquiry will be prosecuted, may be tempered with that calmness and moderation which should ever accompany philosophical researches.

With the greatest regard,

I remain

Yours, very sincerely,

EDWARD JENNER.

Berkeley, Gloucestershire,
5th April, 1799.

FURTHER

OBSERVATIONS,

&c., &c.

ALTHOUGH it has not been in my power to extend the Inquiry into the causes and effects of the Variolæ Vaccinæ much beyond its original limits, yet, perceiving that it is beginning to excite a general spirit of investigation, I think it of importance, without delay, to communicate such facts as have since occurred, and to point out the fallacious sources from whence a disease resembling the true Variolæ Vaccinæ might arise, with the view of preventing those who may inoculate from producing a spurious disease; and further, to enforce the precaution suggested in the former Treatise on the subject, of subduing the inoculated pustule as soon as it has sufficiently produced its influence on the constitution. From a want of due discrimination of the real existence of the disease either in the brute or in the human subject, and also of that stage of it in which it is capable of producing the change in the animal economy, which renders it unsusceptible of the contagion of the Small Pox, unpleasant consequences might ensue, the source of which, perhaps, might not be suspected by one inexperienced in conducting such experiments.

My late publication contains a relation of most of the facts which had come under my own inspection at the time it was written, interspersed with some conjectural observations. Since then Dr. G. Pearson has established an inquiry into the validity of my principal assertion, the result of which cannot but be highly flattering to my feelings. It contains not a single case which

vas so firmly
uman body
ome further
also bear
spectability
into
farmer
wing
was
table.
was

me
ts
ture-
te
re
e
ng
y

n
d
d
te

ate

ear to

of the

specific
putre-
ses
-tage,

ntact

—To
s of
but

tain it is, that these parts of the animal are subject to some riety of maladies of this nature; and as many of these eruptions robably all of them) are capable of giving a disease to the man body, would it not be discreet for those engaged in this vestigation to suspend controversy and cavil until they can certain with precision what *is* and what *is not* the genuine ow Pox?

For example.—A farmer who is not conversant with any of these maladies, but who may have heard of the Cow Pox in general terms, may acquaint a neighbouring surgeon that the distemper appears at his farm. The surgeon, eager to make an experiment, takes away matter, inoculates, produces a sore, uneasiness in the axilla, and perhaps some affection of the system. This is a way in which a fallacious idea of security both in the mind of the inoculator and the patient may arise; for a disease may thus have been propagated from a simple eruption only.

One of the first objects then of this pursuit, as I have observed, should be, to learn how to distinguish with accuracy between that peculiar pustule which is the *true* Cow Pox, and that which is *spurious*. Until experience has determined this, we view our object through a mist. Let us for instance suppose, that the Small Pox and the Chicken Pox were at the same time to spread among the inhabitants of a country which had never been visited by either of these distempers, and where they were quite unknown before; what confusion would arise! The resemblance between the symptoms of the eruptive fever and between the pustules in either case would be so striking, that a patient, who had gone through the Chicken Pox to any extent, would feel equally easy with regard to his future security from the Small Pox, as the person who had actually passed through that disease. Time and future observation would draw the line of distinction.

So I presume it will be with the Cow Pox, until it is more generally understood. All cavilling therefore on the mere report of those who *tell us* they have had this distemper, and are afterwards found to be susceptible of the Small Pox, should be suspended. To illustrate this, I beg leave to give the following history:

SARAH MERLIN, of the parish of Eastington in this county, when about thirteen or fourteen years of age, lived as a servant with Farmer Clarke, who kept a dairy, consisting of about eighteen cows, at Stonehouse, a neighbouring village. The nipples and udders of three of the cows were extensively affected [illegible] the girl milked daily, and [illegible] two others, in milking the rest [illegible] the disease was communicated [illegible] escaped the infection, although [illegible] the three above specified had [illegible] udders, and even after the [illegible] others who were engaged in [illegible] indiscriminately, received [illegible] of the girl's hands there [illegible] she supposes about three or [illegible] arms inflamed and swelled, [illegible] followed. The sores were [illegible] and got well without

[illegible] Pox, and recorded as such [illegible] regardless of the Small Pox; [illegible] afterwards, she was infected,

[illegible] the habits of the disease [illegible] no hesitation in pronounc- [illegible] considering its deviation in the [illegible] girl's hands; their termin- [illegible] more generally contagious [illegible] those employed in milking; [illegible] *no general indisposition,* [illegible]

[illegible] form in which an eruptive [illegible] the cow, and it certainly [illegible] nating it. The most perfect [illegible] may be guided, is perhaps that [illegible] cattle. These white blisters [illegible] *the fleshy parts* like those [illegible] and which constitute the [illegible] skin only, quickly end in [illegible]

[illegible] cause of spurious eruptions, I [illegible] treatise, namely, the transi- [illegible] from a poor to a nutritious [illegible] this time more vascular than [illegible] there is another source of [illegible] is not uncommon in all [illegible] A cow intended to be [illegible] udder, is previously for a day or two neither milked artificially, nor is her calf suffered to have access to her. Thus the milk is preternaturally accumulated, and the udder and nipples become greatly distended. The consequences frequently are, inflammation and eruptions, which maturate.

Whether a disease generated in this way has the power of affecting the constitution in any *peculiar* manner, I cannot presume positively to determine. It has been conjectured to have been a cause of the true Cow Pox, though my inquiries have not led me to adopt this supposition in any one instance; on the contrary, I have known the milkers affected by it, but always found that an affection thus induced left the system as susceptible of the Small Pox as before.

What is advanced in my second position, I consider also of very great importance, and I could wish it to be strongly impressed on the minds of all who may be disposed to conclude hastily on my observations, whether engaged in their investigation by experiments or not.—To place this in its clearest point of view (as the similarity between the action of the Small Pox and the Cow Pox matter is so obvious) it will be necessary to consider what we sometimes observe to take place in inoculation for the Small Pox when imperfect variolous matter is made use of. The concise history on this subject that was brought forward respecting what I had observed in this neighbourhood,* I perceive by a reference since made to the *Memoirs of the Medical Society of London*, may be considered as no more than a corroboration of the facts very clearly detailed by Mr. Kite.† To this copious evidence I have to add still more in the following communications from Mr. Earle, surgeon, of Frampton-upon-Severn, in this county, which I deem the more valuable, as he has with much candour permitted me to make them public.

"Sir,

"I have read with satisfaction your late publication on the Variolæ Vaccinæ, and being, among many other curious circumstances, particularly struck with that relating to the inefficacy of Small Pox matter in a particular state, I think it proper to lay before you the following facts which came within my own knowledge, and which certainly tend to strengthen the opinions advanced in page 26 of your Treatise.

* *Inquiry into the Causes and Effects of the Variolæ Vaccinæ*, page 51.

† See an account of some anomalous appearances consequent to the inoculation of the Small Pox, by Charles Kite, Surgeon, of Gravesend, in the *Memoirs of the Medical Society of London*. Vol. iv. page 114.

"In March, 1784, a general inoculation took place at Arlingham in this county. I inoculated several patients with active variolous matter, all of whom had the disease in a favourable way; but my matter being all used, and not being able to procure any more in the state I wished, I was under the necessity of taking it from a pustule which, experience has since proved, was advanced too far to answer the purpose I intended. Of five persons inoculated with this last matter, four took the Small Pox afterwards in the natural way; one of whom died, three recovered, and the other, being cautioned by me to avoid as much as possible the chance of catching it, escaped from the disease through life. He died of another disorder about two years ago.

"Although one of these cases ended unfortunate, yet I cannot suppose that any medical man will think me careless or inattentive in their management; for I conceive the appearances were such as might have induced any one to suppose that the persons were perfectly safe from future infection. Inflammation in every case took place in the arm, and fever came on with a considerable degree of pain in the axilla. In some of their arms the inflammation and suppuration were more violent than is commonly observed when perfect matter is made use of; in one there was an ulcer which cast off several large sloughs. About the ninth day eruptions appeared, which died away earlier than common without maturation.—From these circumstances I should suppose that no medical practitioner would scarcely have entertained a doubt but that these patients had been infected with a true Small Pox; yet I must confess that some small degree of doubt presented itself to me at the speedy disappearance of the eruptions; and in order, as far as I could, to ascertain their safety, I sent one of them to a much older practitioner than myself. This gentleman, on hearing the circumstances of the case, pronounced the patient perfectly secure from future infection.

"The following facts are also a striking proof of the truth of your observations on this subject:

"In the year 1789 I inoculated three children of Mr. Coaley, of Hurst-farm in this county. The arms inflamed properly, fever and pain in the axilla came on precisely the same as in the former cases, and in ten days eruptions appeared, which disappeared in the course of two days. I must observe that the matter here made use of was procured for me by a friend: but no doubt it was in an improper state; for, from the similarity of these cases to those which happened at Arlingham five years before, I was somewhat alarmed for their safety, and desired to inoculate them again; which being permittéd, I was particularly careful to procure matter in its most perfect state. All the children took the Small Pox from this second inoculation, and all had a very full burthen. These facts I conceive strikingly corroborate your opinion relative to the different states of matter; for in both the instances that I have mentioned it was capable of producing something strongly resembling the true Small Pox, although it afterwards proved not to be so.

"As I think the communication of these Cases is a duty I owe to the Public, you are at liberty to make what use you please of this letter.

"I remain, etc.,

"JOHN EARLE.

"Frampton-upon-Severn, Gloucestershire,
"November 10, 1798.

"P.S.—I think it necessary to observe, that I can pronounce with the greatest certainty, that the matter with which the Arlingham patients were inoculated was taken from a true Small Pox pustule. I took it myself from a subject that had a very full burthen."

Certain then it is that variolous matter may undergo such a change from the putrefactive process, as well as from some of the more obscure and latent processes of nature, as will render it incapable of giving the Small Pox in such a manner as to secure the human constitution from future infection, although we see at the same time it is capable of exciting a disease which bears so strong a resemblance to it, as to produce inflammation and matter in the incised skin (frequently indeed more violent than when it produces its effects perfectly), swelling of the axillary glands, general indisposition, and eruptions. So strongly persuaded was the gentleman, whose practice I have mentioned in page 28 of the late Treatise, that he could produce a mild Small Pox by his mode of managing the matter, that he spoke of it as a useful discovery, until convinced of his error by the fatal consequence which ensued.

After this ought we to be in the smallest degree surprised to find, among a great number of individuals who, by living in dairies, have been casually exposed to the Cow Pox virus when in a state analogous to that of the Small Pox above described, some who may have had the disease so imperfectly, as not to render them secure from variolous attacks? For the matter, when burst from the pustules on the nipples of the Cow, by being exposed, from its lodgment there, to the heat of an inflamed surface, and from being, at the same time, in a situation to be occasionally moistened with milk, is often likely to be in a state conducive to putrefaction; and thus, under some modification of decomposition, it must of course sometimes find access to the hand of the milker in such a way as to infect him. What confusion should we have, were there no other mode of inoculating the Small Pox than such as would happen from handling the diseased skin of a person labouring under that distemper in some of its advanced and loathsome stages! It must be observed, that every case of Cow Pox in the human species, whether communicated by design or otherwise, is to be considered as a case of inoculation. And here I may be allowed to make an observation on the case of the farmer, communicated to me by Dr. Ingenhousz. That he was exposed to the matter when it had undergone the putrefactive change, is highly probable from the Doctor's observing that the sick cows at the farm gave out an *offensive stench from their udders.* However, I must remark, that it is unusual for cattle to suffer to such an extent, when disordered with the Cow Pox, as to make a by-stander sensible of any ill smell. I have often stood among a herd which had the distemper without being conscious of its presence from any particular effluvia. Indeed, in this neighbourhood it commonly receives an early check from escharotic applications of the *cow leech*. It has been conceived to be contagious among cows without contact; but this idea cannot be well founded, because the cattle in one meadow do not infect those in another (although there may be no other partition than a hedge) unless they be handled or milked by those who bring the infectious matter with them; and of course the smallest particle imaginable, when applied to a part susceptible of its influence, may produce the effect. Among the human species it appears to be very clear, that the disease is produced by contact only. All my attempts, at least, to communicate it by effluvia have hitherto proved ineffectual.

As well as the perfect change from that state in which variolous matter is capable of producing full and decisive effects on the constitution, to that wherein its specific properties are entirely lost, it may reasonably be supposed that it is capable of undergoing a variety of intermediate changes. The following singular occurrences in cases of Inoculation, obligingly communicated to me by Mr. Freer, Surgeon to the Infirmary at Gloucester, seem to indicate that the variolous matter previously to its being taken from the patient for the intended purpose was beginning to part with some of its original properties; or, in other words, that it had suffered a partial decomposition. Mr. Trye says, "I inoculated ten children with matter taken at one time, and from the same subject. I observed no peculiarity in any of them previously to their inoculation, nor did anything remarkable appear in their arms till after the decline of the disease. Two infants of three months old had erysipelas about the incisions, in one of them extending from the shoulders to the fingers' ends. Another infant had abscesses in the cellular substance in the neighbourhood of the incisions, and five or six of the rest had axillary abscesses. The matter was taken from the distinct Small Pox late in its progress, and when some pustules had been dried. It was received upon glass, and slowly dried by the fire. All the children had pustules which maturated, so that I suppose them all secure from future infection; at least, as secure as any others whom I have ever inoculated. My practice never afforded a sore arm before."

In regard to my former observation on the improper and dangerous mode of preserving variolous matter, I shall here remark, that it seems not to have been clearly understood. Finding that it has been confounded with the more eligible modes of preservation, I will explain myself further. When the matter is taken from a fit pustule, and properly prepared for preservation, it may certainly be kept without losing its specific properties a great length of time; for instance, when it is previously dried in the open air on some compact body, as a quill or a piece of glass, and afterwards secured in a small vial.* But when kept several days in a state of moisture, and during that time exposed to a warm temperature, I do not think it can be relied upon as capable of giving a *perfect disease*, although, as I have before observed, the progress of the symptoms arising from the action of the imperfect matter bears so strong a resemblance to the Small Pox when excited completely.

3dly. That the first formed virus, or what constitutes the true Cow-Pock pustule, invariably possesses the power I have ascribed to it, namely, that of affecting the constitution with a specific disease, is a truth that no subsequent occurrence has yet led me to doubt. But as I am now endeavouring to guard the public as much as possible against erroneous conclusions, I shall observe, that when this pustule has degenerated into an ulcer (to which state it is sometimes disposed to pass, unless timely checked) I

* Thus prepared, the Cow Pox virus was found perfectly active, and possessing all its specific properties, at the end of three months.

[illegible]

... ... of the farmer ... was ... the ... at the farm ... their udders. ... however ... must ... an extent ... sensible ... which ... from any part ... commonly ... of the cow ... cows without ... because the cattle ... though there may ... be handled or ... them ; and ... applied to a part ... Among the huma[n] ... the disease ... produce ... at least, to communicate ... contagious.

... well as the perfect ... matter is capable of pro[ducing] ... constitution, to that whe[n] ... lost it may reasonably ... going a variety of interna[l] ... occurrences ... cases ... me by ... seem to indicate that the ... taken from the patient ... to part with some of ...

[illegible]

... matter ... small ... mitted ... produce a disease ... generally, yet ... obtaining the ... of Mary Miller ... to, it appears ... culated arm were ... underwent ... which appears ... with the natural Small ... Some of the ... confirm this ... on the inoculated part

... cutaneous disease ... veyed to the animal ... which, though ... shall digress ... give my reasons ... has appeared ... though not amounting ... of so forcible a kind ... person have made the ... the imputation of

... from observing that ... the dairies here (unless ... infected cow or servant) ... diseased in the manner ... attended by some of the

... throughout this ... insisted on by those who

Thirdly. From the total absence of the disease in those countries, where the men servants are not employed in the dairies.*

Fourthly. From having observed that morbid matter generated by the horse frequently communicates, in a casual way, a disease to the human subject so like the Cow Pox, that in many cases it would be difficult to make the distinction between one and the other.†

Fifthly. From being induced to suppose, from experiments, that some of those who had been thus affected from the horse resisted the Small Pox.

Sixthly. From the progress and general appearance of the pustule on the arm of the boy whom I inoculated with matter taken from the hand of a man infected by a horse; and from the similarity to the Cow Pox of the general constitutional symptoms which followed.‡

I fear it would be trespassing too far to adduce the general testimony of our farmers in support of this opinion; yet I beg leave to introduce an extract of a letter on this subject from the Rev. Mr. Moore, of Chalford Hill, in this county.

"In the month of November, 1797, my horse had diseased heels, which was certainly what is termed the grease; and at a short subsequent period my cow was also affected with what a neighbouring farmer (who was conversant with the complaints of cattle) pronounced to be the Cow Pox, which he at the same time observed my servant would be infected with: and this proved to be the case; for he had eruptions on his hands, face, and many parts of the body, the pustules appearing large, and not much unlike the Small Pox, for which he had been inoculated a year and a half before, and had then a very heavy burthen. The pustules on the face might arise from contact with his hands, as he had a habit of rubbing his forehead, where the sores were the largest and thickest.

---

* This information was communicated to me from the first authorities.

† The sound skin does not appear to be susceptible of this virus when inserted into it, but, when previously diseased from little accidents, its effects are often conspicuous. See Plate No. 2.

‡ This Case (on which I laid no inconsiderable stress in my late Treatise, as presumptive evidence of the fact adduced) seems to have been either mistaken or overlooked by those who have commented upon this subject.—See Case xviii., page 21. The boy unfortunately died of a fever at a parish workhouse before I had an opportunity of observing what effects would have been produced by the matter of Small Pox. The experiments published by Mr. Simmons of Manchester, and others, on the subject, with the view of refuting this Theory, appear to have but little weight, as even the Cow Pock virus itself, when repeatedly introduced into the sound nipples of cows by means of a lancet, was found to produce no effect.

"The boy associated with the farmer's sons during the continuance of the disease, neither of whom had had the Small Pox, but they felt no ill effects whatever. He was not much indisposed, as the disease did not prevent him from following his occupations as usual. No other person attended the horse or milked the cow, but the lad above mentioned. I am firmly of opinion that the disease in the heels of the horse, which was a virulent grease, was the origin of the servant's and the cow's malady."

But to return to the more immediate object of this proposition.

From the similarity of symptoms, both constitutional and local, between the Cow Pox and the disease received from morbid matter generated by a horse, the common people in this neighbourhood, when infected with this disease, through a strange perversion of terms, frequently called it the Cow Pox. Let us suppose then such a malady to appear among some of the servants at a farm, and at the same time that the Cow Pox were to break out among the cattle; and let us suppose too that some of the servants were infected in this way, and that others received the infection from the cows. It would be recorded at the farm, and among the servants themselves, wherever they might afterwards be dispersed, that they had all had the Cow Pox. But it is clear that an individual thus infected from the horse would neither be for a certainty secure himself, nor would he impart security to others, were they inoculated by virus thus generated. He still would be in danger of taking the Small Pox. Yet were this to happen before the nature of the Cow Pox be more maturely considered by the public, my evidence on the subject might be depreciated unjustly. For an exemplification of what is here advanced relative to the nature of the infection when received directly from the horse, see *Inquiry into the Causes and Effects of the Variolæ Vaccinæ*, pages 17, 18, and page 21; and by way of further example, I beg leave to subjoin the following intelligence received from Mr. Fewster, Surgeon, of Thornbury, in this county, a gentleman perfectly well acquainted with the appearances of the Cow Pox on the human subject.

"WILLIAM MORRIS, aged thirty-two, servant to Mr. Cox of Almonsbury, in this county, applied to me the 2nd of April, 1798. He told me, that four days before he found a stiffness and swelling in both his hands, which were so painful, it was with difficulty he continued his work; that he had been seized with pain in his head, small of the back, and limbs, and with frequent chilly fits succeeded by fever. On examination I found him still affected with these symptoms, and that there was a great prostration of strength. Many parts of his hands on the inside were chapped, and on the middle joint of the thumb of the right hand there was a small phagedenic ulcer, about the size of a large pea, discharging an ichorous fluid. On the middle finger of the same hand there was another ulcer of a similar kind. These sores were of a *circular* form, and he described their first appearance as being somewhat like blisters arising from a burn. He complained of excessive pain, which extended up his arm into the axilla. These symptoms and appearances of the sores were so exactly like the Cow Pox, that I pronounced he had taken the distemper from milking cows. He assured me he had not milked a cow for more than half a year, and that his master's cows had nothing the matter with them. I then asked him if his master had a *greasy* horse? which he answered in the affirmative; and further said, that he had constantly dressed him twice a day for the last three weeks or more, and remarked that the smell of his hands was much like that of the horse's heels. On the 5th of April I again saw him, and found him still complaining of pain in both his hands, nor were his febrile symptoms at all relieved. The ulcers had now spread to the size of a seven-shilling gold coin, and another ulcer, which I had not noticed before, appeared on the first joint of the forefinger of the left hand, equally painful with that on the right. I ordered him to bathe his hands in warm bran and water, applied escharotics to the ulcers, and wrapped his hands up in a soft cataplasm. The next day he was much relieved, and in something more than a fortnight got well. He lost his nails from the thumb and fingers that were ulcerated."

The sudden disappearance of the symptoms in this case, after the application of the escharotics to the sores, is worthy of observation; it seems to shew that they were kept up by the irritation of the ulcers.

The general symptoms which I have already described of the Cow Pox, when communicated in a casual way to any great extent, will, I am convinced, from the many Cases I have seen, be found accurate; but from the very slight indisposition which ensues in cases of inoculation, where the pustule, after affecting the constitution, quickly runs into a scab spontaneously, or is artificially suppressed by some proper application, I am induced to believe that the violence of the symptoms may be ascribed to the inflammation and irritation of the ulcers (when ulceration takes place to any extent, as in the casual Cow Pox), and that the constitutional symptoms which appear during the presence of the sore, while it assumes the character of a pustule only, are felt but in a very trifling degree. This mild affection of the system happens when the disease makes but a slight local impression on those who have been accidentally infected by cows; and, as far as I have seen, it has uniformly happened among those who have been inoculated, when a pustule only, and no great degree of inflammation or any ulceration, has taken place from the inoculation. The following cases will strengthen this opinion:

The Cow Pox appeared at a farm in the village of Stonehouse, in this county, about Michaelmas last, and continued gradually to pass from one cow to another till the end of November. On the 26th of that month some ichorous matter was taken from a cow, and dried upon a quill. On the 2nd of December some of it was inserted into a scratch, made so superficial that no blood appeared, on the arm of Susan Phipps, a child seven years old. The common inflammatory appearances took place in consequence, and advanced till the fifth day, when they had so much subsided, that I did not conceive anything further would ensue.

6th. Appearances stationary.

7th. The inflammation began to advance.

8th. A vesication perceptible on the edges, forming, as in the inoculated Small Pox, an appearance not unlike a grain of wheat, with the cleft or indention in the centre.

9th. Pain in the axilla.

10th. A little headache; pulse 110; tongue not discoloured; countenance in health.

11th—12th. No perceptible illness; pulse about 100.

13th. The pustule was now surrounded by an efflorescence, interspersed with very minute confluent pustules, to the extent of about an inch. Some of these pustules advanced in size and maturated. So exact was the resemblance of the arm at this stage to the general appearance of the inoculated Small Pox, that Mr. D., a neighbouring surgeon, who took some matter from it, and who had never seen the Cow Pox before, declared he could not perceive any difference.* The child's arm now showed a disposition to scab, and remained nearly stationary for two or three days, when it began to run into an ulcerous state; and *then*

* That the Cow Pox was a supposed guardian of the constitution from the action of the Small Pox, has been a prevalent idea for a long time past; but the similarity in the constitutional effects between one disease and the other could never have been so accurately observed, had not the inoculation of the Cow Pox placed it in a new and stronger point of view. This practice too has shown us what before lay concealed, the rise and progress of the pustule formed by the insertion of the virus, which places in a most conspicuous light its striking resemblance to the pustule formed from the inoculated Small Pox.

commenced a febrile indisposition, accompanied with an increase of axillary tumour. The ulcer continued spreading near a week, during which time the child continued ill, when it increased to a size nearly as large as a shilling. It began now to discharge pus; granulations sprung up, and it healed. This child had before been of a remarkably sickly constitution, but is now in very high health.

MARY HEARN, twelve years of age, was inoculated with matter taken from the arm of Susan Phipps.

6th day. A pustule beginning to appear, slight pain in the axilla.

7th. A distinct vesicle formed.

8th. The vesicle increasing; edges very red; no deviation in its appearance at this time from the inoculated Small Pox.

9th. No indisposition; pustule advancing.

10th. The patient felt this evening a slight febrile attack.

11th. Free from indisposition.

12th—13th. The same.

14th. An efflorescence of a faint red colour, extending several inches round the arm. The pustule beginning to shew a disposition to spread, was dressed with an ointment composed of *hydrarg. nit. rub.* and *ung. ceræ.* The efflorescence itself was covered with a plaster of *ung. hydr. fort.*—In six hours it was examined, when it was found that the efflorescence had totally disappeared. The application of the ointment with the *hydr. nit. rub.* was made use of for three days, when the state of the pustule remaining stationary, it was exchanged for the *ung. hydr. nit.* This appeared to have a more active effect than the former, and in two or three days the virus seemed to be subdued, when a simple dressing was made use of; but the sore again shewing a disposition to inflame, the *ung. hydr. nit.* was again applied, and soon answered the intended purpose effectually. The girl after the tenth day, when, as has been observed, she became a little ill, shewed not the least symptom of indisposition. She was afterwards exposed to the action of variolous matter, and completely resisted it. Susan Phipps also went through a similar trial. Conceiving these cases to be important, I have given them in detail; first, to urge the precaution of using such means as may stop the progress of the pustule; and secondly, to point out (what appears to be the fact) that the most material indisposition, or at least that which is felt most sensibly, *does not arise primarily from the first action of the virus on the constitution, but that it often comes on, if the pustule is left to chance, as a secondary disease.* This leads me to conjecture, what experiment must finally determine, that they who have had the Small Pox are not afterwards susceptible of the primary action of the Cow Pox virus; for seeing that the simple virus itself, when it has not passed beyond the boundary of a vesicle, excites in the system so little commotion, is it not probable the trifling illness thus induced may be lost in that which so quickly, and oftentimes so severely, follows in the *casual Cow Pox* from the presence of corroding ulcers? This consideration induces me to suppose that I may have been mistaken in my former observation on this subject.

In this respect, as well as many others, a parallel may be drawn between this disease and the Small Pox. In the latter, the patient first feels the effect of what is called the absorption of the virus. The symptoms then often nearly retire, when a fresh attack commences different from the first, and the illness keeps pace with the progress of the pustules through their different stages of maturation, ulceration, etc.

Although the application I have mentioned in the case of Mary Hearn proved sufficient to check the progress of ulceration, and prevent any secondary symptoms, yet, after the pustule has duly exerted its influence, I should prefer the destroying it quickly and effectually to any other mode. The term caustic to a tender ear (and I conceive none will feel more interested in this Inquiry than the anxious guardians of a nursery) may sound harsh and unpleasing, but every solicitude that may arise on this account will no longer exist, when it is understood that the pustule in a state fit to be acted upon is then quite superficial, and that it does not occupy the space of a silver penny.*

As a proof of the efficacy of this practice, even before the virus had fully exerted itself on the system, I shall lay before my reader the following history.

By a reference to the Treatise on the Variolæ Vaccinæ, it will be seen that, in the month of April 1798, four children were inoculated with the matter of Cow Pox; and that in two of these cases the virus on the arm was destroyed soon after it had produced a perceptible sickening. Mary James, aged seven years, one of the children alluded to, was inoculated in the month of December following with fresh variolous matter, and at the same time was exposed to the effluvia of a patient affected with

* I mention escharotics for stopping the progress of the pustule, because I am acquainted with their efficacy; probably more simple means might answer the purpose quite as well, such as might be found among the mineral and vegetable astringents.

the Small Pox. The appearance and progress of the infected arm was, in every respect, similar to that which we generally observe when variolous matter has been inserted into the skin of a person who has not previously undergone either the Cow Pox or the Small Pox. On the eighth day, conceiving there was infection in it, she was removed from her residence among those who had not had the Small Pox. I was now anxiously waiting the result, conceiving from the state of the girl's arm she would fall sick about this time. On visiting her on the evening of the following day (the ninth), all I could learn from the woman who attended her was, that she felt somewhat hotter than usual during the night, but was not restless; and that in the morning there was the faint appearance of a rash about her wrists. This went off in a few hours, and was not at all perceptible to me on my visit in the evening. Not a single eruption appeared, the skin having been repeatedly and carefully examined. The inoculated arm continued to make the usual progress to the end, through all the stages of inflammation, maturation, and scabbing.

On the eighth day matter was taken from the arm of this girl, (Mary James), and inserted into the arms of her mother and brother, (neither of whom had had either the Small Pox or the Cow Pox,) the former about fifty years of age, the latter six.

On the eighth day after the insertion, the boy felt indisposed, and continued unwell two days, when a measles-like rash appeared on his hands and wrists, ana was thinly scattered over his arms. The day following his body was marbled over with an appearance somewhat similar, but he did not complain, nor did he appear indisposed. A few pustules now appeared, the greater part of which went away without maturating.

On the ninth day the mother began to complain. She was a little chilly, and had a head-ache for two days, but *no pustule appeared on the skin*, nor had she any appearance of a rash.

The family was attended by an elderly woman as a nurse, who in her infancy had been exposed to the contagion of the Small Pox, but had resisted it. This woman was now infected, but had the disease in the slightest manner, a very few eruptions appearing, two or three of which only maturated.

From a solitary instance like that adduced of Mary James, whose constitution appears to have resisted the action of the variolous virus, after the influence of the Cow Pox virus had been so soon arrested in its progress, no positive conclusion can be fairly drawn; nor from the history of the three other patients who were subsequently infected; but nevertheless the facts collectively may be deemed interesting.

That one mild variety of the Small Pox has appeared, I have already plainly shown;* and by the means now mentioned we probably may have it in our power to produce at will another.

At the time when the pustule was destroyed in the arm of Mary James, I was informed she had been indisposed about twelve hours; but I am now assured, by those who were with her, that the space of time was much less. Be that as it may, in Cases of Cow Pox inoculation, I would not recommend any application to subdue the action of the pustule, until convincing proofs had appeared of the patient's having felt its effects at least twelve hours. No harm indeed could ensue, were a longer period to elapse before the application was made use of. In short, it should be suffered to have as full an effect as it could, consistently with the state of the arm.

As the cases of inoculation multiply, I am more and more convinced of the extreme mildness of the symptoms arising merely from the primary action of the virus on the constitution, and that those symptoms, which (as in the accidental Cow Pox) affect the patient with severity, are entirely secondary, excited by the irritating processes of inflammation and ulceration; and it appears to me that this singular virus possesses an irritating quality of a peculiar kind; but as a single Cow Pox pustule is all that is necessary to render the variolous virus ineffectual, and as we possess the means of allaying the irritation, should any arise, it becomes of little or no consequence.

It appears then (as far as an inference can be drawn from the present progress of Cow Pox inoculation) that it is an accidental circumstance only, which can render this a violent disease, and a circumstance of that nature, which fortunately it is in the power of almost every one to avoid. I allude to the communication of the disease from cows. In this case, should the hands of the milker be affected with little accidental sores to any extent, every sore would become the *nidus* of infection, and feel the influence of the virus; and the degree of violence in the constitutional symptoms would be in proportion to the number and to the state of these local affections. Hence it follows that a person, either by accident or design, might be so filled with these wounds from contact with the virus, that the constitution might sink under the pressure.

* See *Inquiry into the Causes and Effects of the Variolæ Vaccinæ*, page 27.

Seeing that we possess the means of rendering the action of the sores mild, which, when left to chance, are capable of producing violent effects; and seeing too that these sores bear a resemblance to the Small Pox, especially the confluent, should it not encourage the hope that some topical application might be used with advantage to counteract the fatal tendency of that disease, when it appears in this terrific form? At what stage or stages of the disease this may be done with the most promising expectation of success, I will not pretend now to determine. I only throw out this idea as the basis of further reasoning and experiment.

I have often been foiled in my endeavours to communicate the Cow Pox by inoculation. An inflammation will sometimes succeed the scratch or puncture, and in a few days disappear without producing any further effect. Sometimes it will even produce an ichorous fluid, and yet the system will not be affected.* The same thing we know happens with the Small Pox virus.

Four or five servants were inoculated at a farm contiguous to this place, last summer, with matter just taken from an infected cow. A little inflammation appeared on all their arms, but died away without producing a pustule; yet all these servants caught the disease within a month afterwards from milking the infected cows, and some of them had it severely. At present, no other mode than that commonly practised for inoculating the Small Pox has been used for giving the Cow Pox; but it is probable this might be varied with advantage. We should imitate the casual communication more clearly, were we first, by making the smallest superficial incision or puncture on the skin, to produce a little scab, and then, removing it, to touch the abraded part with the virus. A small portion of a thread imbrued in the virus (as in the old method of inoculating the Small Pox), and laid upon the slightly incised skin, might probably prove a successful way of giving the disease; or the cutis might be exposed in a minute point by an atom of blistering plaster, and the virus brought in contact with it. In the Cases just alluded to, where I did not succeed in giving the disease constitutionally, the experiment was made with matter taken in a purulent state from a pustule on the nipple of a cow.†

Is *pure pus*, though contained in a Small Pox pustule, ever

* At this period of the Inquiry, I had not discovered the importance of inoculating with virus newly formed in the pustule. The Reader will find this explained as he proceeds.

† The cause of these disappointments will be explained.

capable of producing the Small Pox perfectly? I suspect it is not.—Let us consider that it is always preceded by the limpid fluid, which, in constitutions susceptible of variolous contagion, is always infectious; and though, on opening a pustule, its contents may appear perfectly purulent, yet a given quantity of the limpid fluid may at the same time be blended with it, though it would be imperceptible to the only test of our senses, the eye. The presence then of this fluid, or its mechanical diffusion through pus, may at all times render active what is apparently *mere pus*, while its total absence (as in stale pustules) may be attended with the imperfect effects we have seen.

It would be digressing too widely to go far into the doctrine of secretion, but as it will not be quite extraneous, I shall just observe, that I consider both the pus and the limpid fluid of the pustule as secretions, but that the organs established by nature to perform the office of secreting these fluids may differ essentially in their mechanical structure. What but a difference in the organization of glandular bodies, constitutes the difference in the qualities of the fluids secreted? From some peculiar derangement in the structure, or, in other words, some deviation in the natural action of a gland destined to secrete a mild, innoxious fluid, a poison of the most deadly nature may be created: for example—That gland, which in its sound state secretes pure saliva, may, from being thrown into diseased action, produce a poison of the most destructive quality. Nature appears to have no more difficulty in forming minute glands among the vascular parts of the body, than she has in forming blood vessels, and millions of these can be called into existence, when inflammation is excited, in a few hours.*

In the present early stage of the Inquiry (for early it certainly must be deemed), before we know for an absolute certainty how soon the virus of the Cow Pox may suffer a change in its specific properties, after it has quitted the limpid state it possessed when forming a pustule, it would be prudent for those who have been inoculated with it to submit to variolous inoculation. No injury or inconvenience can accrue from this; and were the same method practised among those who, from inoculation, have felt the Small Pox in an unsatisfactory manner at any period of their lives, it might appear that I had not been too officious in offering a cautionary hint, in recommending a second inoculation with matter in its most perfect state.

* Mr. Home, in his excellent dissertation on pus and mucus, justifies this assertion.

And here let me suppose, for argument's sake (not from conviction), that one person in an hundred, after having had the Cow Pox, should be found susceptible of the Small Pox, would this invalidate the utility of the practice? For, waiving all other considerations, who will deny that the inoculated Small Pox, though abstractedly it may be considered as harmless, does not involve in itself something that in numberless instances proves baneful to the human frame?

That in delicate constitutions it sometimes excites scrophula, is a fact that must generally be subscribed to, as it is so obvious to common conversation. This consideration is important.

As the effects of the Small Pox inoculation on those who have had the Cow Pox, will be watched with the most scrupulous eye by those who prosecute this Inquiry, it may be proper to bring to their recollection some facts relative to the Small Pox, which I must consider here as of consequence, but which hitherto seem not to have made a due impression.

It should be remembered that the constitution cannot by previous infection be rendered totally unsusceptible of the variolous poison; neither the casual nor the inoculated Small Pox, whether it produces the disease in a mild or in a violent way, can perfectly extinguish the susceptibility. The skin, we know, is ever ready to exhibit, though often in a very limited degree, the effects of the poison when inserted there; and how frequently do we see among nurses, when much exposed to the contagion, eruptions, and these sometimes preceded by sensible illness! yet should any thing like an eruption appear, or the smallest degree of indisposition, upon the insertion of the variolous matter on those who have gone through the Cow Pox, my assertions respecting the peculiarities of the disease might be unjustly discredited.

I know a gentleman, who many years ago was inoculated for the Small Pox, but having no pustules, or scarcely any constitutional affection that was perceptible, he was dissatisfied, and has since been repeatedly inoculated. A vesicle has always been produced in the arm in consequence, with axillary swelling and a slight indisposition: this is by no means a rare occurrence. It is probable that the fluid thus excited upon the skin would always produce the Small Pox.

On the arm of a person who had gone through the Cow Pox, many years before, I once produced a vesication by the insertion of variolous matter, and with a little of the fluid inoculated a young woman, who had a mild, but very efficacious, Small Pox in consequence, although no constitutional effect was produced on the patient from whom the matter was taken. The following communication from Mr. Fewster affords a still clearer elucidation of this fact.—Mr. Fewster says, "On the 3rd of April, 1797, I inoculated Master H——, aged fourteen months, for the Small Pox. At the usual time he sickened, had a plentiful eruption, particularly on his face, and got well. His nursemaid, aged twenty-four, had many years before gone through the Small Pox in the natural way, which was evident from her being much pitted with it. She had used the child to sleep on her left arm, with her left cheek in contact with his face, and during his inoculation he had mostly slept in that manner. About a week after the child got well, she (the nurse) desired me to look at her face, which she said was very painful. There was a plentiful eruption on the left cheek; *but not on any other part of the body*, which went on to maturation.

"On inquiry I found, that three days before the appearance of the eruption, she was taken with slight chilly fits, pain in her head and limbs, and some fever. On the appearance of the eruption these pains went off, and now (the second day of the eruption) she complains of a little sore throat. Whether the above symptoms are the effects of the Small Pox or a recent cold, I do not know. On the fifth day of the eruption I charged a lancet from two of the pustules, and on the next day I inoculated two children, one two years, the other four months old, with the matter. At the same time I inoculated the mother and eldest sister with variolous matter taken from Master H——. On the fifth day of their inoculation, *all* their arms were inflamed alike; and on the eighth day, the eldest of those inoculated from the nurse sickened, and the youngest on the eleventh. They had both a plentiful eruption, from which I inoculated several others, who had the disease very favourably. The mother and the other child sickened about the same time, and likewise had a plentiful eruption.

"Soon after a man in the village sickened with the Small Pox, and had a confluent kind. To be convinced that the children had had the disease effectually, I took them to his house and inoculated them in both arms with matter taken from him, but without effect."

These are not brought forward as uncommon occurrences, but as exemplifications of the human system's susceptibility of the variolous contagion, although it has been previously sensible of its action.

Happy is it for mankind that the appearance of the Small Pox a second time on the same person, beyond a trivial extent, is so extremely rare, that it is looked upon as a phenomenon. Indeed, since the publication of Dr. Heberden's paper on the *Varicellæ*, or Chicken Pox, the idea of such an occurrence, in deference to authority so truly respectable, has been generally relinquished. This I conceive has been without just reason ; for after we have seen, among many others, so strong a Case as that recorded by Mr. Edward Withers, Surgeon, of Newbury, Berks, in the Fourth Volume of the *Memoirs of the Medical Society of London* (from which I take the following Extracts), no one I think will again doubt the fact.

"Mr. RICHARD LANGFORD, a farmer of West Shefford, in this county, (Berks,) about fifty years of age, when about a month old had the Small Pox at a time when three others of the family had the same disease, one of whom, a servant man, died of it. Mr. Langford's countenance was strongly indicative of the malignity of the distemper, his face being so remarkably pitted and seamed, as to attract the notice of all who saw him, so that no one could entertain a doubt of his having had that disease in a most inveterate manner." Mr. Withers proceeds to state that Mr. Langford was seized a second time, had a bad confluent Small Pox, and died on the twenty-first day from the seizure: and that four of the family, as also a sister of the patient's, to whom the disease was conveyed by her son's visiting his uncle, falling down with the Small Pox, fully satisfied the country with regard to the nature of the disease, which nothing short of this would have done:—the sister died.

"This case was thought so extraordinary a one, as to induce the rector of the parish to record the particulars in the parish register."

It is singular, that in most cases of this kind the disease in the first instance has been confluent ; so that the extent of the ulceration on the skin (as in the Cow Pox) is not the process in nature which affords security to the constitution.

As the subject of the Small Pox is so interwoven with that which is the more immediate object of my present concern, it must plead my excuse for so often introducing it. At present it must be considered as a distemper not well understood. The Inquiry I have instituted into the nature of the Cow Pox, will probably promote its more perfect investigation.

The Inquiry of Dr. Pearson into the History of the Cow Pox, having produced so great a number of attestations in favour of my assertion that it proves a protection to the human body from the Small Pox, I have not been assiduous in seeking for more ; but as some of my friends have been so good as to communicate the following, I shall conclude these observations with their insertion.

Extract of a Letter from Mr. Drake, Surgeon, at Stroud, in this county, and late Surgeon to the North Gloucester Regiment of Militia.

"In the spring of the year 1796, I inoculated men, women, and children, to the amount of about seventy. Many of the men did not receive the infection, although inoculated at least three times, and kept in the same room with those who actually underwent the disease during the whole time occupied by them in passing through it. Being anxious they should in future be secure against it, I was very particular in my inquiries to find out whether they ever had previously had it, or at any time been in the neighbourhood of people labouring under it. But after all, the only satisfactory information I could obtain was, that they had had the Cow Pox. As I was then ignorant of such a disease affecting the human subject, I flattered myself what they imagined to be the Cow Pox was in reality the Small Pox in a very slight degree. I mentioned the circumstance in the presence of several of the officers, at the same time expressing my doubts if it were not Small Pox; and was not a little surprised when I was told by the Colonel, that he had frequently heard you mention the Cow Pox as a disease endemial to Gloucestershire, and that if a person were ever affected by it, you supposed him afterwards secure from the Small Pox. This excited my curiosity, and when I visited Gloucestershire I was very inquisitive concerning the subject; and from the information I have since received, both from your publication, and from conversation with medical men of the greatest accuracy in their observations, I am fully convinced that what the men supposed to be the Cow Pox was actually so, and I can safely affirm that they effectually resisted the Small Pox."

Mr. Fry, Surgeon, at Dursley, in this county, favours me with the following communication:

"During the spring of the year 1797, I inoculated fourteen hundred and seventy-five patients, of all ages, from a fortnight old to seventy years; amongst whom there were many who had previously gone through the Cow Pox. The exact number I cannot state; but if I say they were near thirty, I am certainly within the number. There was not a single instance of the variolous matter producing any constitutional effect on these people, nor any greater degree of local inflammation than it would have done in the arm of a person who had before gone through the Small Pox, notwithstanding it was invariably inserted four, five, and sometimes six different times, to satisfy the minds of the patients. In the common course of inoculation previous to the general one, scarcely a year passed without my meeting with one or two instances of persons who had gone through the Cow Pox, resisting the action of the variolous contagion. I may fairly say, that the number of people I have seen inoculated with the Small Pox, who at former periods had gone through the Cow Pox, are not less than forty;* and in no one instance have I known a patient receive the Small Pox, notwithstanding they invariably continued to associate with other inoculated patients during the progress of the disease, and many of them purposely exposed themselves to the contagion of the natural Small Pox; whence I am fully convinced, that a person who had *fairly* had the Cow Pox, is no longer capable of being acted upon by the variolous matter.

"I also inoculated a very considerable number of those who had had a disease which ran through the neighbourhood a few years ago, and was called by the common people the *Swine Pox*, not one of whom received the Small Pox.†

"There were about half a dozen instances of people who never had either the Cow or Swine Pox, yet did not receive the Small Pox, the system not being in the least deranged, or the arms inflamed, although they were repeatedly inoculated, and associated with others who were labouring under the disease; one of them was the son of a farrier."

Mr. Tierny, Assistant Surgeon of the South Gloucester Regiment of Militia, has obliged me with the following information:

"That in the summer of the year 1798, he inoculated a great number of the men belonging to the Regiment, and that among them he found eleven, who, from having lived in dairies, had gone through the Cow Pox. That all of them resisted the Small Pox, except one; but that, on making the most rigid and scrupulous inquiry at the farm in Gloucestershire, where the man said he lived when he had the disease, and among those with whom at the same time he declared he had associated, and particularly of a person in the parish, whom he said had dressed his fingers, it most clearly appeared that he aimed at an imposition,

* The greater part of these people must of course have had the Cow Pox many years before this trial was made upon them with the matter of Small Pox.—E. J.

† This was that mild variety of the Small Pox which I have noticed in the late Treatise on the Cow Pox, page 27.

and that he never had been affected with the Cow Pox.* Mr. Tierny remarks, that the arms of many who were inoculated, after having had the Cow Pox, inflamed very quickly, and that in several a little ichorous fluid was formed."

Mr. Cline, who in July last was so obliging, at my request, as to try the efficacy of the Cow Pox virus, was kind enough to give me a letter on the result of it, from which the following is an extract:

"My dear Sir,

"The Cow Pox experiment has succeeded admirably. The child sickened on the seventh day, and the fever, which was moderate, subsided on the eleventh. The inflammation arising from the insertion of the virus extended to about four inches in diameter, and then gradually subsided, without having been attended with pain or other inconvenience. There were no eruptions.†

"I have since inoculated him with Small Pox matter in three places, which were slightly inflamed on the third day, and then subsided.

"Dr. Lister, who was formerly Physician to the Small Pox Hospital, attended the child with me, and he is convinced that it is not possible to give him the Small Pox. I think the substituting the Cow Pox poison for the Small Pox, promises to be one of the greatest improvements that has ever been made in medicine; and the more I think on the subject, the more I am impressed with its importance.

"With great esteem,

"I am, &c.,

"Henry Cline.

"Lincoln's-Inn Fields,
"August 2, 1798."

From communications, with which I have been favoured from Dr. Pearson, who has occasionally reported to me the result of his private practice with the vaccine virus in London, and from Dr. Woodville, who has also favoured me with an account of his more extensive inoculation with the same virus at the Small Pox

* The public cannot be too much upon their guard respecting persons of this description.

† [The statement "*There were no eruptions*" does not exist in the original letter, but was here substituted for the following, "*The ulcer was not large enough to contain a pea, therefore I have not converted it into an issue as I intended.*" Vide copy of Mr. Cline's letter, vol. i., p. 140.– E.M.C.]

Hospital, it appears that many of their patients have been affected with eruptions, and that these eruptions have maturated in a manner very similar to the variolous. The matter they made use of was taken, in the first instance, from a cow belonging to one of the great milk farms in London. Having never seen maturated pustules produced either in my own practice among those who are casually infected by cows, or those to whom the disease had been communicated by inoculation, I was desirous of seeing the effect of the matter generated in London, on subjects living in the country. A thread imbrued in some of this matter was sent to me, and with it two children were inoculated, whose Cases I shall transcribe from my notes.

STEPHEN JENNER, three years and a half old.

3d day. The arm shewed a proper and decisive inflammation.

6th. A vesicle arising.

7th. The pustule of a cherry colour.

8th. Increasing in elevation.—A few spots now appear on each arm near the insertion of the inferior tendons of the biceps muscles. They are very small, and of a vivid red colour. The pulse natural; tongue of its natural hue; no loss of appetite, or any symptom of indisposition.

9th. The inoculated pustule on the arm this evening began to inflame, and gave the child uneasiness: he cried, and pointed to the seat of it, and was immediately afterwards affected with febrile symptoms. At the expiration of two hours after the seizure, a plaster of *ung. hydrarg. fort.* was applied, and its effect was very quickly perceptible; for in ten minutes he resumed his usual looks and playfulness. On examining the arm about three hours after the application of the plaster, its effects in subduing the inflammation were very manifest.

10th. The spots on the arms have disappeared, but there are three visible in the face.

11th. Two spots on the face are gone; the other barely perceptible.

13th. The pustule delineated in the second plate in the Treatise on the Variolæ Vaccinæ, is a correct representation of that on the child's arm, as it appears at this time.

14th. Two fresh spots appear on the face. The pustule on the arm nearly converted into a scab. As long as any fluid remained in it, it was limpid.

JAMES HILL, four years old, was inoculated on the same day, and with part of the same matter which infected Stephen Jenner. It did not appear to have taken effect till the fifth day.

7th. A perceptible vesicle: this evening the patient became a little chilly: no pain or tumour discoverable in the axilla.

8th. Perfectly well.

9th. The same.

10th. The vesicle more elevated than I have been accustomed to see it, and assuming more perfectly the variolous character than is common with the Cow Pox at this stage.

11th. Surrounded by an inflammatory redness, about the size of a shilling, studded over with minute vesicles. The pustule contained a limpid fluid till the fourteenth day, after which it was incrusted over in the usual manner; but this incrustation or scab being accidentally rubbed off, it was slow in healing.

These children were afterwards fully exposed to the Small Pox contagion without effect.

Having been requested by my friend Mr. Henry Hicks, of Eastington, of this county, to inoculate two of his children, and at the same time some of his servants and the people employed in his manufactory, matter was taken from the arm of this boy for the purpose. The numbers inoculated were eighteen. They all took the infection, and either on the fifth or sixth day a vesicle was perceptible on the punctured part. Some of them began to feel a little unwell on the eighth day, but the greater number on the ninth. Their illness, as in the former Cases described, was of short duration, and not sufficient to interrupt, but at very short intervals, the children from their amusements, or the servants and manufacturers from following their ordinary business.

Three of the children, whose employment in the manufactory was in some degree laborious, had an inflammation on their arms beyond the common boundary about the eleventh or twelfth day, when the feverish symptoms, which before were nearly gone off, again returned, accompanied with increase of axillary tumour. In these Cases (clearly perceiving the symptoms were governed by the state of the arms) I applied on the inoculated pustules, and renewed the application three or four times within an hour, a pledget of lint, previously soaked in *aqua lythargyri acetati*,* and covered the hot efflorescence surrounding them with cloths dipped in cold water.

The next day I found that this simple mode of treatment had succeeded perfectly. The inflammation was nearly gone off, and with it the symptoms which it had produced.

* Goulard's Extract of Saturn.

Some of these patients have since been inoculated with variolous matter without any effect beyond a little inflammation on the part where it was inserted.

Why the arms of those inoculated with the vaccine matter in the country should be more disposed to inflame than those inoculated in London, it may be difficult to determine. From comparing my own Cases with some transmitted to me by Dr. Pearson and Dr. Woodville, this appears to be the fact: and what strikes me as still more extraordinary with respect to those inoculated in London is, the appearance of maturating eruptions. In the two instances only which I have mentioned, (the one from the inoculated, the other from the casual Cow Pox), a few red spots appeared, which quickly went off without maturating. The Case of the Rev. Mr. Moore's servant may indeed seem like a deviation from the common appearances in the country, but the nature of these eruptions was not ascertained beyond their not possessing the property of communicating the disease by their effluvia. Perhaps the difference we perceive in the state of the arms may be owing to some variety in the mode of action of the virus upon the skin of those who breathe the air of London, and those who live in the country. That the erysipelas assumes a different form in London from what we see it put on in the country, is a fact very generally acknowledged. In calling the inflammation, that is excited by the Cow Pox virus, erysipelatous, perhaps I may not be critically exact, but it certainly approaches near to it. Now, as the diseased action going forward in the part infected with the virus may undergo different modifications, according to the peculiarities of the constitution on which it is to produce its effect, may it not account for the variation which has been observed?

To this it may probably be objected, that some of the patients inoculated, and who had pustules in consequence, were newly come from the country; but I conceive that the changes wrought in the human body through the medium of the lungs, may be extremely rapid. Yet, after all, further experiments made in London with vaccine virus generated in the country, must finally throw a light on what now certainly appears obscure and mysterious.

The principal variation perceptible to me in the action of the vaccine virus generated in London, from that produced in the country, was its proving more certainly infectious, and giving a less disposition in the arm to inflame. There appears also a greater elevation of the pustule above the surrounding skin. In my former

Cases, the pustule produced by the insertion of the virus was more like one of those which are so thickly spread over the body in a bad kind of confluent Small Pox. This was more like a pustule of the distinct Small Pox, except that I saw no instance of pus being formed in it, the matter remaining limpid till the period of scabbing.

Wishing to see the effects of the disease on an infant newly born, my nephew, Mr. Henry Jenner, at my request, inserted the vaccine virus into the arm of a child about twenty hours old. His report to me is, that the child went through the disease without apparent illness, yet that it was found effectually to resist the action of variolous matter with which it was subsequently inoculated.

I have had an opportunity of trying the effects of the Cow Pox matter on a boy who, the day preceding its insertion, sickened with the measles. The eruption of the measles, attended with cough, a little pain in the chest, and the usual symptoms accompanying that disease, appeared on the third day, and spread all over him. The disease went through its course without any deviation from its usual habits; and, notwithstanding this, the Cow Pox virus excited its common appearances, both on the arm and on the constitution, without any sensible interruption; on the sixth day there was a vesicle.

8th. Pain in the axilla, chilly, and affected with head-ache.

9th. Nearly well.

12th. The pustule spread to the size of a large split pea, but without any surrounding efflorescence. It soon afterwards scabbed, and the boy recovered his general health rapidly. But it should be observed, that before it scabbed, the efflorescence, which had suffered a temporary suspension, advanced in the usual manner.

Here we see a deviation from the ordinary habits of the Small Pox, as it has been observed that the presence of the measles suspends the action of variolous matter. However, the suspension of the efflorescence is worthy of observation.

The very general investigation that is now taking place, chiefly through inoculation (and I again repeat my earnest hope that it may be conducted with that calmness and moderation which should ever accompany a philosophical research), must soon place the vaccine disease in its just point of view. The result of all my trials with the virus on the human subject has been uniform. In every instance, the patient who has felt its influence has completely lost the susceptibility for the variolous contagion; and as these instances are now become numerous, I conceive that, joined to the observations in the former part of this paper, they sufficiently preclude me from the necessity of entering into controversies with those who have circulated reports adverse to my assertions, on no other evidence than what has been casually collected.

AN

ADDRESS TO THE PUBLIC

ON THE ADVANTAGES OF

VACCINE INOCULATION.

AN

ADDRESS TO THE PUBLIC

ON THE ADVANTAGES OF

VACCINE INOCULATION:

WITH THE

OBJECTIONS TO IT REFUTED.

By HENRY JENNER, Surgeon, F.L.S., &c.

" ——————————'Tis evidence so full—
If the last Trumpet sounded in my ear,
Undaunted I should meet the Saints half way,
And in the face of Heav'n maintain the fact."
DRYDEN.

BRISTOL:
PRINTED AND SOLD BY W. BULGIN, WINE-STREET;
SOLD ALSO BY S. HAZARD, BATH; J. AND W. RICHARDSON,
ROYAL EXCHANGE; AND CADELL AND DAVIES,
STRAND, LONDON.

ADDRESS.

I TRUST that the importance of the subject will be a sufficient apology for making this (I hope my final) Appeal to the Candour and good Sense of the Public. Confident of the strength of the foundation on which I stand, I fear not the blasts of baseless detraction. Conscious of no motives which an honest and a feeling mind would blush to avow, I would wish seriously to impress the importance of VACCINE INOCULATION.

I shall commence, according to the mode adopted by Dr. JENNER, by fairly stating, in the way of comparison, the peculiar differences which mark the Small-Pox and Cow-Pox; at the same time premising, that I can with the utmost confidence affirm, that the statement is in every particular confirmed by very extensive experience.

SMALL-POX.	COW-POX.
VERY frequently calls latent diseases into action; in these are included the various species of Scrofula.	WE may safely conclude, from a long and careful observation of this disease, as communicated from the Cow, and from no limited experience in its Inoculation, that it excites no disposition to other complaints. It is a pure disease, proceeding from the healthiest and the most cleanly of all animals, the Heifer.—The Scrofula cannot be generated, as that animal is never affected by it.
Is contagious and communicable by effluvia.	Numerous experiments testify, that this never happens in the Cow-Pox.
Cannot be communicated with safety to children when cutting teeth.	This circumstance forms no objection to inoculate with Vaccine Matter. — Numerous experiments justify the assertion.
In sickening with the Small-Pox, children are *frequently* afflicted with alarming fits; and when their constitutions are delicate, they suffer materially in their health during life.	Nothing of this kind has ever appeared in this disease; and the constitutions of children have been improved by its communication.
Is oftentimes fatal.	No instance of the kind has ever happened.

SMALL-POX.	COW-POX.
Is attended with Eruptions, and very often disfigures the Countenance.	In this disease (even in the natural way) I never observed any pustules.
Persons afflicted with this disease cannot mingle with those who have never been affected by it.	This objection does not apply to the Cow-Pox, as it is neither contagious, nor communicable by effluvia.
Medicines are necessary to be administered.	Here no medicines are required.
Notwithstanding the present improved state of Inoculation, parents and friends must feel a considerable degree of anxiety for the safety of relatives, &c.	Little anxiety can be felt in this disorder, as it is never attended with the least danger.
Requires a Nurse.	This disease does not.

The above comparison of the advantages which are to be derived from the substitution of the Vaccine Disease for the Small-Pox, is founded upon principles which experience has proved to be fixed upon the solid basis of truth. I am certainly entitled to speak with confidence on the subject; as, in conjunction with my uncle, Dr. JENNER (who, with indefatigable industry, has completely investigated the nature of Cow-Pox) I have had a very extensive acquaintance in this part of medical practice; but prejudice and illiberality will ever be on the watch to stop the progress of improvement, and to overturn the edifice of well-earned fame. The history of the advancement of Science exhibits this truth in every page, but the same detail will inform us that succeeding ages have never failed to place in its proper nook, in the Temple of Fame, the discoverer of any thing beneficial to human kind. Ignorant as we are what place may be consigned to Dr. JENNER by the present age, he may confidently appeal, by the justice of his claims, to unprejudiced, impartial posterity.

It is perfectly consistent with my present design, briefly to notice the most popular objections which have been urged against the introduction of Cow-Pox.

It has been called a bestial humour, and by a fallacious association of ideas, it is supposed to introduce an *unnatural* disease into the constitution.

If this very weak and futile objection were worthy of reply, we might observe, that the Cow is of all others the most healthy and the most cleanly of our domestic animals, and might also remark, that no females are so healthy as our dairy maids, whose morning and evening hours are spent amongst the cows; and we should not forget that the most eminent Physicians recommend invalids to avail themselves of the salubrious effects of the breath of the Heifer. How void of foundation then must be the objection to the insertion of an atom of matter taken from the teat of the cow, once in the life only, when every person is in the daily habit of introducing into his stomach various parts of the same animal. The human stomach revolts not at beef, butter, cheese, and cream; yet every one, acquainted with the animal economy, must know, that these aliments are quickly mingled with the constitution.

It may not be irrelevant to remark, that cheese, which constitutes so considerable a part of human food, may very frequently contain a sufficient quantity of vaccine matter for the inoculation of thousands.

Nor may it, perhaps, be too hypothetical to suppose, that the Cow-Pox may possibly be the Small-Pox in its original unadulterated state, before it became contaminated by passing through the impure and scrofulous habits of human constitutions. Is not this idea, in some measure, supported by the fact, that Cow-Pox never excites Scrofula, for the simple reason, that heifers have never this disease? And may it not appear after Small-Pox, as the matter may have passed through diseased habits?

Another grand objection (which indeed is the only one that strikes at the *foundation* of our theory) is, that persons are liable to be affected with Small-Pox after having been inoculated with the Cow-Pox.

A very extensive practice, and an equally extensive communication of the experience of medical friends of the first reputation, would almost warrant a short, abrupt answer to this question; an answer conveyed in terms unaccommodated to the feelings of the present age. After this objection, which has been refuted as often as it has been urged, a laconic reply, conveyed in no polite language, would by no means be improper, as it would harmonize with the general mode of such objections; and by all laws, the answer ought to be of the colour of the question: But what is not owing to cavilling individuals, is a just debt due to a candid and judicious Public.

Every case that has been brought forward to undermine the theory we defend, we can prove to a demonstration was not one of the *genuine* kind. There are *three* diseases which have indiscriminately been termed Cow-Pox, only *one* of which is the real preventive of Small-Pox. In the Spring season particularly, Cows are frequently sent to market for sale: The farmer omits to milk them in the morning, previous to their setting out, that their udders may appear full, and the animals on that account become more valuable. The frequent consequence is, that inflammation ensues, which terminates in eruptions on the teats and udder, and affects the milker with a loathsome disease on the hands, arms, and shoulders. The forehead sometimes does not escape, from the circumstance of the servant's leaning against the udder in milking. This disease may affect the same person several times, but it will *never* prove a preventive for Small-Pox: A case of this kind occurs in the city of Bristol. A Mr. JACOBS, attorney at law, was extensively affected *twice* with this disease (which, from his total ignorance of *real* Cow-Pox, he has called by that name), but it did not prevent his being afflicted with a subsequent severe Small-Pox.

Much stress has been laid on this case of Mr. JACOBS, as militating against the validity of the arguments adduced in support of the superior claim of the Vaccine Inoculation over the Variolous. Were fifty such cases to arise, they could make no impression on the minds of those who have studied the nature of the Cow-Pox. For the satisfaction of those who have not, I will explain the nature of these cases. But which evidence are we to look upon as the true one? That which Mr. JACOBS laid before Dr. SIMS in London, and was afterwards published by that Gentleman in the first Number of the *Medical and Physical Journal;* or that which he gave to Dr. BEDDOES, and which was published in his *Contributions to Physical and Medical Knowledge?* For be it known, these evidences differ most essentially.* However, as it may be more accommodating to those who live in the neighbourhood of Bristol, I will take the latter. He tells us, that the disease shewed itself by producing pustules on every finger, but that he does not recollect their producing any indisposition or fever; consequently, including the thumbs, Mr. JACOBS had at least twenty Cow-pock sores. Now I appeal to any of my medical neighbours in the Vale of Glocester, whether a person who

* In the extract of the letter published by Dr. SIMS, it is stated, that he (meaning Mr. JACOBS) "describes the Cow-Pox as the most loathsome of diseases, and adds, that his right arm was in a state of eruption, *both the first and second time*, from one extremity to the other."—But in his answer to Dr. BEDDOES's query, he mentions the *second* infection to have been slight.

had had the tenth part of the number of true Cow-pock sores on such irritable parts as the fingers, would not have felt so much indisposition as never to have forsaken his recollection of it?

This case may be supposed to have received some additional weight by the comment of Dr. BEDDOES at the conclusion of the dialogue. But it is very probable that at that time Dr. BEDDOES had never seen the Cow-Pox in *any* form, otherwise he would not have risked such an opinion. In short, the case of Mr. JACOBS very clearly appears to be one of those which Dr. JENNER has defined to be a *spurious* Cow-Pox, that is, one not capable of producing any specific change in the constitution, but leaving it as susceptible of the Small-Pox as after any other common eruption.

I hope therefore it will not be expected I should come forward to prove *again* to the public, that every such case of eruptive disorder, improperly called Cow-Pox (because it arises from a disease on the Cow's udder, which has been, and always may be, succeeded by Small-Pox), is actually of the spurious kind, and has no more to do with Small-Pox than the Hooping-Cough or Measles. But it is certainly the *duty* of those persons who bring forward such spurious cases for the true and genuine Cow-Pox, fully to investigate and give a minute description of every particular symptom, with which such disease is attended, to medical practitioners conversant with the disorders in question, and suffer *them* first to determine whether it be the true or the spurious kind, before they attempt to prejudice the public mind by giving an absolute determination of their own.

Every case of my *own* inoculation for Cow-Pox, and of every *genuine* natural case I shall have mentioned to be such, I do here assert, and will answer for the result of it, that it shall withstand every effort that can be devised, either by inoculation or otherwise, to introduce the contagion or infection of the Small-Pox into the system, at all ages and at any distant period from their having had the Cow-Pox. But as the spurious disease frequently shews an exact similarity in many of its appearances to the true species, it will require the discrimination of the exercised practitioner to distinguish one disease from the other, so that I can only ensure *my own* cases, or those cases inoculated with the vaccine matter *immediately* from myself; and I beg leave to ask the parents and relatives of those patients inoculated by me, whether every thing I have herein stated respecting the Cow-Pox, as far as they are capable of judging, be not strictly true?

The other sort of spurious Vaccine Disease is occasioned by flies of a particular species biting or stinging the teats of the Heifer; but this has no effect in preventing the attack of Small-Pox.

The third, or genuine Cow-Pox, affects the teats of the animal generally in the spring. It is conveyed by the milker from Cow to Cow, until the whole stock becomes infected, together with the milkers themselves; a wound or two appears on the hands, which swell considerably; the glands under the arms become enlarged, and the constitution is sensibly affected, unless the patient has previously gone through the Small-Pox, in which case it proves very mild.

After a person has had this disease or *true* Cow-Pox, he will never afterwards be liable to receive the infection of Small-Pox, either by contagion or inoculation, as I have before stated. And as I have produced a case of the spurious Cow-Pox which occurred in Bristol, I shall here introduce one of the *genuine* kind, which may be referred to in the same city, and will as clearly demonstrate the existence of the same complaint, as Mr. Jacobs's case does that of the other.

Mr. John Stinchcombe, broker, St. James's-back, was infected with the Cow-Pox, about thirty years ago, by milking at Mr. Coxe's Farm at Stone, near Berkeley. He had one pustule on each thumb, with some degree of soreness and swelling of the glands under the arms; but upon the whole the disease proved milder than the natural Cow-Pox generally does. Since that period he has resided many years in Bristol, and has lost four children in the natural Small-Pox, all of whom he attended and *slept* with during their illness. He was never inoculated for the Small-Pox, being fully assured that the Cow-Pox had sufficiently shielded his constitution against the influence of that disease.

A case also occurs in the town of Berkeley, where nearly *sixty* years have elapsed since the person had the Vaccine Disease, but he cannot be infected with Small-Pox. The person in question (Mr. John Phillips, barber) is now healthy, and will, if required, readily appear to verify my assertions, and give any person the liberty of infecting him with the Small-Pox, if he possibly can: but he has already thoroughly stood the test, both by frequent inoculations and exposure to variolous effluvia.

Another person, in the parish of Berkeley, who for many years past has been in the habit of nursing Small-Pox patients, and washing their linen, had the Cow-Pox more than *thirty* years ago; and although I have several times inoculated her, and she has been so frequently exposed to Small-Pox contagion, yet she has always resisted its infection.

Were it necessary, I could produce "Volumes of Evidences and Clouds of Witnesses" to prove the truth of the facts which I have adduced. I could refer the Public to Medical Gentlemen of the first character and highest eminence in their profession, whose repeated experiments corroborate my assertions respecting the peculiar properties of the Vaccine Disease. But waiving this reference for the present, I cannot avoid observing that I should consider myself as the grand enemy of Society if I were to recommend the general introduction of the practice, if experience, the test of theory, and the only sure guide of conduct, did not fully warrant its highest recommendation. Nay, in what light should I consider myself as a professional man, and I trust an honest member of Society, if I were to enforce a practice which involves in itself the dearest interests of Society, which comprehends in its influence the healths and *lives* of my fellow creatures, if I were not assured of its inevitable safety, and its numerous advantages? These advantages will doubtless be embraced by the serious and reflective. The mind of feeling, anxious for the health and safety of relatives and friends, will pause and consider before the Small-Pox be admitted, while so mild and so efficacious a substitute is offered. The imminent danger, the disfigured skin, the subsequent scrofula of the one will be contrasted with the unmarked countenance and the perfect safety of the other. But if prejudice should still continue to operate on the general mind, I am confident a time will come when those who have neglected to take advantage of the present opportunity will lament their conduct, and possibly lament it with unavailing sorrow—For sorrow must be unavailable for breathless friends, nor can a fruitless recollection soothe the miseries of continual disease.

Conscious as I equally am of the purity of my intentions, and of the truth of my assertions, I leave these remarks with the candid judgment of the Public, to whom I would recommend this concluding observation, that if by a good-natured stretch of its opinion, the illiberality of my opposers may be overlooked, their ignorance cannot be unnoticed; for I must be bold enough to affirm, that not one case of *genuine* Cow-Pox has ever come under their inspection.

HENRY JENNER.

Berkeley, Glocestershire,
December 26, 1799.

POSTSCRIPT.

To give the poor, and persons of indigent circumstances, the opportunity of escaping the Small-Pox, and of reaping the benefit of this discovery in common with other persons, I will with pleasure inoculate, *gratis*, for the Vaccine Disease, any such families, or individuals, who shall come forward with a proper recommendation from any reputable person.

A CONSCIOUS VIEW OF CIRCUMSTANCES AND PROCEEDINGS RESPECTING VACCINE INOCULATION, &c., &c.

"EGO AMPLIUS DELIBERANDUM CENSEO;
"RES MAGNA EST."

TERENCE.

BATH, PRINTED BY R. CRUTTWELL;
AND SOLD BY
T. HURST, PATER-NOSTER-ROW, LONDON.
1800.

PREFACE.

WHEN so much ill-blood and animosity appear, at times, to be excited by a mere difference of opinion in medical matters and pursuits, the Author of the following sheets would fain hope the well-meant intentions of one, who has devoted nearly thirty years of his past life to close observation, and a faithful discharge of the duties of his profession, may, at the present advanced period of it, be allowed to shield him from personalities, that could lead to no useful purpose, and to submit his thoughts to others as unknown to him as he is desirous of being to them; for, if the things he has to relate be true, it can be but very little matter or concern who spake them, whether PETER, PAUL, or JOHN. Besides, their being anonymous is less a proof of their being apocryphal, than that they were dictated by views of aggrandisement or motives of self-interest; whilst, as to personal reflections, they never once entered into the head or heart of the writer, who professes to be at enmity with no man living. And if, after so many years of practical experience, he has not hitherto sought for fame in print (farther than his occasional mite of contribution to different periodical publications), it would scarcely be expected that he should run his head into controversy now, upon a subject too which none of its abettors could possibly have entered upon, without some degree of enthusiasm, whilst not a few of them might (without offence, he conceives) be termed very bigots; so, the Author, knowing himself to be not altogether a body *papyral*, chooses not to hazard the risk of receiving quite so many darts as the zodiaco-chartaceous man in RYDER's Almanack.* Yet, a sincere regard for his fellow-creatures, a due respect for the medical character, and, above all, a conscientious discharge of that duty he owes to himself and to his fellow-creatures, forbad him any longer to be silent.

Now it so happens, that he is not intimately acquainted with

* Who, I always thought, looked like a fool surrounded by hieroglyphic friends, ready to carve (γλυφω) and weigh him out.

any of the leading experimenters in this same *Cow-Pox* business; and, thinking as he does, perhaps he may have no great reason to be sorry, being most decidedly of opinion, that the present rage for experiment has absolutely become outrageous; but his meaning at present is, to confine himself chiefly to that wanton exercise of it so indiscriminately and daringly practised, in endeavouring to incorporate the *diseases of brutes* with those of mankind; as though poor human nature had not already a sufficient catalogue of afflictions. What next the professional presumption of some men may lead them to, the Author of the present lines shudders even to conjecture; and "although diseases of bestial origin" may, by some, be maintained to be already in existence, yet, God be thanked, the laws of our country have wisely forbidden——and more especially since so great a disregard to God's holy ordinances has manifested itself; for surely, it is not alone the suddenly depriving another of life, that constitutes murder, but he also who rashly administers poison, whether in the form of pill or potion, from the point of Indian arrow or well-polished lancet, be its action remote or sudden, is equally the cause of death.

Now as in opposition to this remark it may be said, that many of our most active remedies might be classed in the rank of poisons, therefore practitioners should be forbad the use of them, so, no doubt, the unskilful ought; nor should the rash experimenter be a whit more tolerated. What availment is it to any man, whether he suffer loss of limb, life, or property, through the ignorance or temerity of another? And should any appeal be made to this doctrine, it need but be carried before the Court of King's Bench, where the present Lord Chief Justice would, I fancy, not only approve himself a learned doctor, but an upright judge.

ON

COW-POX, &c.

HOW any idea of such a subject as the one now under consideration could ever have entered into the mind of a rational being, is still a matter of wonder to me, notwithstanding the apparent corroborations and acknowledged respectability of several adjuncts in this extraordinary business; betwixt whom, however, a strong difference of opinion has already manifested itself, not only in regard to the most elaborately strained origin of this same Cow-Pox, but likewise as to its subsequent appearance and effects, when applied to the human frame.

But as it is intended in the following sheets that each approver should speak for himself, I shall only beg leave to follow as a fair Expositor, or rather Expostulator; adding, as circumstances and occasion may seem to admit, some few remarks also from the writings of others, who may, perhaps, appear to be not a little inclined towards my own way of thinking; but amongst whom will most assuredly be found characters of truly-deserved excellency, and of justly-approved integrity.*

As plain and candid discussion, however, needs not the proemial aids of an occult science, and in order that this view may be rendered as concise as possible, I shall proceed at once to the consideration of this most extraordinary subject; the first or grand ostensible promulgator of which appears to be Dr. JENNER, who, by a most wonderful kind of *Metastasis*, or rather ***Μεταπτωσις*** has, in a manner equally sublime as peculiar to himself, contrived the means—first of commixing, and then of transferring or communicating, the diseases of one animal to another—aye, and to another after that, of a quite different species; and all this under the humane idea of benefiting mankind: the more rational part of whom, however, it is humbly conceived, would not ill befit them-

* No small support, by-the-bye, to an anonymous author.

selves by enquiring som
cannot be other than prod
only to the present but t
plain thinking man be su
whether in physic or di
existence—the only safe a
And unless this same
amongst that "prolific s
man from the state in w
has brought upon us,"*
observation was intend
the indulgences of luxu
be sure, by a slight st
what infectious. But
that inoculation would
though the matter sh
and as to any new m
number of animals, v
for our associates," I
the smallest concept
lately-revived practi
in a Cow-house, wh
to produce the m
means could be d
Hygæieneal vapou
would certainly a

But in order t
ness I at first in
loath," to the g
noses, gentle re
for your own g

* Vide Introdu
† Perhaps I ou
present day for
fear if they are
the Disciples of
when it may),
lungs to know
seem to stand
when they h
a state of ca
powerful en
approved of
in the dark,
foul at the
he was in

practitioners in general, that no care, no skill, ever did, or ever can, tame that dreadful Hydra—the Small Pox."

> "Who shall decide when Doctors disagree?
> Sickness, sorrow, time, or eternity!"

Dr. M. further says, "We all know from experience, *that* disease, properly treated,* leaves nothing after it injurious to the constitution." Mr. R. replies, "that we do not all know it, is certain; if Dr. M. has been so happy as to discover the secret, I hope his humanity will prompt him to disclose it."

Confessing myself decidedly of opinion with Dr. M. in this respect, and conceiving his humanity to be inferior to that of no man living, I have no hesitation, even without his permission, to disclose this mighty secret; which solely consists in a due attention to the rise and progress of the disorder (*semeiotica*), with a proper deference to the good old practice, through its different stages. I mean here to be understood as speaking more particularly of the Small Pox in the natural way; but the observations and the practice might, no doubt, go a good way towards rendering the inoculated Small Pox what it was at first proposed to be, viz. "a safe expedient against the ravages of Small Pox." How far it has proved effectual in this point, or contributed to introduce other alarming disorders into the system, will become tolerably apparent by the discussions which the New Inoculation has already given birth to.

Mr. R. himself says, "It is well known, that the Small Pox, whether natural or inoculated, is one of the most common causes of *scrophula*." Now to this observation I feel no repugnance in repeating what I have, in part, before declared, viz., That I do really and truly consider the Small Pox, when properly treated, not only to act as a probable cure for *strumas*, but likewise for other disorders which may have possibly pre-existed in the habit: and am still further of opinion, that to improper treatment of Small Pox alone (whether casually appearing or produced by artificial insertion) we may chiefly ascribe the late frequent appearance not only of scrophulous, but of many other equally unseemly and alarming disorders.

Dr. M. has also taken upon him (but whether with or without the consent of Dr. Herschel, is not, I believe, mentioned) to

* But [illegible] care [illegible] ask [illegible] the majority of inoculated patients [illegible] properly treated? Are not scores and hundreds seated [illegible] scratchings, punctures and threadings, with[illegible] and whether they [illegible] is sometimes just as little known [illegible]

denominate the Cow Pox "*a new star* in the Esculapian System;" declaring, at the same time, that "in this Cow Mania it is not enough for reason to concede that the Cow Pox may lessen, for a time, the disposition in the habit to receive the infection of the Small Pox," whilst "all cutaneous determinations, catarrhal fevers, and every disease of the lymphatics, and medicine tending to what SYDENHAM would call depurating that system, do the same. Surgeons know that the first inflammation of any membrane is the most violent, and that reiterated inflammation deadens sensibility. The Small Pox does not destroy the disposition in the habit to receive the Cow Pox, neither are they analogous, but radically dissimilar."

"Can any person say," Dr. MOSELY asks, "what may be the consequence of introducing a bestial humour (the Cow Pox, he hopes, does not deserve the name of disease) into the human frame, after a long lapse of years?"

To which, after passing the retort courteous of "Cow-Phobia," Mr. RING "begs leave to ask, in his turn, if any person can say, what may be the consequence, after a long lapse of years, of introducing into the human frame cow's milk, beef-stakes, or a mutton-chop?"

No very difficult question to solve, I should imagine, for though a man must "every day grow older," he might, no doubt, at the same time hope, like Mr. R., to grow somewhat wiser too; at least wise enough not to cast reflections on such goodly cheer, especially in these dear times!

"The doctrine of engrafting distempers," continues Dr. M., "is not yet understood by the wisest men; and I wish to guard parents against suffering their children becoming victims to experiments. What miseries may be brought on a family after many years of imaginary security!"*

It was a part of my intention to have replied to *all* or most of the queries, which had been proposed by the several favourers of this new practice, that had come to my knowledge; but, for brevity sake, I shall now confine my observations to a few of them only. The following are among the Queries as proposed by Dr. PEARSON, in the *London Medical Review* for April 1799:—

3*d*. "Is the same cow liable to the disease more than once?"

Ans. I have not the smallest doubt but she is, if the same mode

* Now how soon the late pretended modes of subduing syphilitic affections by means of the nitric or citric acids may excite an equal dread, I will not pretend to say; but the proofs of their fallaciousness are daily manifesting, and are neither more nor less than what I expected at their first introduction.

of treatment be pursued at the same period and condition of the cow.

4th. "Has any cow ever appeared to die of this disease?"

Ans. I have never heard of one, which, if the disease had possessed all or any of that wide-spreading contagion and malignity it was so alarmingly announced to be fraught with, must, I think, have been the case pretty often. But viewing the complaint to be merely local, and the nature of it such as to forbid a continuation of the same rude action which first excited the injury, kinder treatment, or kind Nature herself, has generally proved the happy *medicatrix.*

7th. "Have cows, in a state of pregnancy, been observed to be affected with this distemper?"

Ans. Never to my knowledge; nor do I think them susceptible of it, even by inoculation, nor by any means short of the violence above reprobated; but which their condition for a while exempts them, most fortunately, from undergoing.

Queries with respect to Human Creatures.

8th. "Has it been observed, that a person has ever taken the Small Pox after having gone through the Cow Pox?"

Ans. Yes!*

9th. "Does the Cow Pox render the human constitution unsusceptible of any other disease besides the Small Pox; or, on the contrary, increase its susceptibility to any particular disease?"

Ans. The former part of this query being considered as highly problematical, and no time having as yet been allowed to ascertain or furnish a precise answer to the latter, I would just beg leave to ask in my turn, whether the introduction of any disease whatever could be reasonably supposed to "better" a good constitution?

10th. "What are the effects of Cow Pox on pregnant women?"

To this query I were almost inclined to answer, "*pregnant* with mischief must the mind of that man be, who should make the experiment;" nor would I alter one tittle in the expression, were the attempt to be made without the free and unbiassed consent of the woman. Who that has any pretensions to medical knowledge can be ignorant of the danger attending pregnant women, when attacked with measles, etc.?

* Vide pp. 215, 226, 227, 228, 229, 230, 231, 232.

In an account of the Vaccine Institution, as given in the *London Medical Review* for January 1800, it is said, "Those who are more extensively acquainted with the history of the Small Pox, know that it is productive of a great *deal of mischief*, notwithstanding the *advantage of inoculation;* for,

"*1st.* Under the *best treatment* a certain proportion of persons die in the inoculated Small Pox."

Now this being the case, how miserable must have been the condition of such as meet with no treatment at all? Or more deplorable those, who fall under *bad treatment*, from ignorant pretenders? Horrid dilemma!

"*2ndly.* It seems fair to calculate, that in the inoculated Small Pox one in twenty-five undergoes a severe disease."

Do they so? The first promoters of this practice allured mankind (and the successive encouragers of it have said nothing to the contrary) with a very different account; announcing nothing but perfect safety. Should any one doubt my assertion, they need only amuse themselves by looking over a host of writers on the subject, too numerous for us to mention even by name; but all found agreeing in the main point—namely, the propagation of disorders.

"*3rdly.* The numerous sources of the Small Pox infection now preclude every prospect of extinguishing this disease."

Now I would just beg leave to ask, who we have to thank for this sad calamity, but the inoculators themselves; than for whose avidity to propagate and keep up, as it were, both the terror and *fomes* of this disease, we might, with no small degree of probability, have known, and consequently have dreaded, as little about Small Pox as (I have before hinted) we now do, thank God, about the plague, scurvy, or sweating-sickness.

"*4thly.* A certain proportion of inoculated cases of Small Pox produce deformities of the skin, which no practitioner can be answerable for preventing in any instance."

This, by-the-bye, is somewhat more than I can readily concede to, especially after what has been already stated.

"Diseases, also, are frequently excited by inoculation, to which a pre-disposition pre-existed in the constitution."

Why then rouse them into action? And here again let me ask, may not this renowned Cow Pox do the same, or something worse perhaps?

"Now, according to the justest calculation," it is said in Dr. Woodville's Reports, that "about one in two hundred dies of the variolous inoculation." And in p. 613 of the *London Medical*

Review for August 1799, Dr. PEARSON observes, "to those inoculators who boast of never having lost a patient, that no advantage on the score of life will be allowed from the Cow Pox. But he begs leave to say farther, that more persons have died from inoculation within a few years, than did in the same time twenty years ago."

Enough, one would think, to point out its baneful influence, as "*twenty years ago*" inoculation might be considered as being very little more than in its infancy, as it were; and then, perhaps, as now, most shamefully suffered to be conducted by persons wholly unacquainted with the treatment befitting the different states of the human constitution. And happy, no doubt, might it have been for many, had the proposal of Baron DIMSDALE been adopted by our Government, as well as that of Russia, forbidding any, but physicians or surgeons duly licensed, "to inoculate for the Small Pox; for the mischief arising from the practice of inoculation by the illiterate and ignorant is beyond conception."*

Now I own I should like to be satisfied, if any one or all of the Vaccine gentry had been interrogated concerning the inoculated Small Pox only some few years back, whether their declarations then would have at all squared with their opinions now? With several of them I know the pursuit of the latter practice has proved abundantly productive; whilst others, perhaps with a foresight not given to all alike, saw the approaching change, and, unwilling to part with both thread and lancet,† stepped themselves instantly forward into as much public notice as they could; in order, no doubt, to maintain that certain degree of influence they are ever sure to gain when once admitted into a family, where the sad proceeding may happen to have been determined upon.

Here, indeed, I was about to conclude, but perceiving that the greasy-heeled Pegasus had absolutely carried one gentleman to the summit of human wishes, "his being's end and aim," as will appear by the following letter communicated by Dr. PEARSON.‡

"I am *happy* in having it in my power to communicate *forty-three* successful cases of inoculation with Vaccine matter, and to thank you for the matter which you so obligingly sent me. With

* Vide *Thoughts by Baron Dimsdale*, published by Owen, in Fleet Street, 1776.

† With neither of which, in my opinion, ought a physician at all to intermeddle whilst there is a regular-bred surgeon at hand.

‡ Vide *Medical and Physical Journal*, p. 234.

the *lancet* you received from Dr. PEARSON I inoculated the first case, but in no instance could I succeed with the *thread.**

" I shall do myself the honour, at some future period, to transmit two cases, which go far to prove, that Cow Pock contagion cannot be communicated by effluvia."

Now could not the good gentleman contrive to add a case or two to prove the like in regard to variolous contagion ? I think he might, if he would ; and by so doing make some few as happy, perhaps, in the old pursuits as he appears to be in the new ; having declared himself "firmly of opinion, that the Cow Pox inoculation is attended with many advantages, sufficiently to *force* its way into general practice here, notwithstanding the *opposition* and *crafty insinuations* of *interested practitioners.*"

Now with all those opposing on such principles, if any such there should be, I not only disclaim even the most distant league or connection, but am puzzled even to conjecture what sort of interest that can be, which could hope to derive any advantage from such unworthy means.

"But," continues this happy gentleman, " to obviate the evil intentions of such men,† the following history is subjoined.

" 'JOHN M'GUBBIN's child, aged *two days*, on account of his mother being ill with the *Small Pox when he was born*, was *inoculated* with Vaccine matter on Tuesday, January 21st.

" 'Saturday, 4th day, as it was doubtful whether or not the infection had taken place, it was determined to inoculate him a second time with recent matter, which could not in the course of this day be easily procured.

" 'Sunday, 5th day, the punctured part of the right arm slightly inflamed and of a pustular form.

" 'Monday, 6th day, the child was very ill all night, with frequent vomiting and bleeding at the nose, and other symptoms, denoting much constitutional disease. From the bleeding at the nose, alteration of the countenance, etc., we suspected the seat of the disease to be in the head ; there was not, however, the slightest mark of injury to be perceived externally. He died about one o'clock this afternoon ; upon inspecting his head, in presence of Dr. H., we found that by pressing on the fontanelle and back part of the *os frontis*, blood issued from the nose. The scalp covering

* "The thread was impregnated with matter, and the lancet was stained at the same time from the same pustule."—Dr. PEARSON.

† The letter, I observe, is dated Plymouth, 13th January, 1800, where, since the much-lamented departure of MUDGE and GEACH, I know not that I have a single medical acquaintance.

the left parietal bone and the corresponding part of the occipital was thickened and discoloured, the subjacent part of the pericranium to a greater extent was much inflamed; the occipital and left parietal bones which it covered, were of a dark red colour. Between the *dura mater* and skùll of the same side, there was a great quantity of extravasated blood, and the brain itself underneath was also slightly inflamed.'

"That the morbid appearances above described were the consequences of external violence, though that could not be ascertained, will not be doubted; nor is it material, whether we suppose the inflammation or the extravasation of blood to have been the immediate cause of his death, as this case is not communicated with any practical view, but merely that the *unbiassed* and intelligent part of the profession may judge how much, or rather how little, the Cow Pox had in occasioning it. As a report has been spread abroad, evidently for the purpose of discouraging the progress of the Cow Pox, that the child died of this disease, it was judged necessary to describe the morbid appearances which we discovered on dissection."

"I am, etc., etc."

In the useful publication from which the above is extracted, follows another letter from Plymouth,* replete with conclusions as extraordinary as some of the remarks appear to be illiberal; I have not my quoting dictionary at hand, or I would certainly have copied out a stanza or two in return for the author's *exegi monumentum* from the odes of HORACE. Now the dogmatical writer of this letter seems to me to be not a little eager to make a figure in the Cow Poxing calendar, as you shall hear:—

"GENTLEMEN,—The introduction of the Cow Pox into practice, as a substitute for the Small Pox, having been found to be *expedient*, in the most extensive sense of the word, the discussion of the subject will of course be considered *as closed*."

GOD help the good gentleman, that is to say, the learned doctor, for he certainly has just claim to be considered as such, notwithstanding the encomiastic adulations he has been pleased to bestow on Doctors JENNER, PEARSON, and WOODVILLE; or the sad state of degradation to which he has thought fit to reduce all those not immediately of his own way of thinking, calling us "reptiles, that plant (ourselves) in the high road of improvement, and try to hiss back all that would advance."

* But not with the same signature, though of the same date.

Now, methinks, the good Doctor might have *let us down* somewhat more gradually, as well as more philosophically, by a sort of a kind of a quadrupedal assimilation, which, for aught he knows, may be going forward at this very moment through the introduction of this same matter into our bodies, an idea or conjecture which, I am told, has been typically anticipated already.

"When I hear," continues this same gentleman, "of medical men ridiculing the Cow Pox, seemingly with the view of preventing its advantages from being experimentally ascertained by that part of the community who have been *wheedled* into a mistaken confidence in their candour, I cannot help suspecting the *opposition* of *such men* to proceed from motives other than those of conviction; especially if their professional rank does not allow us to impute to them *ignorance* or *want of discernment.* What medical man of candour or professional information would attempt *to resist the force of so great and incontrovertible a mass of evidence* of the utility of the new practice, or *the high authorities on which it has been so strongly* recommended?"

That I am one still to doubt the permanent efficacy of this same *new practice* is as true as that I continue most seriously to deplore the mischief occasioned by the indiscriminate proceedings, and too frequent mismanagement, in the variolous inoculation. And being of that opinion, I am utterly regardless of what may be said or thought of me by those so enthusiastically engaged in the present pursuit; nor am I disposed to bow down to recommendations from *any authority, however high,* touching matters of which they cannot be supposed to know any thing but from the representation of others; or feel myself at all inclined to admit the conclusions drawn by the writer of this article, as knowing nothing myself about "the *wheedling arts,*" or what purposes they could possibly be expected to answer in the opposers of the business. I own I am unwilling to believe that any such attempts have ever been seriously made. To all fair and candid experiments, which may tend to meliorate the condition of my fellow-creatures, I am as staunch an advocate, as I am a foe decided against all presumptuous precipitation in *forcing down a matter,* or rather, in the language of Dr. JENNER, *a wide-spreading contagion;* the casual benefits arising from which could neither, in reasoning natural or physical, be satisfactorily ascertained for a considerable time yet to come.

It is now many years since the Small Pox has appeared epidemic in Great Britain, it may be full as many more before it appears so again. But I will hazard no predictions; I will content myself with saying, that experiments enough have already been made, and that a reasonable time ought to be allowed to observe their effects; and if such a reasonable time be not allowed, then, I think, the *reflections* on the score of *present personal interest* will very justly revert where they most certainly ought to attach.

A remark or two more and I shall lay down my pen.

"None of my patients," says Dr. H.,* "except the woman before-mentioned, had a single troublesome symptom after the fever had gone off; nor were any of them likely to be afflicted with *scrophula, etc.*, which has been known to follow the Small Pox, even under its mildest form." So here's another *kick* at the *Variolous* from the *heels* of the *Vaccine*. But I should be glad to be informed, what time the scrophula generally takes before it makes its appearance after the *mildest form* of Small Pox? A much easier thing to do, I fancy, than it would be to tell me what time scrophula, or consumption, takes to show itself after recovery from the *confluent Small Pox*, when it has been judiciously treated.

"Another advantage of the Cow Pox, as we learn from Dr. JENNER,† but which, in the present state of its progress, must not yet be counted upon, is, that it is never communicated by effluvia; therefore it would appear from this, that however similar in their appearance, etc., the Variolous and Vaccine are, they are really *different* specific diseases.‡ Some of the readers of this Journal, who are of the same opinion, may, perhaps, consider the confidence with which the contrary has been so roundly affirmed (*Monthly Magazine* for June last) as bordering upon presumption. It has been asserted, and that without the least shadow of proof, that the Cow Pox is only the Small Pox having undergone a certain modification, alias conjuration, by passing through the quadruped; and that it will degenerate into Small Pox again, by passing a *series of times from one human being to another* without interruption. The author of this opinion, however, not satisfied with the grounds on which he rests it, intends, he tells us, to determine this point by experiment, the result of which he promises to lay before the public." What a grand desideratum to have in expectation!

Towards the conclusion of this letter § (by no means deficient

* *Medical and Physical Journal*, p. 244.

† *Ibid.*

‡ In a pamphlet lately published at Oxford, with a title-page assuming much more than is warranted by the context, we are told, "the *Variolous* and *Vaccine* are considered as terms synonymous."

§ I am not certain whether or not this is the same gentleman who, in a "Treatise on Croup" (vide *Medical and Physical Journal*, vol. iii., p. 60), has in sound physiological discussion), I observe two cases preceded by what I consider to be a most prudential caution to inoculators in general. "The inoculation," says Dr. H., "though, from the simple manner in which it can be performed, it appears so trivial a circumstance, yet it may be of the last importance to the feelings and safety of an individual, as well as the reputation of the surgeon, that it be performed so as to insure the infection taking place. A patient of mine was inoculated twice by means of a thread inserted into each arm without effect, and a third time by puncture; on the following day the Small Pox appeared.

"D. C., seventeen months old, was inoculated by puncture with Vaccine matter, taken from a pustule in the state of suppuration, and dried; on the 6th day the first inflammation had not subsided, on the 7th it was less, and on the 8th had almost entirely disappeared.

"He was again inoculated (Dec. 25th) with recent matter in its fluid state; on Saturday the infection had evidently taken place; that evening the child, who had been seemingly unwell the day before, was taken very ill; and on Sunday the Small Pox appeared, of the confluent kind; on Monday, the pustules in each arm, from the inoculation, coming forward; on the 31st they contain matter; the child's body is covered with petechial spots, not a hope of his recovery is entertained. It will, perhaps, in general be found, that if the first inflammation continues beyond the 5th day, the infection will not take place. Now, from the event of this case, as the child is since dead, which might perhaps have been prevented, if the matter used in the first inoculation had been taken earlier from the patient, and in a more fluid state, as the child was not unsusceptible of the disease, the propriety of Dr. PEARSON's suggestions on this part of the subject will appear evident."

And here I can but again remark, that scarce any two of the Cow Pox inoculators agree, either upon the true mode of operations or upon the precise appearance of the disease they wish to produce.

drawn the following most extraordinary conclusion respecting the use of venesection in the practice of medicine; viz.—"That it is never safe, often hurtful, and sometimes fatal;" nor do I pretend to know what the grey-bearded phlebotomists will say to it. But there is so much of apparent applicability to this my view of the present subject, in a preceding remark of his (p. 57), that I cannot deny myself the pleasure of transcribing it:—"It surely is not enough that we can with certainty prognosticate the ultimate event of a disease to be favourable; it is undoubtedly as much our duty in the choice of our measures for that purpose to weigh well not only their immediate, but all possible remote consequences which may follow the use of them, as the future health or comfort of our patients, that neither may be endangered."

Nor is it at all clear to me, that any of the cases already adduced deserve, in any shape, to be considered as fully and fairly conclusive in this business; as what may have been considered by many as previous affections of Cow Pox, may, no doubt, have proved truly Small Pox. And this will serve to account for many of those subsequent attempts to inoculate the latter being so repeatedly resisted, whilst in cases of simple or genuine Vaccine infection, as it is called, there are sufficient instances on record already to show their states of insecurity against future attacks of the Variolous infection.

So far, however, as this new introduction of the Vaccine (I am almost sick of the term) may contribute to lessen the practice of the Variolous inoculation, it possibly may, in that case, prove a sort of preponderance against some of its own future mischiefs; but how soon they shall become manifest, or to what lengths they may extend previous to a detection of them, I shall not hazard even a single conjecture, but wait with all imaginable solicitude until circumstances shall arise to confirm the utility, or declare at least the harmlessness of the measure. And, perhaps, if some of those now so very active in the present *pursuit* were to "*hold-hard*" for a little while only, they might, like *good sportsmen*, not be quite so liable to *overrun* the *scent*, and thence lose an opportunity of *preserving the game* it was neither their wishes nor their interest to have wholly destroyed; or, in other words (for I am but a so-so hand at a simile), if somewhat less eagerness had been shown in so presumptuously pushing forward this new-fangled business, taking the whole world, as it were, by surprise; or in fine, had a little more deference been shown to the feelings of those who, with nearly equal discernment perhaps, and with no less deserving caution, were not in a state quite so prone to be led away by the *vanities* of *innovation*, the prejudices of *fashion*, or the bolder enterprises of some men (however highly they might conceive themselves to be apparently sanctioned); and by which they could, in my humble opinion, have lost nothing in the just estimation of the physiologist or the philosopher.

CONCLUSION.

Whether these, my feeble exertions, may have any effect in checking the further progress of a matter fraught with so much indecisiveness, and also of apparent danger, is not for me to say, much less determine; whilst I trust, nay, I know, whatever I may have said has been conscientiously written. My aim has been neither at the exaltation nor depreciation of any one of my brethren—No! let them take their airy flights, so as they do but return in due time to the discharge of their chief and best duty, viz. *the cure of diseases,* and give up at once all vain preventive presumptions to quacks and quackery; as *these,* together with the *causes natural* and advenient, *will,* most assuredly, continue as heretofore to furnish sufficient employment for *minds* the *most active,* and for intentions the *most honourable,* in every branch of *our liberal profession.*

FINIS.

A CONTINUATION OF

FACTS AND OBSERVATIONS

RELATIVE TO THE

VARIOLÆ VACCINÆ.

A

CONTINUATION

OF

FACTS AND OBSERVATIONS

RELATIVE TO THE

VARIOLÆ VACCINÆ,

OR

COW POX.

By EDWARD JENNER, M.D., F.R.S., &c.

London:

PRINTED FOR THE AUTHOR,

BY D. N. SHURY, NO. 7, BERWICK STREET, SOHO.

1801.

ADVERTISEMENT.

THE foregoing pages[1] contain the whole of my first Treatise on the Variolæ Vaccinæ, published in June, 1798. The importance of the Inquiry to the whole human race naturally excited universal attention. Ingenuity and industry were set in motion: but as physiological discussions are ever liable to error, from the complicated nature of their character, I soon clearly perceived that this theory, so beneficial to mankind, was liable to fall into disrepute, and to be wholly discredited by the force of hasty conclusions unfounded on experiment.

To guard the public mind from prejudice, and to enforce the necessity of a scrupulous precaution in the conduct of inoculation with vaccine matter, I was induced to offer to the world *Further Observations* on the disease, which were published in the beginning of the year 1799.[2] These Treatises I have here combined, together with some additions,[3] which the continuance of the Inquiry has enabled me to submit to the public.

---

[1] [Vide pp. 3-33.--E.M.C.]

[2] [Vide pp. 155-189.—E.M.C.]

[3] [*A Continuation of Facts and Observations.* Vide the following pages 251-274.—E.M.C.]

A CONTINUATION OF

FACTS AND OBSERVATIONS,

&c., &c.

SINCE my former publications on the Vaccine Inoculation, I have had the satisfaction of seeing it extend very widely. Not only in this country is the subject pursued with ardour, but from my correspondence with many respectable medical gentlemen on the Continent (among whom are *Dr. De Carro* of Vienna, and *Dr. Ballhorn* of Hanover), I find it is as warmly adopted abroad, where it has afforded the greatest satisfaction. I have the pleasure too of seeing that the feeble efforts of a few individuals to depreciate the new practice, are sinking fast into contempt beneath the immense mass of evidence which has risen up in support of it.

Upwards of six thousand persons have now been inoculated with the virus of Cow Pox, and the far greater part of them have since been inoculated with that of Small Pox, and exposed to its infection in every rational way that could be devised, without effect.

It was very improbable that the investigation of a disease so analogous to the Small Pox, should go forward without engaging the attention of the Physician of the Small Pox Hospital in London.

Accordingly, Dr. Woodville, who fills that department with so much respectability, took an early opportunity of instituting an Inquiry into the nature of the Cow Pox. This Inquiry was begun in the early part of the present year, and in May Dr. Woodville published the result, which differs essentially from mine in a point of much importance. It appears that three-fifths of the patients inoculated were affected with eruptions, for the most part so perfectly resembling the Small Pox, as not to be distinguished from them. On this subject it is necessary that I should make some comments.

When I consider that out of the great number of Cases of casual inoculation immediately from cows, which have from time to time presented themselves to my observation, and the many similar instances which have been communicated to me by medical gentlemen in this neighbourhood; when I consider too that the matter with which my inoculations were conducted in the years 1797, 98, and 99, was taken from different cows, and that in no instance any thing like a variolous pustule appeared, I cannot feel disposed to imagine that eruptions, similar to those described by Dr. Woodville, have ever been produced by the *pure, uncontaminated Cow Pock virus:* on the contrary, I do suppose that those which the Doctor speaks of, originated in the action of variolous matter, which crept into the constitution with the vaccine. And this I presume happened from the inoculation of a great number of the patients with variolous matter (some on the third, others on the fifth day) after the vaccine had been applied; and it should be observed, that the matter thus propagated became the source of future inoculations in the hands of many medical gentlemen who appeared to have been previously unacquainted with the nature of the Cow Pox.

Another circumstance strongly, in my opinion, supporting this supposition, is the following: the Cow Pox has been known among our dairies time immemorial. If pustules then, like the variolous, were to follow the communication of it from the cow to the milker, would not such a fact have been known, and recorded at our farms? Yet neither our farmers nor the medical people of the neighbourhood have noticed such an occurrence.

A few scattered pimples I have sometimes, though very rarely, seen, the greater part of which have generally disappeared quickly, but some have remained long enough to suppurate at their apex. That local cuticular inflammation, whether springing up spontaneously, or arising from the application of acrid substances, such, for instance, as *Cantharides, Pix Burgundica, Antimonium Tartarizatum*, etc., will often produce cutaneous affections, not only near the seat of the inflammation, but on some parts of the skin far beyond its boundary, is a well-known fact. It is, doubtless, on this principle that the inoculated Cow Pock pustule and its concomitant efflorescence may, in very irritable constitutions, produce this affection. The eruption I allude to has commonly appeared some time in the third week after inoculation. But this appearance is too trivial to excite the least regard.

The change which took place in the general appearance during the progress of the vaccine inoculation at the Small Pox Hospital should likewise be considered.

Although at first it took on so much of the variolous character, as to produce pustules in three Cases out of five, yet in Dr. Woodville's last report, published in June, he says, "Since the publication of my reports of inoculations for the Cow Pox, upwards of three hundred Cases have been under my care; and out of this number, only thirty-nine had pustules that suppurated: viz. out of the first hundred, nineteen had pustules; out of the second, thirteen; and out of the last hundred and ten, only seven had pustules. Thus it appears that the disease has become considerably milder; which I am inclined to attribute to a greater caution used in the choice of the matter with which the infection was communicated; for lately, that which has been employed for this purpose has been taken only from those patients in whom the Cow Pox proved very mild and well characterised."*

The inference I am induced to draw from these premises is very different. The decline, and finally the total extinction nearly of these pustules, in my opinion, are more fairly attributable to the Cow Pox virus, assimilating the variolous,† the former probably being the original, the latter the same disease under a peculiar, and at present an inexplicable modification.

One experiment, tending to elucidate the point under discussion, I had myself an opportunity of instituting. On the supposition of its being possible that the cow which ranges over the fertile meadows in the vale of Gloucester, might generate a virus differing in some respects in its qualities from that produced by the animal artificially pampered for the production of milk for the metropolis, I procured, during my residence there in the spring, some Cow Pock virus from a cow at one of the London milk farms.‡ It was immediately conveyed into Gloucestershire

* In a few weeks after the Cow Pox inoculation was introduced at the Small Pox Hospital, I was favoured with some virus from this stock. In the first instance it produced a few pustules which did not maturate; but in the subsequent cases none appeared.

† In my first publication on this subject I expressed an opinion that the Small Pox and the Cow Pox were the same diseases under different modifications. In this opinion Dr. Woodville has concurred. The axiom of the immortal Hunter, that *two diseased actions cannot take place at the same time in one and the same part*, will not be injured by the admission of this theory.

‡ It was taken by Mr. Tanner, then a student at the Veterinary College, from a cow at Mr. Clark's farm at Kentish Town.

to Dr. Marshall, who was then extensively engaged in the inoculation of the Cow Pox, the general result of which, and of the inoculation in particular with this matter, I shall lay before my Readers in the following communication from the Doctor.

"Dear Sir,

"My neighbour, Mr. Hicks, having mentioned your wish to be informed of the progress of the inoculation here for the Cow Pox, and he also having taken the trouble to transmit to you my minutes of the Cases which have fallen under my care, I hope you will pardon the further trouble I now give you in stating the observations I have made upon the subject. When first informed of it, having two children who had not had the Small Pox, I determined to inoculate them for the Cow Pox whenever I should be so fortunate as to procure matter proper for the purpose. I was therefore particularly happy when I was informed that I could procure matter from some of those whom you had inoculated. In the first instance, I had no intention of extending the disease further than my own family, but the very extensive influence which the conviction of its efficacy in resisting the Small Pox has had upon the minds of the people in general, has rendered that intention nugatory, as you will perceive by the continuation of my Cases inclosed in this letter,* by which it will appear, that since the 22nd of March, I have inoculated an hundred and seven persons; which, considering the retired situation I reside in, is a very great number. There are also other considerations which, besides that of its influence in resisting the Small Pox, appear to have had their weight; namely, the peculiar mildness of the disease, the known safety of it, and its not having in any instance prevented the patient from following his ordinary business. In all the Cases under my care, there have only occurred two or three which required any application owing to the erysipelatous inflammation on the arm, and they immediately yielded to it. In the remainder the constitutional illness has been slight but sufficiently marked, and considerably less than I ever observed in the same number inoculated with the Small Pox. In only one or two of the cases have any other eruptions appeared than those around the spot where the matter was inserted, and those near the infected part. Neither does there appear in the Cow Pox to be the least exciting cause to any other disease, which in the Small

* Dr. Marshall has detailed these cases with great accuracy, but their publication will [illegible] be deemed superfluous.—E. J.

Pox has been frequently observed, the constitution remaining in as full health and vigour after the termination of the disease as before the infection. Another important consideration appears to be the impossibility of the disease being communicated, except by the actual contact of the matter of the pustule, and consequently the perfect safety of the remaining part of the family, supposing only one or two should wish to be inoculated at the same time.

"Upon the whole, it appears evident to me, that the Cow Pox is a pleasanter, shorter, and infinitely more safe disease than the inoculated Small Pox, when conducted in the most careful and approved manner; neither is the local affection of the inoculated part, or the constitutional illness, near so violent. I speak with confidence on the subject, having had an opportunity of observing its effects upon a variety of constitutions, from three months old to sixty years; and to which I have paid particular attention. In the Cases alluded to here you will observe that the removal from the original source of the matter has made no alteration or change in the nature or appearance of the disease, and that it may be continued, *ad infinitum* (I imagine), from one person to another (if care be observed in taking the matter at a proper period), without any necessity of recurring to the original matter of the cow.

"I should be happy if any endeavours of mine could tend further to elucidate the subject, and shall be much gratified in sending you any further observations I may be enabled to make.

"I have the pleasure to subscribe myself,

"Dear Sir, &c.,

"JOSEPH H. MARSHALL.

"Eastington, Gloucestershire,
"April 26th, 1799."

The gentleman who favoured me with the above account has continued to prosecute his inquiries with unremitting industry, and has communicated the result in another letter, which at his request I lay before the public without abbreviation.

DR. MARSHALL'S SECOND LETTER.

"DEAR SIR,

"Since the date of my former letter, I have continued to inoculate with the Cow Pox virus. Including the cases before enumerated, the number now amounts to four hundred and twenty-three. It would be tedious and useless to detail the progress of the disease in each individual—it is sufficient to observe, that I noticed no deviation in any respect from the Cases I formerly adduced. The general appearances of the arm exactly corresponded with the account given in your first publication. When they were disposed to become troublesome by erysipelatous inflammation, an application of equal parts of vinegar and water always answered the desired intention. I must not omit to inform you, that when the disease had duly acted upon the constitution, I have frequently used the vitriolic acid. A portion of a drop applied with the head of a probe or any convenient utensil upon the pustule, suffered to remain about forty seconds, and afterwards washed off with sponge and water, never fail to stop its progress, and expedite the formation of a scab.

"I have already subjected two hundred and eleven of my patients to the action of the variolous matter, *but every one resisted it.*

"The result of my experiments (which were made with every requisite caution) has fully convinced me that the *true Cow Pox* is a safe and infallible preventive from the Small Pox; that in no case which has fallen under my observation has it been in any considerable degree troublesome, much less have I seen any thing like danger; for in no instance were the patients prevented from following their ordinary employments.

"In Dr. Woodville's publication on the Cow Pox, I notice an extraordinary fact. He says that the generality of his patients had pustules. It certainly appears extremely extraordinary that in all my Cases there never was but one pustule, which appeared on a patient's elbow on the inoculated arm, and maturated. It appeared exactly like that on the incised part.

"The whole of my observations, founded, as it appears, on an extensive experience, leads me to these obvious conclusions; that those Cases which have been or may be adduced against the preventive powers of the Cow Pox, could not have been those of the true kind, since it must appear to be absolutely impossible that I should have succeeded in such a number of Cases without a single exception, if such a preventive power did not exist. I cannot entertain a doubt that the inoculated Cow Pox must quickly supersede that of Small Pox. If the many important advantages which must result from the new practice are duly considered, we may reasonably infer that public benefit, the sure test of the real merit of discoveries, will render it generally extensive.

"To you, Sir, as the discoverer of this highly-beneficial practice, mankind are under the highest obligations. As a private individual, I participate in the general feeling; more particularly as you have afforded me an opportunity of noticing the effects of a singular disease, and of viewing the progress of the most curious experiment that ever was recorded in the History of Physiology.

"I remain, Dear Sir, &c.,

"JOSEPH H. MARSHALL.

"P.S.—I should have observed, that of the patients I inoculated and enumerated in my letter, one hundred and twenty-seven were infected with the matter you sent me from the London cow. I discovered no dissimilarity of symptoms in these cases, from those which I inoculated from matter procured in this county. No pustules have occurred, except in one or two cases, where a single one appeared on the inoculated arm. No difference was apparent in the local inflammation. There was no suspension of ordinary employment among the labouring people, nor was any medicine required.

"I have frequently inoculated one or two in a family, and the remaining part of it some few weeks afterwards. The uninfected have slept with the infected during the whole course of the disease without feeling it; so that I am fully convinced the disease cannot be taken but by actual contact with the matter.

"A curious fact has lately fallen under my observation, on which I leave you to comment.

"I visited a patient with the confluent Small Pox, and charged a lancet with some of the matter. Two days afterwards I was desired to inoculate a woman and four children with the Cow Pox, and I inadvertently took the vaccine matter on the same lancet which was before charged with that of Small Pox. In three days I discovered the mistake, and fully expected that my five patients would be infected with Small Pox; but I was agreeably surprised to find the disease to be the genuine Cow Pox, which proceeded without deviating in any particular from my former cases. I afterwards inoculated these patients with variolous matter, but all of them resisted its action.

"I omitted mentioning another great advantage that now occurs to me in the inoculated Cow Pox; I mean the safety with which pregnant women may have the disease communicated to them. I have inoculated a great number of females in that situation, and never observed their cases to differ in any respect from those of my other patients. Indeed the disease is so mild, that it seems as if it might at all times be communicated with the most perfect safety."

I shall here take the opportunity of thanking Dr. Marshall and those other gentlemen who have obligingly presented me with the result of their inoculations; but, as they all agree in the same point as that given in the above communication, namely, the security of the patient from the effects of the Small Pox after the Cow Pox, their perusal, I presume, would afford 'us'[1] satisfaction that has not been amply given already. Particular occurrences I shall of course detail. Some of my correspondents have mentioned the appearance of Small Pox-like eruptions at the commencement of their inoculations; but in these cases the matter was derived from the original stock at the Small Pox Hospital.

I have myself inoculated a very considerable number from the matter produced by Dr. Marshall's patients, originating in the London cow, without observing pustules of any kind, and have dispersed it among others who have used it with a similar effect. From this source, Mr. H. Jenner informs me, he has inoculated above an hundred patients without observing eruptions. Whether the nature of the virus will undergo any change from being farther removed from its original source, in passing successively from one person to another, time alone can determine. That which I am now employing has been in use near eight months, and not the least change is perceptible in its mode of action either locally or constitutionally. There is therefore every reason to expect that its effects will remain unaltered, and that we shall not be under the necessity of seeking fresh supplies from the cow.

The following observations were obligingly sent me by Mr. Tierny, Assistant-Surgeon to the South Gloucester Regiment of Militia, to whom I am indebted for a former Report on this subject:

"I inoculated with the Cow Pox matter, from the 11th to the latter part of April, twenty-five persons, including women and children. Some on the 11th were inoculated with the matter Mr. Shrapnell (Surgeon to the Regiment) had from you, the others with matter taken from these. The progress of the puncture was accurately observed, and its appearance seemed to differ from the Small Pox in having less inflammation around its basis on the first days, that is, from the third to the seventh; but after this the inflammation increased, extending on the tenth or eleventh day to a circle of an inch and a half from its centre, and threatening very sore arms; but this, I am happy to say, was not the case; for, by applying mercurial ointment to the inflamed part, which was

[1] ["*no*"?—E.M.C.]

repeated daily until the inflammation went off, the arm got well without any further application or trouble. The constitutional symptoms which appeared on the eighth or ninth day after inoculation scarcely deserved the name of disease, as they were so slight as to be barely perceptible, except that I could connect a slight headache and languor with a stiffness and rather painful sensation in the axilla. This latter symptom was the most striking; it remained from twelve to forty-eight hours. In no case did I observe the smallest pustule, or even discolouration of the skin like an incipient pustule, except about the part where the virus had been applied.

"After all these symptoms had subsided, and the arms were well, I inoculated four of this number with variolous matter taken from a patient in another regiment. In each of these it was inserted several times under the cuticle, producing slight inflammation on the second or third day, and always disappearing before the fifth or sixth; except in one who had the Cow Pox in Gloucestershire before he joined us, and who also received it at this time by inoculation. In this man the puncture inflamed, and his arm was much sorer than from the insertion of the Cow Pox virus; but there was no pain in the axilla, nor could any constitutional affection be observed.

"I have only to add, that I am now fully satisfied of the efficacy of the Cow Pox in preventing the appearance of the Small Pox, and that it is a most happy and salutary substitute for it.

"I remain, etc.,

"M. J. Tierny."

Although the susceptibility of the virus of the Cow Pox is for the most part lost in those who have had the Small Pox, yet in some constitutions it is only partially destroyed, and in others it does not appear to be in the least diminished.

By far the greater number on whom trials were made resisted it entirely; yet I found some on whose arms the pustule, from inoculation, was formed completely, but without producing the common efflorescent blush around it, or any constitutional illness; while others have had the disease in the most perfect manner. A case of the latter kind having been presented to me by Mr. Fewster, Surgeon, of Thornbury, I shall insert it.

"Three children were inoculated with the vaccine matter you obligingly sent me. On calling to look at their arms three days after, I was told that John Hodges, one of the three, had been inoculated with the Small Pox when a year old, and that he had a full burthen, of which his face produced plentiful marks, a circumstance I was not before made acquainted with. On the sixth day the arm of this boy appeared as if inoculated with variolous matter, but the pustule was rather more elevated. On the ninth day he complained of violent pain in his head and back, accompanied with vomiting and much fever. The next day he was very well, and went to work as usual. The punctured part began to spread, and there was the areola around the inoculated part to a considerable extent.

"As this is contrary to an assertion made in the *Medical and Physical Jounal*, No. 8, I thought it right to give you this information, and remain,

"Dear Sir, etc.,
"J. Fewster."

It appears then that the animal economy, with regard to the action of this virus, is under the same laws as it is with respect to the variolous virus, after previously feeling its influence, as far as comparisons can be made between the two diseases.

Some striking instances of the power of the Cow Pox in suspending the progress of the Small Pox, after the patients had been several days casually exposed to the infection, have been laid before me by Mr. Lyford, surgeon, of Winchester, and my nephew, the Rev. G. C. Jenner. Mr. Lyford, after giving an account of his extensive and successful practice in the vaccine inoculation in Hampshire, writes as follows:

"The following Case occurred to me a short time since, and may probably be worth your notice. I was sent for to a patient with the Small Pox, and on inquiry found that, five days previous to my seeing him, the eruption began to appear. During the whole of this time, two children, who had not had the Small Pox, were constantly in the room with their father, and frequently on the bed with him. The mother consulted me on the propriety of inoculating them, but objected to my taking the matter from their father, as he was subject to erysipelas. I advised her by all means to have them inoculated at that time, as I could not procure any variolous matter elsewhere. However, they were inoculated with vaccine matter; but I cannot say I flatter myself with its proving successful, as they had previously been so long, and still continued to be, exposed to the variolous infection. Notwithstanding this, I was agreeably surprised to find the vaccine disease advance and go through its regular course; and, if I may be allowed the expression, to the total extinction of the Small Pox."

Mr. Jenner's Cases were not less satisfactory. He writes as follows:

"A son of Thomas Stinchcomb, of Woodford, near Berkeley, was infected with the natural Small Pox at Bristol, and came home to his father's cottage. Four days after the eruptions had appeared upon the boy, the family (none of which had ever had the Small Pox), consisting of the father, mother, and five children, were inoculated with vaccine virus. On the arm of the mother it failed to produce the least effect, and she of course had the Small Pox;* but the rest of the family had the Cow Pox in the usual mild way, and were not affected with the Small Pox, although they were in the same room, and the children slept in the same bed with their brother, who was confined to it with the natural Small Pox; and subsequently with their mother.

"I attended this family with my brother, Mr. H. Jenner."

The following cases are of too singular a nature to remain unnoticed.

Miss R——, a young lady about five years old, was seized, on the evening of the eighth day after inoculation with vaccine virus, with such symptoms as commonly denote the accession of violent fever. Her throat was also a little sore, and there were some uneasy sensations about the muscles of the neck. The day following a rash was perceptible on her face and neck, so much resembling the efflorescence of the *Scarlatina Anginosa*, that I was induced to ask whether Miss R—— had been exposed to the contagion of that disease. An answer in the affirmative, and the rapid spreading of the redness over the skin, at once relieved me from much anxiety respecting the nature of the malady, which went through its course in the ordinary way, but not without symptoms which were alarming both to myself and Mr. Lyford, who attended with me. There was no apparent deviation in the ordinary progress of the pustule to a state of maturity, from what we see in general; yet there was a total suspension of the *Areola*, or florid discolouration around it, until the *Scarlatina* had retired from the constitution. As soon as the patient was freed from this disease, this appearance advanced in the usual way.†

* Under similar circumstances, I think it would be advisable to insert the matter into each arm, which would be more likely to insure the success of the matter.—E. J.

† I witnessed a similar fact in a case of Measles.[1] The pustule from the Cow Pock virus advanced to maturity, while the Measles existed in the constitution, but no *efflorescence* appeared around it until the measles had ceased to exert its influence.

[1] See page 188.

The Case of Miss H—— R—— is not less interesting than that of her sister above related. She was exposed to the contagion of the *Scarlatina* at the same time, and sickened almost at the same hour. The symptoms continued severe about twelve hours, when the Scarlatine rash showed itself faintly upon her face, and partly upon her neck. After remaining two or three hours it suddenly disappeared, and she became perfectly free from every complaint. My surprise at this sudden transition from extreme sickness to health, in great measure ceased, when I observed that the inoculated pustule had occasioned, in this case, the common efflorescent appearance around it, and that as it approached the centre, it was nearly in an erysipelatous state. But the most remarkable part of this history is, that on the fourth day afterwards, as soon as the efflorescence began to die away upon the arm, and the pustule to dry up, the *Scarlatina* again appeared, her throat became sore, the rash spread all over her. She went fairly through the disease, with its common symptoms.

That these were actually Cases of *Scarlatina*, was rendered certain by two servants in the family falling ill at the same time with the distemper, who had been exposed to the infection with the young ladies.

Some there are who suppose the security from the Small Pox obtained through the Cow Pox will be of a temporary nature only. This supposition is refuted, not only by analogy with respect to the habits of diseases of a similar nature, but by incontrovertible facts, which appear in great numbers against it. To those already adduced in the former part of my first Treatise,* many more might be added were it deemed necessary; but among the Cases I refer to, one will be found of a person who had the Cow Pox fifty-three years before the effect of the Small Pox was tried upon him. As he completely resisted it, the intervening period I conceive must necessarily satisfy any reasonable mind. Should further evidence be thought necessary, I shall observe, that among the Cases presented to me by Mr. Fry, Mr. Darke, Mr. Tierny, Mr. H. Jenner, and others, there were many whom they inoculated ineffectually with variolous matter, who had gone through the Cow Pox many years before this trial was made.

It has been imagined that the Cow Pox is capable of being communicated from one person to another by effluvia without the intervention of inoculation. My experiments, made with the design of ascertaining this important point, all tend to establish

* See pp. 10, 11, 12, 15, etc.

my original position, that it is not infectious, except by contact. I have never hesitated to suffer those on whose arms there were pustules exhaling the effluvia, from associating or even sleeping with others who never had experienced either the Cow Pox or the Small Pox. And further, I have repeatedly, among children, caused the uninfected to breathe over the inoculated vaccine pustules during their whole progress; yet these experiments were tried without the least effect. However, to submit a matter so important to a still further scrutiny, I desired Mr. H. Jenner to make any further experiments which might strike him as most likely to establish or refute what had been advanced on this subject. He has since informed me, "that he inoculated children at the breast, whose mothers had not gone through either the Small Pox or the Cow Pox; that he had inoculated mothers whose sucking infants had never undergone either of these diseases; that the effluvia from the inoculated pustules, in either case, had been inhaled from day to day during the whole progress of their maturation, and that there was not the least perceptible effect from these exposures. One woman he inoculated about a week previous to her *accouchement*, that her infant might be the more fully and conveniently exposed to the pustule; but, as in the former instances, no infection was given, although the child frequently slept on the arm of its mother, with its nostrils and mouth exposed to the pustule in the fullest state of maturity. In a word, is it not impossible for the Cow Pox, whose *only* manifestation appears to consist in the pustules *created by contact*, to produce *itself* by effluvia?

In the course of a late inoculation, I observed an appearance which it may be proper here to relate. The punctured part on a boy's arm (who was inoculated with fresh limpid virus) on the the sixth day, instead of shewing a beginning vesicle, which is usual in the Cow Pox at that period, was encrusted over with a rugged amber-coloured scab. The scab continued to spread and increase in thickness for some days, when at its edges a vesicated ring appeared, and the disease went through its ordinary course, the boy having had soreness in the axilla, and some slight indisposition. With the fluid matter taken from his arm, five persons were inoculated. In one it took no effect. In another it produced a perfect pustule without any deviation from the common appearance; but in the other three the progress of the inflammation was exactly similar to the instance which afforded the virus for their inoculation; there was a creeping scab of a loose texture, and subsequently the formation of limpid fluid at its edges. As these people were all employed in laborious exercises, it is possible that these anomalous appearances might owe their origin to the friction of the clothes on the newly-inflamed part of the arm. I have not yet had an opportunity of exposing them to the Small Pox.

In the early part of this Inquiry I felt far more anxious respecting the inflammation of the inoculated arm than at present; yet that this affection will go on to a greater extent than could be wished, is a circumstance sometimes to be expected. As this can be checked, or even entirely subdued, by very simple means, I see no reason why the patient should feel an uneasy hour, because an application may not be absolutely necessary. About the tenth or eleventh day, if the pustule has proceeded regularly, the appearance of the arm will almost to a certainty indicate whether this is to be expected or not. Should it happen, nothing more need be done than to apply a single drop of the *Aqua Lythargyr. Acetati* * upon the pustule, and having suffered it to remain two or three minutes, to cover the efflorescence surrounding the pustule with a piece of linen dipped in the *Aqua Lythargyr. Compos.*† The former may be repeated twice or thrice during the day; the latter as often as it may feel agreeable to the patient.

When the scab is prematurely rubbed off (a circumstance not unfrequent among children and working people), the application of a little *Aqua Lythargyri Acet.* to the part immediately coagulates the surface, which supplies its place, and prevents a sore.

In my former Treatises on this subject, I have remarked that the human constitution frequently retains its susceptibility of the Small Pox contagion (both from effluvia and contact) after previously feeling its influence. In further corroboration of this declaration, many facts have been communicated to me by various correspondents. I shall select one of them.

"Dear Sir,

"Society at large must I think feel much indebted to you for your *Inquiries and Observations on the Nature and Effects of the Variolæ Vaccinæ*, &c., &c. As I conceive what I am now about to communicate to be of some importance, I imagine it cannot be uninteresting to you, especially as it will serve to corroborate your assertion of the susceptibility of the human system

---

* Extract of Saturn.

† Goulard Water. For further information on this subject see the first *Treatise on the Var. Vac.*, Dr. Marshall's Letters, etc.

of the variolous contagion, although it has previously been made sensible of its action. In November 1793, I was desired to inoculate a person with the Small Pox. I took the variolous matter from a child under the disease in the natural way, who had a large burden of distinct pustules. The mother of the child being desirous of seeing my method of communicating the disease by inoculation, after having opened a pustule, I introduced the point of my lancet in the usual way on the back part of my own hand, and thought no more of it until I felt a sensation in the part, which reminded me of the transaction. This happened upon the third day; on the fourth there were all the appearances common to inoculation, at which I was not at all surprised; nor did I feel myself uneasy, upon perceiving the inflammation continue to increase to the sixth and seventh day, accompanied with a very small quantity of fluid, repeated experiments having taught me it might happen so with persons who had undergone the disease, and yet would escape any constitutional affection: but I was not so fortunate; for on the eighth day I was seized with all the symptoms of the eruptive fever, but in a much more violent degree than when I was before inoculated, which was about eighteen years previous to this, when I had a considerable number of pustules. I must confess I was now greatly alarmed, although I had been much engaged in the Small Pox, having at different times inoculated not less than two thousand persons. I was convinced my present indisposition proceeded from the insertion of the variolous matter, and therefore anxiously looked for an eruption. On the tenth day I felt a very unpleasant sensation of stiffness, and heat on each side of my face near my ear, and the fever began to decline. The affection in my face soon terminated in three or four pustules attended with inflammation, but which did not maturate, and I was presently well.

"I remain, Dear Sir, etc.,

"THOMAS MILES."

This Inquiry is not now so much in its infancy as to restrain me from speaking more positively than formerly on the important point of Scrophula, as connected with the Small Pox.

Every practitioner in medicine, who has extensively inoculated with the Small Pox, or has attended many of those who have had the distemper in the natural way, must acknowledge that he has frequently seen scrophulous affections, in some form or another, sometimes rather quickly showing themselves after the recovery of the patients. Conceiving this fact to be admitted, as I presume it must be by all who have carefully attended to the subject, may I not ask whether it does not appear probable that the general introduction of the Small Pox into Europe has not been among the most conducive means in exciting that formidable foe to health? Having attentively watched the effects of the Cow Pox in this respect, I am happy in being able to declare, that the disease does not appear to have the least tendency to produce this destructive malady.

The scepticism that appeared even among the most enlightened of medical men, when my sentiments on the important subject of the Cow Pox were first promulgated, was highly laudable. To have admitted the truth of a doctrine, at once so novel and so unlike any thing that had ever appeared in the Annals of Medicine, without the test of the most rigid scrutiny, would have bordered upon temerity; but now, when that scrutiny has taken place, not only among ourselves, but in the first professional circles in Europe, and when it has been uniformly found in such abundant instances, that the human frame, when once it has felt the influence of the genuine Cow Pox in the way that has been described, is never afterwards, at any period of its existence, assailable by the Small Pox, may I not with perfect confidence congratulate my country and society at large on their beholding, in the mild form of the Cow Pox, an antidote that is capable of extirpating from the earth a disease which is every hour devouring its victims; a disease that has ever been considered as the severest scourge of the human race?

FINIS.

THE ORIGIN OF THE VACCINE INOCULATION.

By EDWARD JENNER, M.D., F.R.S., &c.

LONDON:

PRINTED BY D. N. SHURY, BERWICK STREET, SOHO.

1801.

I AM induced to give the History of the Origin of Vaccine Inoculation from my frequently observing that those who only consider the subject cursorily, confound the casual Cow Pox with the disease when excited by inoculation.

EDWARD JENNER.

BOND STREET,
May 6th, 1801.

ON

THE ORIGIN

OF THE

VACCINE INOCULATION.

MY inquiry into the nature of Cow Pox commenced upwards of twenty-five years ago. My attention to this singular disease was first excited by observing, that among those whom in the country I was frequently called upon to inoculate, many resisted every effort to give them the Small Pox. These patients I found had undergone a disease they called the Cow Pox, contracted by milking cows affected with a peculiar eruption on their teats. On inquiry, it appeared that it had been known among the dairies time immemorial, and that a vague opinion prevailed that it was a preventive of the Small Pox.

This opinion I found was, comparatively, new among them; for all the older farmers declared that they had no such idea in their early days—a circumstance that seemed easily to be accounted for, from my knowing that the common people were very rarely inoculated for the Small Pox, till that practice was rendered general by the improved method introduced by the Suttons. So that the working people in the dairies were seldom put to the test of the preventive powers of the Cow Pox.

In the course of the investigation of this subject, which, like all others of a complex and intricate nature, presented many difficulties, I found that some of those *who seemed to have undergone the Cow Pox*, nevertheless, on inoculation with the Small Pox, felt its influence just the same as if no disease had been communicated to them by the cow. This occurrence led me to inquire among the medical practitioners in the country around me, who all agreed in this sentiment, that the Cow Pox was not to be relied upon as a certain preventive of the Small Pox. This for a while damped, but did not extinguish my ardour; for as

I proceeded, I had the satisfaction to learn that the cow was subject to some varieties of spontaneous eruptions upon her teats; that they were all capable of communicating sores to the hands of the milkers; and that whatever sore was derived from this animal, was called in the dairy the Cow Pox.

Thus, I surmounted a great obstacle, and in consequence, was led to form a distinction between these diseases, one of which only I have denominated the *true*, the others the *spurious* Cow Pox, as they possess no specific power over the constitution.

This impediment to my progress was not long removed, before another, of far greater magnitude in its appearances, started up. There were not wanting instances to prove, that when the true Cow Pox broke out among the cattle at a dairy, a person who had milked an infected animal, and had thereby apparently gone through the disease in common with others, was liable to receive the Small Pox afterwards. This, like the former obstacle, gave a painful check to my fond and aspiring hopes; but reflecting that the operations of nature are generally uniform, and that it was not probable the human constitution (having undergone the Cow Pox) should in some instances be perfectly shielded from the Small Pox, and in many others remain unprotected, I resumed my labours with redoubled ardour.

The result was fortunate; for I now discovered that the virus of Cow Pox was liable to undergo progressive changes, from the same causes precisely as that of Small Pox, and that when it was applied to the human skin in its degenerated state, it would produce the ulcerative effects in as great a degree as when it was not decomposed, and sometimes far greater; but having lost its *specific properties*, it was incapable of producing that change upon the human frame which is requisite to render it unsusceptible of the variolous contagion; so that it became evident a person might milk a cow one day, and having caught the disease, be for ever secure; while another person milking the same cow the next day, might feel the influence of the virus in such a way as to produce a sore or sores, and in consequence of this might experience an indisposition to a considerable extent; yet, as has been observed, the specific quality being lost, the constitution would receive no peculiar impression.

Here the close analogy between the virus of Small Pox and of the Cow Pox becomes remarkably conspicuous; since the former, when taken from a recent pustule, and immediately used, gives the perfect Small Pox to the person on whom it is inoculated; but when taken in a far advanced stage of the disease, or when (although taken early), previously to its insertion, it be exposed to such agents as, according to the established laws of nature, cause its decomposition, it can no longer be relied on as effectual. This observation will fully explain the source of those errors which have been committed by many inoculators of the Cow Pox. Conceiving the whole process to be so extremely simple as not to admit of a mistake, they have been heedless about the state of the vaccine virus; and finding it limpid, as part of it will be, even in an advanced stage of the pustule, when the greater portion has been converted into a scab, they have felt an improper confidence, and sometimes mistaken a spurious pustule, which the vaccine fluid in this state is capable of exciting, for that which possesses the perfect character.

During the investigation of the casual Cow Pox, I was struck with the idea that it might be practicable to propagate the disease by inoculation, after the manner of the Small Pox, first from the Cow, and finally from one human being to another. I anxiously waited some time for an opportunity of putting this theory to the test. At length the period arrived. The first experiment was made upon a lad of the name of Phipps, in whose arm a little vaccine virus was inserted, taken from the hand of a young woman, who had been accidentally infected by a cow. Notwithstanding the resemblance which the pustule thus excited on the boy's arm bore to variolous inoculation, yet as the indisposition attending it was barely perceptible, I could scarcely persuade myself the patient was secure from the Small Pox. However, on his being inoculated some months afterwards, it proved that he was secure.* This case inspired me with confidence, and as soon as I could again furnish myself with virus from the cow, I made an arrangement for a series of inoculations. A number of children were inoculated in succession, one from the other; and after several months had elapsed, they were exposed to the infection of the Small Pox; some by inoculation, others by variolous effluvia, and some in both ways; but they all resisted it. The result of these trials gradually led me into a wider field of experiment, which I went over not only with great attention, but with painful solicitude. This became universally known through a treatise published in June 1798. The result of my further experience was also brought forward in subsequent publications in the two succeeding years, 1799 and 1800. The distrust and scepticism

* This boy was inoculated nearly at the expiration of five years afterwards with variolous matter, but no other effect was produced beyond a local inflammation around the punctured part of the arm.

which naturally arose in the minds of medical men, on my first announcing so unexpected a discovery, has now nearly disappeared. Many hundreds of them, from actual experience, have given their attestations that the inoculated Cow Pox proves a perfect security against the Small Pox; and I shall probably be within compass if I say, thousands are ready to follow their example; for the scope that this inoculation has now taken is immense. A hundred thousand persons, upon the smallest computation, have been inoculated in these realms. The numbers who have partaken of its benefits throughout Europe and other parts of the globe are incalculable; and it now becomes too manifest to admit of controversy, that the annihilation of the Small Pox, the most dreadful scourge of the human species, must be the final result of this practice.

AN ACCOUNT OF SOME EXPERIMENTS ON THE ORIGIN OF THE COW-POX.

By JOHN G. LOY, M.D.

Whitby:
PRINTED BY THOMAS WEBSTER.

SOLD BY G. PHILLIPS, GEORGE YARD, LOMBARD STREET, LONDON;
WILSON AND SPENCE, YORK; AND BY THE BOOKSELLERS IN WHITBY.

1801.

TO

EDWARD JENNER, M.D., F.R.S., F.L.S., &c.

SIR,

As an acknowledgment of the high sense of gratitude I entertain towards you for the introduction of a discovery which has already produced extensive benefits to mankind, permit me to present you with the following pages, devoted to a subject which cannot but be particularly interesting to you.

I am, Sir, with the utmost respect,

Your most obedient servant,

JOHN G. LOY.

AISLABY,

October 13*th*, 1801.

AN ACCOUNT OF SOME EXPERIMENTS

ON THE

ORIGIN OF THE COW-POX.

AFTER the publication of Dr. Woodville's Reports, wherein he mentions several unsuccessful attempts made, both by himself and Mr. Coleman, Professor at the Veterinary College, to produce the Cow-pox from inoculation with the matter of Grease upon the udder or teats of the cow, Dr. Jenner's opinion, concerning the origin of this disease, was pretty generally considered fallacious; and the experiments of Mr. Simmons tended still further to refute it.

The experiments, however, of which I shall give an account, were attended with a result very different from that of the experiments related by Dr. Woodville or Mr. Simmons; but, before entering upon them, it is proper to mention the circumstances which gave rise to them.

Early in the spring of the year 1801, Mr. Loy, Surgeon at Pickering, in Yorkshire, had an opportunity of observing a disease which had been before noticed in the western counties only, where it is supposed to originate from the Grease in horses.

His first patient was a farrier, who applied to him with an eruption on his hands, which was composed of distinct pustules containing a thin fluid, and surrounded by an inflamed ring. The vesicles had an appearance similar to those arising from a burn; but were all regularly circumscribed, and a small dark speck could be discovered in the middle of each, which appeared to be the remains of some slight injury. . . . This person had been in the custom of dressing the heels of a horse affected with the Grease, and he had never been subject to any such affection previous to that employment. He had no general fever, and had had the small-pox.

The origin of this person's complaint was rendered more

probable, by the appearance of the following, which was detected by the same gentleman.

A young man, a butcher at Middleton, near Pickering, was affected with painful sores on both his hands, particularly about the roots of the nails. These sores in a few days became inflamed, and a vesicle formed upon each. Soon after the appearance of the vesicles, a number of red painful lines, which appeared to be inflamed lymphatics, extended from the pustules to the arm-pit, where a tumor formed; he had also a pustule, of the same appearance as those on his hands, upon one eyebrow, which, he said, had been affected with an itching, inducing him frequently to scratch it; and the pustule had no doubt been communicated in that manner from his fingers. He had a considerable degree of fever, which continued obstinate till the absorption from the pustules was prevented by destroying them with caustic, when the tumor in the axilla also dispersed. This patient, like the former, had been for some time employed in applying remedies to the heels of a horse affected with the grease, and was continuing to do so at the time he begun to be indisposed. He had never undergone the small-pox.

In order to satisfy himself whether or not this disease could be communicated by inoculation, he took a quantity of matter from the pustules of the last patient, and inserted it into the arm of his brother, who had also never had the small-pox. He gave me the following account of the effects of the inoculation :—

"In a few days some degree of inflammation appeared, and on the eighth day a vesicle formed; my patient had now some slight feverish symptoms, which continued a day or two.

"This disease had exactly the appearances of the genuine Cow-pox, and I intended to have tried the effect of the small-pox virus, had not the fears of the boy's parents prevented me."

EXPERIMENT I.

At the time that Mr. Loy performed this experiment, I procured matter from a pustule on the hand of the same patient, with a lancet which had never before been used, part of which I inserted the next day into the udder of a cow, reserving the remainder for trial upon the human subject. For five days the inoculated place offered no appearances, and was not again inspected till the ninth day, when a vesicle, surrounded by a rose-coloured rim, appeared. The udder, to a considerable distance from the wound, was hard, and so painful that the animal would scarcely suffer it to be handled. The vesication continued to spread for several days, but at length a scab formed, and the place healed without any remedy.

EXPERIMENT II.

Matter procured from the udder of the cow on the ninth day of her disease was inserted into a child's arm. The progress of the inoculation was closely watched, and the inflammation, vesication, and scabbing were found to correspond so exactly with those appearances in mild cases of the genuine Cow-pox, that they admitted only of a similar description. On the sixth day of this disease, the child was inoculated with the small-pox virus. The wound into which the small-pox matter was inserted, seemed to be rather inflamed on the third day; but in a few days more it healed, and the child continued free from indisposition.

EXPERIMENT III.

I now inoculated a child on its arm with the remainder of the matter taken from Mr. Loy's patient. On the third day the inoculated part rose above the level of the neighbouring skin ; on the sixth day it was surrounded by a dullish inflammation, and its edges were more elevated than the centre, which on the eighth day presented a vesicle containing a limpid fluid, which soon burst from the vesicle, and on the fourteenth day was converted into a firm scab of a dark brown appearance. As soon as an opportunity offered, this child was carefully inoculated with the matter of small-pox, which produced no effect.

EXPERIMENT IV.

Some of the thin limpid matter that issued from a sore in the heel of a horse affected with the Grease, was inserted, by a perfectly clean lancet, immediately after its being procured, into the teat of a cow. On the fifth day the wound appeared rather elevated, and a faintish redness surrounded it. In a few days a vesicle formed, containing a large quantity of watery fluid, and of a purple tinge. Though the inoculated part was tumefied and painful, the animal did not seem otherwise diseased.

EXPERIMENT V.

A quantity of the limpid matter obtained from the teat of this cow was inserted into the arm of a child. On the third and fourth days the incision appeared without any evident signs of having received the infection, but on the sixth day a considerable degree of redness surrounded the wound, and a vesicle was formed on the ninth day, when the child was inoculated with the small-pox virus in three different places, and in such a manner that there could not be the least doubt of communicating the infection, was the constitution capable of receiving it. The child, however, continued free from any topical or general symptoms of the small-pox.

EXPERIMENT VI.

Some Grease matter, obtained from the same horse, was inserted in the arm of a child. On the third day a small degree of inflammation surrounded the wound. On the fourth the inoculated place was much elevated, and a vesicle, of a purple colour, was formed on the fifth day: on the sixth and seventh the vesicle increased, and the inflammation extended, and became of a deeper colour; on the same day a chilliness came on, attended with nausea and some vomiting. These were soon succeeded by increased heat, pain in the head, and a frequency of breathing; the pulse was very frequent, and the tongue was covered with a white crust. When in bed, the child was much disposed to sweat. By the use of some medicines, and exposure to cool air, the feverish symptoms soon abated, and disappeared entirely on the ninth day. On the sixth day small-pox matter was inserted into the same arm in which the matter of Grease had been placed, but at a considerable distance from it. On the fourth and fifth days of the small-pox inoculation some redness appeared about the wound, and on the sixth a small vesicle. The inflammation now decreased, and on the ninth day the vesicle was converted into a scab.

EXPERIMENT VII.

On the sixth day of the Grease inoculation, and previous to the insertion of the small-pox virus, matter was procured from this child, and five others were inoculated with it. From the remoteness of their situation I had not an opportunity of seeing them till the tenth day of the inoculation; on that day an extensive erysipelatous efflorescence surrounded the vesicles, which were now beginning to dry, but still contained a considerable quantity of limpid matter. On the tenth day they were all inoculated for the small-pox in the arms free from the former inoculation. Nothing appeared from the insertion of the variolous matter except a very small degree of inflammation, which vanished on the fifth day.

From these experiments it appears, . . . That a disease excited in the human body from casual infection of the Grease in the horse is capable of being communicated to the cow by inoculation.

And in this manner of inoculation we have imitated exactly the process by which Dr. Jenner supposes the genuine Cow-pox to be produced. But it was not till after several trials that I was convinced the infection of the Grease could be made to operate upon the cow without having been previously made to pass the action of the human system; for I made several unsuccessful attempts to produce any appearances of the Cow-pox by the application of Grease matter as obtained directly from the heels of the horse. . . . Matter taken from three different horses in the Grease, and at different times of the disease, did not produce, when inserted into the teats or udder of the cow, the least appearance of the Cow-pox. To make a fair trial, various cows were subjected to the experiment, which always failed. The same ill success attended a few trials upon the human subject. At length, however, I had the good fortune to meet with one horse from whose heels I procured the matter of Grease in a more limpid state than that obtained from any of the others, at about the fourteenth day of the disease, and a week from the first appearance of the discharge. The matter from this horse produced the disease in experiments IV. and VI., and also in three cows whose cases I have not particularised, as the appearances were similar to experiment IV., and as no further trials were made from them.

This fact induces me to suspect, that two kinds of Grease exist, differing from each other in the power of giving disease to the human or brute animal; and there is another circumstance which renders this supposition probable. The horses that communicated the infection to their dressers were affected with a general, as well as a topical disease. The animals, at the commencement of their disease, were evidently in a feverish state, from which they were relieved as soon as the complaint appeared at their heels, and an eruption upon the skin. The horse, too, from whom the infectious matter was procured for inoculation, had a considerable indisposition, previous to the disease at his heels, which was attended, as in the others, with an eruption over the greatest part of his body; but those that did not communicate the disease at all, had a local affection only. From this, perhaps, may be explained, the want of success attending the experiments of the gentlemen I have mentioned. The most curious fact that these experiments have discovered, is the property which the matter of Grease possesses, of communicating a disease to the human body which will prevent the action of the small-pox, whether it be used genuine from its original source, or be made to pass a more circuitous route. Thus we have seen it exert this quality, when acted upon by the human and vaccine systems, separately.

We have seen it possess the same power when obtained directly from the heels of the horse.

The opinion, however, which I entertain of the anti-variolous nature of genuine Grease matter, is founded only upon a single experiment; but the result which followed has made me confident of the success of future trials.

Along with one case of casual infection of the Grease, where the small-pox was completely resisted, Dr. Jenner has given two others in which the action of the variolous contagion had considerable effect.

It certainly appears odd that the matter of Grease should exert a specific action upon one person and not upon another; but this want of uniformity in its effects is much more likely to have been produced by the manner of its application than by the irregular nature of the matter itself. The matter issuing from the heels of horses in the Grease is soon converted into a crust, adhering firmly to the hair and epidermis. Under this crust the subsequent fluid is collected till it bursts through it, at a place perhaps considerably distant from its source. In this situation it may undergo those changes inducible by heat and stagnation, and thus be deprived of its original properties before it can be applied to the hands of the dresser; to whom it may sometimes communicate an imperfect disease, sometimes none at all. Also, though a person may have received the infection from genuine matter, by dressing the greased heels of a horse, his hands may be exposed to accidents, from his employment, which may either produce too much inflammation, or burst the vesicles before the commencement of absorption, and thus prevent the infection from entering the system. It is probable that both these circumstances have produced inefficient inoculations for the cow-pox. I believe, however, that whoever may be induced to inoculate with the genuine Grease virus, with attention, will have an opportunity of observing the effects I have mentioned.

The Grease matter which I successfully employed in my experiments, was procured as near as possible to the sore from whence it issued; it was in a perfectly limpid state; and in this respect differed from that used by Mr. Simmons, which was brownish coloured, and ichorous.

I am fully satisfied, that when the disease of Grease has continued long in the horse, it will not give the infection; for matter procured from the horse with the infectious disease, did not communicate the infection, when the disease had continued above a month, and when the appearance and consistence of the matter were changed.

The experiments made for the purpose of proving the origin of the Cow-pox, although not numerous, must be deemed perfectly decisive, as also those made to ascertain whether the Grease matter, after undergoing the action of the human constitution, possessed the same properties as that which had passed the action of the vaccine system.

It is of some consequence to remark the differences observable in these experiments. They consist chiefly in the degree of topical inflammation and general fever; in the colour of the vesicle; and the time of appearance of the vesicle.

The Grease matter seems to produce the greatest and earliest commotion in the human system, when used from its original source, viz., the heels of the horse; for from experiment VI. a disease of considerable violence was produced.

On the vaccine constitution, it does not appear to operate with much violence, when only inserted at one place, nor to produce a disease communicable by effluvia; for, although the cows that had the experiments performed on them, were in the same house with a number of others, the disease did not spread to any of them.

The matter of Grease appears to act with greater mildness, and produce later appearances, when regenerated either in the cow or the human subject; for in experiments I., II., III., and V. the appearances presented later and more mildly than in the others.

In experiments IV. and VI. the purple tinge presented; but it did not appear either in the human or brute animal infected with matter which had been once removed from the horse, whether through the medium of the cow, or the human body.

The vesicle appears earlier from the insertion of pure Grease matter. In experiment VI. the vesicle showed itself as early as the fifth day.

From the two cases of casual infection of the Grease above related, it seems probable, that the small-pox has considerable influence in preventing the action of Grease virus upon the system. The first person had undergone the small-pox, and had the disease from the Grease in a partial manner only: . . . the second, who had not previously had the small-pox, had a general indisposition.

AN

EXAMINATION

OF

THAT PART OF THE EVIDENCE RELATIVE TO

COW-POX,

WHICH WAS DELIVERED TO THE COMMITTEE OF

The House of Commons,

BY TWO OF THE

SURGEONS OF ST. THOMAS'S HOSPITAL.

To which is added

A LETTER TO THE AUTHOR

FROM

JOHN BIRCH, ESQ.,

Surgeon Extraordinary to His Royal Highness the Prince of Wales, &c., &c.

THE SECOND EDITION.

London:

PRINTED FOR J. CALLOW, MEDICAL BOOKSELLER,

CROWN COURT, PRINCES STREET, SOHO; AND

HARRIS, IN ST. PAUL'S CHURCH YARD,

BY W. SMITH AND SON, NO. 49, KING STREET, SEVEN DIALS

1805.

PREFACE

TO

THE SECOND EDITION.

THE favourable reception the first edition of this pamphlet has met with, and the change that has been made in the public mind with respect to Vaccination, lead me to think I have treated the argument with candour. The letter which is annexed to this edition, I have Mr. Birch's permission to print. I trust it will not be unacceptable. His sentiments of the inefficacy of Vaccination, have been uniform from its introduction to the present period. Whenever he favours us with his reasons for dissenting from so many respectable members of the faculty, I am persuaded they will be found to be conclusive.

The confession of some advocates for Vaccination in the Medical Journals of the last month, evince the declining state of the practice. Sincerely do I hope that as the experiment is not found to answer, it will be no longer pursued.

W. R. ROGERS.

Hertfordshire Regiment.

AN

EXAMINATION

OF

THAT PART OF THE EVIDENCE RELATIVE

TO

COW-POX,

&c., &c.

THE mass of evidence which was produced before the Committee of the House of Commons in favour of vaccination, did so influence the public mind, that all opposition to it has been borne down; and the faculty of physic having set the example of transferring it to their own children, has been considered as full proof of the superiority of the practice.

But so many subsequent circumstances have arisen, new in themselves, and contrary to that mass of evidence, and so much has been written on the subject without ascertaining anything clearly, that surely, in some degree, to consider the report of that committee may not be improper nor ill-timed.

Let me be allowed to divide those who have given evidence on this subject into three classes:

Physicians, whose province (it will surely be conceded to me) is not to handle the lancet;

Surgeons, to whose particular line of practice inoculation appertains;

And Men-midwives, who are too much interested in the event to be considered fair evidence in the cause, according to a well-known dictum of the English law.

The College of Physicians, as a body, are of opinion, "that, the practice of vaccination is perfectly safe when properly conducted, and highly deserving the encouragement of the public, on account of the ultimate great advantage expected from it, which can only be fully established by the extended and successful experience of many years."

Much of that caution, which should reside in so learned a body of men, is here apparent.

The College of Surgeons was never applied to for an opinion.

I wish, however, to consider the more prominent parts, which appear in the evidence* of two gentlemen in that profession, who stand high in the public esteem, who have practised many years in the same hospital, who were educated under the same tutors, but whose opinions are directly in contradiction to each other upon the point in question; therefore one of them must be in an error.

"Mr. BIRCH, member of the Royal College of Surgeons, surgeon to St. Thomas's Hospital, and surgeon extraordinary to His Royal Highness the Prince of Wales, has seen vaccine inoculation often, but has never practised it, and does not think that he has seen facts sufficient, under his own inspection, to form a positive judgment, having been frequently deceived by the reports of facts in other matters. A case occurred in St. Thomas's Hospital of a child at the breast, the mother being admitted for fever, which proved to be small-pox; the child was inoculated for the cow-pox (not by the witness, for he objected to this new experiment), and went through the vaccine disorder satisfactorily in the opinion of *those who inoculated him*. After the small-pox had terminated in the mother, her child was taken very ill with fever; but on the appearance of eruption he grew better, and in that state they were dismissed. The witness saw the child afterwards, and believes that the eruption was no other than the small-pox, though it was called at that time an *hybrid* disease. He made no notes, nor can he recollect the day on which the eruption appeared; nor does he know that it was later than in the usual progress of the small-pox. Similar circumstances occurring soon afterwards in the same hospital, in two cases, made it evident that patients, having previously received small-pox infection, were not secured from the consequences of it by vaccine inoculation; none of these cases were fatal. He has no doubt, that in the above cases, the patients were infected with small-pox previous to their inoculation with vaccine matter; but he is of opinion, that if they had been inoculated with small-pox matter, they would have only had the inoculated sort of small-pox, and would have escaped the natural sort. His own practice in small-pox inoculation has *not* † been

* Vide Report of the Committee.

† The omission of the word *not*, in Mr. Birch's evidence, he desires may be rectified here.

extensive, but successful: out of more than two hundred whom he has inoculated for small-pox, he never lost one. He has heard much of spurious cow-pox, and all the failures which have been talked of have been attributed to that. He knows no instance of a person, after having gone through the cow-pox, catching the small-pox upon being exposed to it."

"Mr. Cline (to the splendor of whose talents, on many other occasions, I bow), member of the Royal College of Surgeons, and surgeon to St. Thomas's Hospital, stated that, in July, 1798, he received some vaccine matter from Dr. Jenner, with which he inoculated a boy who had not had the small-pox; when he had gone through the stages of vaccine inoculation, he tried to infect him with small-pox by inoculation, but in vain; this circumstance, together with the communications he received from Dr. Jenner, produced the strongest conviction in his mind of the great utility of this practice, and he therefore recommended it strongly to all his friends, amongst whom was Sir Walter Farquhar; and he perfectly recollects the conversation relative to the emolument Dr. Jenner might derive from the practice of vaccine inoculation; but Dr. Jenner at that time declined settling in London.

"Mr. Cline looks upon it as the greatest discovery ever made in the practice of physic, for the preservation of the human race, as the small-pox has been the most destructive of all diseases. He was consulted upon the case of a child of Mr. Austin, at Clapton, with whom it was said the cow-pox inoculation had failed; but from particular enquiries of the parents and nurse, he was perfectly convinced the child had never received the vaccine disease; and this evidence Mr. Taylor, the surgeon who inoculated it, confirmed. He thinks that experience has sufficiently demonstrated that persons inoculated with the cow-pox are incapable of receiving the small-pox; and he believes that in the instances where the small-pox has been caught, and the patient has, before the coming out of the disease, been inoculated with the cow-pox, it mitigates the virulence of the small-pox. *The vaccine disease is not contagious, nor does it create any blemish on the human frame; nor does it excite scrophula, or any other disease, which is sometimes the case with the inoculated small-pox.* In November, 1800, he performed the operation for the stone on William Bench, a child in Isaac's ward of St. Thomas's Hospital. In a few days after, hearing that this boy was in great danger of catching the small-pox, he directed that he should be inoculated with cow-pox matter, which took effect, and proceeded in the usual manner; but in thirteen days after this inoculation, a few eruptions appeared that seemed to be variolous. Admitting these eruptions were the true small-pox, the time of their appearance shows the infection had been received before the child was inoculated with cow-pox matter; for the natural small-pox frequently does not appear until sixteen or eighteen days after the patient has been exposed to infection. A second case was in November, 1801; the child of Mary Solloway, in Mary's ward of the same hospital: this child was known to have been exposed to the infection of small-pox, and therefore the mother permitted it to be inoculated with cow-pox matter; but in four days after the small-pox appeared, and the disease was very severe; however, the child recovered. A third case was a patient of Dr. Lister's, whose mother had the small-pox. In six days after the complaint had appeared in the mother, the child was inoculated with cow-pox matter, and the complaint from this inoculation proceeded as usual; but in about fifteen days a few eruptions appeared that were of a doubtful nature."

From the most minute enquiry, these are all the cases which have occurred in St. Thomas's Hospital, where variolous eruptions have succeeded the vaccine inoculation, in each of which there can be no doubt that the patients were exposed to the infection of small-pox previous to their being inoculated.

Mr. Birch having taught his pupils the maxim, that experience was preferable to experiment, examines cautiously into facts before he gives them his assent, and therefore admits that his patient, Abraham Howard, should be vaccinated while at the breast of his mother, who was labouring under the natural small-pox; but he refrains doing the operation himself, that the experiment may be most unequivocally relied upon. The event, as he relates it, was, that the vaccine disease passed through its stages to the perfect satisfaction of his colleagues; but *that* being over, the child sickened, had fever and eruption, which he insists was the Small Pox, although his colleagues, with equal firmness, maintained it was an hybrid eruption.*

Two more cases of vaccination in the same hospital, and followed by the same appearance, cleared up the dispute, and it was allowed that if the patient had caught the natural small-pox, the *vaccine* inoculation would not impede its progress.

Now, as it is agreed on all hands, that the inoculation of small-

* Dr. Woodville, physician to the Small-Pox Hospital, supposed the cow-Pox, ingrafted on a patient who had been in the atmosphere of small-pox, would frequently be followed by an eruption of a mulish nature, different from small-pox, which he called the hybrid eruption. It was afterward discovered this was the real small-pox appearing after vaccination.

pox, under similar circumstances, would supersede and destroy the infection naturally received, Mr. Birch took his stand on this ground, and has ever since steadily and firmly maintained that on this account he was satisfied the experiment would not produce the results promised from it.

He named to the committee four practitioners in different parts of the kingdom, who in correspondence with him had related the failure of cases which had been vaccinated: these gentlemen were written to that night, and their answers are printed in the report, recounting four cases where the small-pox has appeared after vaccination.

Mr. Cline, on the other hand, asserts that after trying the experiment in *one* case, he wished Dr. Jenner to settle in London, and communicated his success to several friends, and, upon his opinion alone, they immediately adopted his proposition, in particular Sir Walter Farquhar.

Mr. Cline is of opinion that it is the greatest discovery ever made, because the small-pox is the most destructive of all diseases. He proceeds to say, that it is *sufficiently* demonstrated, that persons who have been vaccinated can never receive the small-pox. He admits, with some reserve, the hospital cases quoted by Mr. Birch, but says the vaccine inoculation, even under such circumstances, though it does not supersede variolous infection, mitigates it; yet in the case of Mary Solloway's child, if I rightly understand him, Mr. C. states "*the disease to have been very severe, but that the child recovered.*" He further declares, the vaccine *creates no blemish, and does not excite scrophula, nor any other disease.*

The contradictory opinions of two such eminent surgeons did not pass unobserved by the committee—the answers returned to the letters of enquiry from Dr. Hope, Mr. Nooth, Mr. Grosvenor, and Mr. Slater—the case of Mary Dyer, of Old Sodbury—together with other opinions, created some doubt; notwithstanding which the committee declare three things (among others) which, if upon enquiry they are found to be erroneous, may tend to invalidate that mass of evidence given in support of this new invented disease.

The first assertion is, that vaccine inoculation has never proved fatal in any one instance.

The second, that it does not excite other humours or disorders in the constitution.

And the third, that it not only is to be relied on as a perfect security against small-pox, but that if it becomes universal, it will absolutely eradicate and extinguish it.

First, I have only to regret, in contradiction to these benevolent *wishes* (rather than *deductions*) of the committee, that I can shew it has proved fatal in more instances than *one:*

That in others it has created a new and undescribed disease:

And that in several the small-pox has followed beyond any dispute.

The first fatal case which was made public was a patient at Islington; the arm ulcerated, and the patient died. Many of the faculty visited this case, among whom were (I am informed) Sir William Blizard and Mr. Cline.

The next was a patient at Clapham, and this is a well-known case.

The third was the infant of Captain B. of the navy. And the last I shall mention was the child of Dr. Smyth Stewart, related by himself in a letter to Dr. Squirrell.

These cases were as favourably palliated and as ingeniously excused as they could be; but it is admitted *that each patient was punctured by a lancet infected with what is called cow-pox; each arm so punctured became inflamed and ulcerated, and each patient died.*

That of Captain B.'s infant was, for a short space of time, concealed; but the anguish of the parents soon caused a disclosure. I forbear, in this instance, to mention names; the practice so strongly patronized, and under the sanction of the legislative body, excuses every one from censure.

The number of children who have died of the natural small-pox, owing to their parents relying on the security of their having been vaccinated, might be added to the fatal catalogue, and be adduced as proofs that *vaccination does not mitigate the virulence of small-pox.* This number might be known by an advertisement; but here are enough to prove the experiment has been fatal in more than *one* instance.

The next point I am to endeavour to establish is, that a new disease, hitherto undescribed, is frequently produced by the insertion of this unnatural fluid into the human frame.

This disease shows itself under three forms.

An eruption, which appears on the face, as well as the body and limbs.

An hasty abscess, which contains a fluid dissimilar to any other; and

Glandular enlargements of the skin; at first the size of a pea, then growing knotty and hard, at length suppurating.

The eruption of the skin is the most frequent. It may be heard of in every parish in London—alas! in too many private families: it is not an *hybrid eruption*, but one *sui generis*.

Mr. Peers, perfumer in Jermyn Street, can exhibit a melancholy instance of it in one of his children.

Rebecca Latchfield, daughter of a workman at Mr. Banck's, Strand, the subject of the print annexed,* was vaccinated when five months old, and the arms proceeded in the usual manner; about a month after a pimple was observed in the middle of her forehead, which was succeeded by several in the arms; at first they felt like peas, they gradually increased in size, and more appeared in the skin on different parts of the body. The child was carried to a surgeon when about twelve months old; he purged it with calomel, and directed the tincture of bark. As its health improved, the knobs advanced to suppuration; that on the forehead first maturated, and was opened; some on the arm slowly followed.† The plate is made from a drawing of one arm only, the whole subject would appear disgusting; but this case, I think, clearly demonstrates a *new disease of the skin*, not at all similar to scrophula, or any other disease I am acquainted with.

A servant belonging to Mr. East, Adelphi, had a child vaccinated while at the breast; the progress of the pustule was regular; about nine days after the scab formed, large superficial abscesses appeared on the nates, thighs, and body of the infant. They suppurated hastily, but the colour of the skin was unlike what it is in common inflammation; it was of a dusky bluish red; the child suffered great pain. They were opened freely with a lancet; their contents were a gelatinous, blue fluid, very similar to a solution of starch, and extremely offensive.

In the last place with grief (but confidently) I assert, that the great advantage which mankind was to have received from this discovery has not been attained, from it being no security, in numerous instances, against the infection of the natural small-pox.

Divers cases to prove this last assertion have been brought forward; but until Mr. Goldson published his they were concealed. Whenever the case pressed strongly, the vaccination was declared imperfect; the matter was taken too soon, or too late, or it was spurious, or the practitioner was informed he had yet a lesson to learn.

Before the committee had made their report (*I believe I am*

* [I have not had this plate re-produced.—E.M.C.]

† This drawing was given to me by Mr. Birch.

accurate in saying) the child of Matthew Montague, Esq., who had been vaccinated in the country, was put to the test of variolous infection. Several eminent practitioners visited the child while under the variolous eruption, and Dr. Denman declared it was not small-pox, because it turned on the sixth day; however, matter was taken from it, by Mr. Walker of St. James's Street, and two *children* of his coachman were infected by that matter with indisputable small-pox.

Dr. Croft saw these children who were inoculated from Mr. Montague's, and I learn he admitted they had the small-pox.

Mr. Gould, at an oyster warehouse in Bow Street, Covent Garden, had a child vaccinated at the Small-Pox Hospital about a year since, and the pustule was considered so perfect, that some were vaccinated from it. The latter end of last January, this child took the natural small-pox, at a time when it was labouring under the hooping cough; it had about two hundred pustules, and the cough proceeded in its course.

The cases of Mr. Hodges's children, in Holborn, have been so accurately drawn up by a medical committee, and confessed indisputable, that I have only to remark, with surprise, how so many persons, pretending to know any thing about small-pox, should for a moment have doubted the nature of the disease.*

If Dr. Wollaston, to whom society (as I have heard it indeed observed) is not a little indebted for a deliberate investigation of these cases, had signed the conclusion annexed to the account of them, we should have been all astonished; as he did not sign it, we are, I believe, all satisfied.

But the case which above all others is the most conclusive, is that of Mr. Bowen's child, at Harrow, which, after being vaccinated, was submitted to the test of variolous inoculation three successive years, without producing any effect. On the fourth inoculation small-pox was made to appear, and matter was taken from one of the pustules, with which another child was successfully inoculated.†

Here, then, is the instance of the child of a medical gentleman, one who heretofore was fully convinced of the security of vaccination, and who boldly submitted his own infant to the test of this experiment (viz., Whether vaccination was an antidote to the small-pox ?), and this he repeated not once nor twice only, but a third

* When so much difference of opinion prevailed among the faculty, whether it was or was not small-pox, it is surprising that Mr. John Hunter's distinction of the slough, lining the bottom of the pustule, should not have been the object of the search.

† See Mr. Bowen's letter to Mr. Birch, in Dr. Moseley's *Lues Bovilla*.

and a fourth time; at length the small-pox takes effect. Here we see the boasted security completely overthrown, and the practitioner, terrified at the event, judiciously putting to the trial all within his circuit, and succeeding in giving the small-pox to many who thought themselves secure from it, they having been previously vaccinated, as it is called.

These cases sounded a fresh alarm. Mr. Bowen was brought to London, and examined by Dr. Pearson and others: nothing could be more clear than the account he gave, or more convincing to those who were interested in investigating the truth.

It is unnecessary at present to bring forward more cases in order to establish the point I proposed: these are certainly sufficient to prove that the report made by the committee, from the mass of evidence they had examined, is not supported by experience, for I think we now demonstrate—

That Cow-pox has in more than one instance proved fatal.

That Cow-pox is productive of new appearances of disease, unknown before in the catalogue of human infirmities.

And that Cow-pox is not by any means to be depended on as a security against the natural small-pox.

Therefore, I conclude that one of these gentlemen is in an error, and I leave the reader to form his own judgment of their evidence.

The question, whether vaccination should be persisted in after what I have stated, comes next into consideration. The order from the medical boards to the surgeons of the army and navy is a matter of very material consequence on this point, and the public mind is so shaken by what has been done, and what is to be feared from it, that I with great diffidence venture to recommend those distinguished gentlemen, who guide and teach the profession of surgery, to consider seriously this matter before the practice of it is further pursued.

The inoculation of the small-pox, in the estimation of any one pcssessing common sensibility, must boast a proud triumph over the cow-pox; for the small-pox exposes the just feelings of the parent to only one conflict, and if not performed till two years after birth, the chances in favour of success are, under proper treatment, become almost a certainty. The change it produces in the absorbent system is in unison with nature; by it destructive consequences are prevented, and the patient is left in perfect security that it cannot attack the system again; a security which seems not to attach to the cow-pox; and what the consequences may be of the revolution produced by cow-pox, when the absorbent system is attacked by scrophula, lues venerea, or cancer, time alone can discover.

When the cases of the Hodges were established, several instances of the small-pox occurring a second time were brought forward; but as Baron Dimsdale took so much pains to enquire into this circumstance, and never could satisfy himself that it had once occurred, I must quote his authority to support my disbelief of such a thing having ever happened: besides, when so many objections were made to inoculation for half a century, surely if this had ever occurred, the enemies to the practice would not have been silent on the subject: yet we hear of no such instance (till now) brought forward.

One rational objection has been urged, I confess, against the inoculation of small-pox, that of spreading the infection, by exposing patients during the maturating process of it in public ways; but this is a practice never followed nor recommended by Baron Dimsdale: it is true that, during the febrile state of the eruption, he insists upon the necessity of external air; but the eruption being completed, his words are "all is over," and from that time it was indeed his practice to keep the patient cool and temperate, not cold; for this purpose a well ventilated chamber, the cool side of the house, a yard, or a garden, were all he required. But I am satisfied his instructions have been misunderstood, and an observance of them would remedy the objection.

One of the striking proofs of the utility and advantage of small-pox inoculation was, in my humble opinion, the safety and certainty with which a whole district, a whole army, a ship's crew, or a regiment, might be insured from the ravages of a pestilential disease, by the artificial method of inflicting it. In this instance art completely triumphs over nature; and I shall here beg to relate a remarkable occurrence, which will fully illustrate this advantage.

Captain Spranger, commander of His Majesty's ship *Crescent*, returning from the East Indies, took a Spanish brig, laden with slaves, many of whom were children from three years old to twelve: to his terror he discovered the natural small-pox had broke out on board this vessel, where much neglect and mismanagement of the disease were evident: the crew were landed on a small uninhabited island, near the Cape of Good Hope, and the sick began to recover surprisingly. This disorder is dreaded at the Cape as much as the plague is in Europe; of course he was directed to perform a strict quarantine, and on consultation with his surgeon he judged it expedient to direct that all the mariners on board the *Crescent*, as well as all persons on board the Spanish brig, who had never had the small-pox, should be inoculated; this was immediately done with complete success, every one so inoculated recovered, notwithstanding they were ill prepared, from a long voyage and salt provisions; many of them were hardly sick at all. During his quarantine he was obliged, by his instructions from the Admiralty, to detain an American vessel which fell in his way; he recommended to the captain to inoculate his crew, lest it should suffer from the infection: the Americans resisted this advice; but the captain being at length persuaded of the danger of the natural disease, and of the safety of inoculation, partly by constraint, and partly by consent, did inoculate as many of the crew as had not previously undergone the small-pox; here also the success was complete, and the favourable returns made to the governor induced Lord Macartney to propose to the colony the introduction of inoculation; but his good intentions were frustrated by the prejudices of the people.

Now, I may fairly ask the advocates for vaccination, whether they are assured, if cow-pox matter had been used, that the success would have been equal?

I believe there are many other places, beside St. Thomas's Hospital, where, upon trial, the small-pox has proceeded without a check, and where inoculation was obliged to be had recourse to before the infection could be cleared away.

But as my rank in the profession does not entitle me to do more than recapitulate remarks, I shall now put an end to them, I trust, before I become either tedious or obtrusive, hoping that I have urged them with becoming decorum, and have offended no one in searching for the truth.

THE END.

A

LETTER

OCCASIONED BY THE MANY FAILURES OF

COW-POX.

FROM JOHN BIRCH, ESQ.

Surgeon to His Royal Highness the Prince of Wales, &c.

ADDRESSED TO

W. R. ROGERS,

Author of the Examination of the Evidence before the House of Commons, &c., &c.

To Mr. W. R. ROGERS.

Herts Regiment, Ipswich.

London, July 6th, 1805.

Dear Sir,

THE able and dispassionate manner in which you have treated the argument concerning Vaccination, seems to have had its proper weight with the thinking part of mankind. I recommend you therefore to reprint your pamphlet. It cannot have too extensive a circulation. I wish it could be sent to every part of the globe in justification of English Surgery. Inoculation has hitherto been considered as distinctly the province of the Surgeon; the success of it, and the alleviation of its distressing symptoms, depend on surgical treatment. It is a melancholy consideration, therefore, to think that this branch of practice should be taken from those who alone ought to exercise it, and transferred to persons, some of whom are totally ignorant of our profession.

The experiment of Vaccination has been carried on from the commencement, to the present period, with a degree of *art*, which does not augur much in favour of the cause.

The number of persons adduced as supporting it when before the Committee of the House of Commons was forty; but the Public has not been told that out of this forty, twenty-three spoke from *hearsay* only, not from any knowledge they had acquired by practice, *while the three persons who spoke against it, corroborated their evidence by proofs.* Strong as this fact is, no one has taken notice of it.

When first Vaccination was recommended to me, it was announced authoritatively to be an absolute security against Small Pox; but the experiment, when tried at St. Thomas's Hospital, failed; and there it was first discovered that in a variolous atmosphere it was not to be depended on.

This in the outset did not prove much in the favour of Vaccination; further difficulties arose from eruptions which appeared, too often in the face; but these were obviated by saying, that observation had proved the vaccine matter to be divided into genuine and spurious, and that its good or ill success depended on the period at which it was taken: on a certain day it would prove innoxious and genuine; before and after that day it could not be depended on. Sometimes the cow was to blame, and sometimes the doctor.

Thus we were left to judge by the event. If the patient should die from the inflammation of the puncture, we might then conclude the matter was not genuine; if the apothecary plunged his lancet too deep, or the infant was not of a proper constitution, the experiment might be fatal. To reason thus was to insult humanity. Alas! how can the constitution of a child be ascertained, when only one month, or six months old? The failures which occurred, instead of operating conviction, seemed but to change the theory of the system; new doctrines, new books, new instructions appeared every month. Even the first principle, of the origin of the disease, could not be settled. Dr. Jenner traced it from the grease of the horse's heel; and the description he gave of it, was alone sufficient to frighten us from adopting it. But this notion was soon found to be erroneous, and it is now conjectured to belong to the cow; yet after all, this animal poison is too mischievous for use, until it has been meliorated by passing through some human body, selected as the victim of the experiment.

But mere uncertainty was not the only evil attendant on Vaccination. New diseases occurred, as in the case, among others, of Rebecca Latchfield. It was studiously represented, indeed, that her affection was nothing more than common boils; but the discriminating colour, the stony hardness, and the continued succession of the tumours, together with the painful sufferings of the afflicted child, marked the novelty of the disease. Many individuals acknowledged this distinction the moment they saw her. As it is important this case should be generally known, I have procured a drawing at full length of this unhappy little sufferer, which may hereafter be presented to the Public.

How far it was well judged, or politic, to direct our soldiers and seamen to become the subjects, whereon a doubtful experiment should be tried, I do not mean to enquire. At all events, it would have been more regular, and more to the interests of Society, as the experiment was surgical, to have consulted the College of Surgeons, and to have had their collected approbation before a parliamentary reward was adjudged. In all cases where

Parliament has neglected to do this, it has committed an error; as in the instance of Mrs. Stevens' medicine for dissolving the stone.

But was it not highly reprehensible to conceal industriously all the cases which occurred to the prejudice of Vaccination, while everything that could tend to lessen the credit of Inoculation was *most artfully* propagated?

The facts which you have adduced are so strong in themselves, and the authority on which they rest so incontrovertible, that they entirely subvert the data laid down by the Committee of the House of Commons. Yet the argument might have been treated in another way, and these questions asked.

I. Is there any disease consequent to Small Pox Inoculation which is not a natural disease, and which may not be produced equally by other exciting causes?

II. Does the puncture of Inoculation ever produce such an inflammation of the arm as to kill the patient?

III. Can the artificial introduction of variolous matter produce any disease but genuine Small Pox?

IV. Are not the symptoms of inoculated Small Pox, after two years old, generally as safe and as mild as those of the kindest Vaccination?

V. Did the justly celebrated Baron Dimsdale, in his extensive practice, both abroad and at home, during the space of forty-five years, ever lose three of his patients?

I affirm that the negative must be replied to each of these questions. What then is there left for Vaccination to do, that may not be done more advantageously by Inoculation?

But the object of the projectors of Vaccination was not, I fear, so much the desire of doing general good, as that of securing to themselves, and to Men-midwives, if the experiment should succeed, the absolute command of the nurseries, to the entire exclusion of the Surgeons.

This being really the state of the case, I must call it an unworthy expedient, to alarm the ignorant multitude with the dangers of Inoculation; an enemy that had been laid at their feet by the firm and steady exertions of the great and good Baron Dimsdale.

A monthly Medical Journal, which has spread the mischief of Vaccination widely, and which, till the last month, has been shut against every statement which could affect its credit, now acknowledges failure upon failure, attested by one practitioner after another. But we are little obliged for these tardy confessions, since the Public has been some time in the possession of the facts, together with many others; and they are now acknowledged, because they can no longer be concealed. I again affirm, that the Public are beforehand with the Medical Journals; they have indeed been too long misled by the charm of novelty, but they perceive their error; and they have loudly called out for regular Inoculation, to prevent the mischiefs of natural Small Pox, which has appeared epidemical in many places, and proved fatal in cases where Vaccination had been relied on.

I forbear to say more on this subject at present. I have collected materials enough to satisfy the Public of the validity of the reasons on which I have uniformly objected to the practice of Vaccination. That I should come forward, is a duty I owe both to them and myself. Should I contribute towards dispelling that mist of prejudice, which has obscured the judgment of many well-intentioned people, and many able practitioners, I shall have just cause to rejoice. To attempt to vindicate truth and expose error, is the noblest exertion of our faculties: to succeed in the attempt, is to obtain the most exalted gratification a reasonable being can desire.

I am,
Dear Sir,
Your faithful friend,
JOHN BIRCH.

Spring Gardens,
July 6th, 1805.

P.S.—Every post brings me accounts of the failures of Vaccination. From Hertfordshire, I have notice of four cases within the last month, two of which were fatal; but as I do not admit *Hearsay* Evidence, I must enquire more particularly before I publish them.—However, I have just seen a child in Orange Court, Swallow Street, vaccinated five years ago by a Man-midwife, who is not only the strongest advocate for Vaccination, but is considered to be one of its most skilful practitioners. By him this child was pronounced to have had the *genuine* sort; and so strong was his conviction of it, that he took matter from him to vaccinate many other patients with; yet this very Child is now full of the *true*, not of the *supposed* Small Pox.

The mother says the Small Pox is not in the Court—and that the child has not been in the way of infection to her knowledge. Add this case to the confessions of the Monthly Journal, and to Dr. Moseley's* list, and what is the conclusion we are to draw?

* *Vide* Moseley on *Lues Bovilla*, 2nd edit.

There is but one; namely, that Vaccination neither secures the patient from catching the Small Pox by variolous infection, nor, when so caught, lessens the danger of disease. For my own part I tremble to think on the perils which await Society, from the prevalence of Vaccination. Unless it be stopped, we shall see Small Pox at no very distant period recur in all the terrors with which it was first surrounded; desolating cities like the plague, and sweeping thousands from the earth, who, lulled into a false security, will have fatally deprived themselves of the only proper means of defence.

ON COW POX

DISCOVERED AT PASSY (NEAR PARIS)

BY

M. BOUSQUET.

[*Mémoires de l'Académie de Médecine, Tome Cinquième, pp.* 600—632.]

TRANSLATED BY THE EDITOR.

1836.

ON COW POX

DISCOVERED AT PASSY (NEAR PARIS),

March 22nd, 1836.

By M. BOUSQUET.

[M. Bousquet introduces this subject with remarks on previous discoveries of Cow Pox, and then proceeds to give the details of his own investigations.—E.M.C.]

ON the 21st of March, 1836, Dame Fleury, living at No. 21, Rue de Longchamps, Passy, went to Chaillot to consult Dr. Perdrau. She had been feeling unwell for some days, and still complained of headache and feverish symptoms. She had three vesicles on the right hand and another on the upper lip. On seeing them, M. Perdrau, struck by their resemblance to vaccinal vesicles, put a few questions to his patient. "What is your occupation?" "I am a milk-woman." "Have you noticed vesicles on the udders of your cows at all like those which you show me?" "Yes, sir; and I feel sure that I have caught them." "Had you chapped hands?" "Yes, sir."

After this explanation, M. Perdrau, putting together what he saw and what he had just heard, felt no doubt that Dame Fleury's vesicles were the result of Cow Pox. With this impression he sent her to M. Nauche, one of the best authorities on vaccination. She promised to go there the same day, but she did not go until the following day. It was none too soon; a few hours more, and all chance would have been lost. M. Nauche paid me the same compliment which he had just received. He sent Dame Fleury to me with a note, in which he mentioned M. Perdrau's opinion and gave me his own, though expressed with more reserve.

Dame Fleury, as I have mentioned, had three vesicles on the right hand: one was situated over the joint of the thumb, the second on the back of the ring finger, and the third (which I have not mentioned in my report of April 12th,) on the inner side of the index finger, close to the pulp; lastly, a fourth was to be seen on the upper lip, at the union of the skin and mucous membrane. These vesicles had the diameter of three to four lines; they were globular or hemispherical, prominent, and well circumscribed. The one on the thumb was different, in that it was longer in one direction than in the other. The other three were perfectly circular. The surface presented a yellowish or purulent appearance while the margin, as well as the areola with which it was surrounded, was violet. Nevertheless the entire vesicle reflected a bluish tint such as I had never seen. This reminded me that Jenner gave this tint as the characteristic feature of Cow Pox, and I was not surprised that the first remove of this eruption preserved something of its original character. It is also worth remarking that Jenner repeatedly mentioned the joints of the fingers and the lips as the parts of the body where the accidental vesicles were commonly found. But for these, there would be difficulty in recognising vaccinia from this description. The most marked characters were absent. There was neither depression in the centre of the pustules, nor that glistening appearance which constitutes the distinctive mark of the vaccinal eruption. But these differences were naturally explained by the advanced state of the vesicles.

Further, we must add that Dame Fleury asserted that she had had Small Pox, although she had no mark, except, perhaps, on her cheek, where there was a little scar, which she pointed out as a proof of the truth of her statement. However this may be, this circumstance was of little moment. At any rate, it was not a reason for abandoning our hopes; there is nothing more common than to see vaccination after Small Pox. The author of this paper is himself an example of this. Nevertheless, we were still in doubt. There was only one way of removing the uncertainty; this was to inoculate the matter of the vesicles.

On the 21st of March, 1836, between twelve and one o'clock, we undertook this operation in the presence of MM. Pariset, Delaberge, Delpech, Boucher, Millet, etc. On puncturing the vesicles with a lancet, thick white purulent matter escaped, as if it were an abscess discharging. From the first I resolved to make a double inoculation, and to devote one arm to each virus. Thus, if I exposed the children, the subjects of my investigation, to a useless experiment, I at least assured them of the benefits of vaccination which they had come for, and I provided for myself, in case of success, a means of comparison which was not to be despised.

Lastly, to leave no doubt about the nature and origin of the results of my inoculations, I employed two lancets. The one which I used for inoculating the matter to be tested was quite new; it came straight from the cutler's,—an absolutely essential precaution in experiments of this nature. Otherwise it would, or at least it could, be said that while imagining that a special virus was inoculated, only the ordinary virus with which the instrument was still charged had been inoculated.

The operation being over, M. Pariset begged me to detain Dame Fleury, and to bring her before the Council of the Royal Academy of Medicine, which met that day. The good woman was kind enough to wait. She was seen by MM. Louyer-Villermay, Marc, Mérat, Roche, Baron, and all the members of the council, except one, who was absent. All of them examined her hands, and all of them heard from her a part of what I have just related.

I had that day to vaccinate nine children, two from the foundling hospital, and seven from the town. They were all inoculated by three punctures on each arm; that is to say, with ordinary vaccine on the right arm, and with matter from Dame Fleury's pustules on the left arm. In all fifty-four punctures.

If, out of the nine children we except one foundling hardly three days old, on whom the two viruses failed equally, only eight remain.

All the punctures of the right arm took, except on the child Brocard, No. 29, Rue Guénégaud, who had only a single vesicle on this arm and none on the other—that is to say, twenty-four punctures gave twenty-two vesicles of typical vaccinia.

The inoculation of the left arm was much less successful; twenty-four punctures gave only three vesicles—that is to say, one vesicle on Dubief, 24, Rue Joubert; one vesicle on Coussinet, 60, Rue du Temple; and one vesicle on Denis, 7, Rue du Mont-Saint-Hiliare. It is remarkable that these three vesicles appeared on three different children, and that each of those having a vesicle on the left arm had three on the right arm. In the order of inoculation these children were the first, the fifth, and the eighth.

As regards age, the first was ten months old, the second seven, and the third three.

Of these three children, one only was brought again to the vaccination station, on the 29th. This was Denis, the youngest of all; a child, slender, puny, and of wretched appearance. All the vesicles were colourless, and weakly like himself; but that of the left arm was unquestionably the feeblest and most ill-developed. However, I took, in the presence of MM. Drs. Requin and Gaultier de Claubry, the matter of this vesicle, and I transferred it to four other children, always taking care to utilise one arm for each virus, and to change the lancet. We shall see directly the result of this inoculation.

However, being anxious to learn the results of all my experiments, I went myself on the 29th, to visit the nine children that I had vaccinated on the 22nd, of whom the greater number were quietly at home, kept in by the bad weather. It was during this tour of inspection that I discovered the two vesicles which have been referred to.

Up to this time I had only obtained as witnesses of my experiments those persons who had come to me by chance. But now I thought it was time to call together the Vaccine Commission, and after arranging with the Secretary, the Commission was convoked on Wednesday morning, the 30th, for the same day at three o'clock.

I showed them two of the children with single vesicles on their left arms, and I gave the address of the third, who in spite of my entreaties had refused to leave home.

The vesicles of Dubief and Coussinet were, in truth, not so puny as that of Denis, but they showed nothing remarkable, nothing which would suggest their origin; in a word, they were altogether exactly like those of the right arm. In calling together the Vaccine Commissioners, I had not only the intention of showing them vesicles from a new source; I wished to transfer the product in their presence to two children whom I held in reserve; one of them, Josserand, was hardly three months old; the other, Flottet, was thirteen months old. On this occasion, the Commissioners appeared to wish that instead of impregnating the system with the two lymphs, only the one we desired to test should be inoculated, doubtless to deprive it of the influence of the other. The inoculation was made in the manner which had been suggested, by three punctures on the right arm and four on the left arm. Further, before the meeting separated, the secretary drew up a report of this experiment.

The results of the experiments of which the details have been given may now be described. It will be remembered how ill-developed and puny was the vesicle of Denis, from which four children were inoculated on the left arm. Of these four children two only can be described; there was no opportunity of seeing the others.

These two children, Brisart, 12, Rue du Dragon, and Duterne, 63, Vielle Rue du Temple, had three vesicles on each arm. In this respect there is a parallel between the two lymphs. Up to the sixth day it appeared to me that there was also a perfect similarity between the vesicles. From the seventh, I thought I was able to observe a difference, all in favour of the new vesicles. These vesicles were in general better formed, that is to say, flatter, more depressed in the centre, more brilliant, and firmer than the vesicles from the old source. The lymph which issued from them had all the transparency of the purest crystal. However, these characters were not equally well-marked in the two children ; in this respect Brisart was far superior to Duterne.

Having been vaccinated on the 29th of March, Brisart and Duterne were, on the 5th of April, at the eighth day of their vaccination.

Being curious to follow the progress to the end, we saw them again on Saturday, the 9th. The difference between the two arms appeared to us still greater. The vesicles on the left side were flat, at least four lines in width, firm at the margin, prominent, and still full of strength and vitality. On the other hand, the pustules of the right arm were already reduced to a small, dry, bulging, entirely inert crust.

We were so struck by this contrast, that, in conjunction with the Secretary, we thought that we ought at once to call together the Vaccination Commission to witness this fact, and we took upon ourselves to invite a certain number of the members of the Academy to meet the Commission, feeling sure that our boldness would be excused on the ground of the motive which inspired us.

How are we to explain the fact of such feeble and miserable vesicles producing such splendid results ? It will be remembered that when Dame Fleury came to me her vesicles were in full suppuration ; now it is well known that in this state vaccine has lost the greater part of its energy. I beg you also to observe, that it produced only three vesicles in twenty-four punctures. But as the quality of this vaccine was in reality excellent, it was only necessary to take it at the right time to restore its native activity.

I now come to the two children vaccinated on the 30th of March in the presence of the Vaccination Commission.

I have stated that in this experiment, only the new virus was used. It so happened that the lymph was nearly the same as the vaccine in use, at least the results were very inferior in appearance to the above described vesicles, especially those of Brisart and Duterne. What was the cause of this difference? Was it only accidental, or must we conclude that the old virus, when used with the new, impressed upon it an excess of vigour which abandoned it when left to its own resources? The result soon cleared up our doubts on this point. Without doubt the new virus does not manifest an equal intensity on all constitutions; but these variations are not peculiar to it; they are met with much more strikingly in the old virus. It is one of the characters of living bodies that they do not always respond equally to the same impressions; and although viruses in general, and the vaccine virus in particular, are perhaps, of all causes, those whose effects are the most constant and the best proportioned, still they have their varieties. The facts, then, of which we are speaking can therefore only be considered as exceptions. However, at this period we were making our first trials, and we thought that we could not be too reserved in our language.

Taught by experience, we do not now hesitate to state that the new virus has no need of the support of the old to exhibit its full strength.

The Old Vaccine.	The New Vaccine.
1stly. The two first days after the operation there is nothing visible at the punctures.	1stly. The day following the operation a red spot is, as a rule, to be distinguished, indicating its commencement to take.
2ndly. From the third to the fourth, a small pink spot is perceptible, more apparent to the finger than to the eye.	2ndly. This spot, of a brighter red, is as apparent to the eye as to the touch.
3rdly. On the fifth, the vaccinal vesicle begins to be visible with all its characters; already, flat at the summit, slightly depressed at the centre On the following day, these features only became more marked. On the seventh day, the entire vesicle reflects the silvery lustre which characterises it, and begins to be surrounded by a small red areola. Its consistency is so soft that however slightly it is touched with the lancet it empties itself, and the lymph which escapes is already a little turbid.	3rdly. The same characters, except that they are more distinct; the depression is more marked; the lustre more brilliant; the consistence much firmer. The lymph is perfectly limpid. There is as yet no trace of areola.
4thly. On the eighth day, the areola increases, on the ninth it disappears; the pustule, larger and higher, gets soft again, rounds itself off, and gets	4thly. The vesicle is never finer, firmer, or more brilliant. The areola commences to form.

The Old Vaccine.	The New Vaccine.
yellow. The middle is surmounted by a brown spot, a certain sign of the commencement of desiccation. The lymph becomes more and more turbid.	The lymph preserves its transparency and its purity.
5thly. From the tenth to the twelfth day, the desiccation makes rapid progress. The entire vesicle is covered by a soft yellowish crust, which gets more and more brown, and shrinks as it becomes denser. There is no longer any lymph.	5thly. The vesicle develops in every way without changing its character. The areola is large and vivid, the subjacent tissue much infiltrated. The glands of the axilla are often painful, swollen, especially in adults. Nevertheless, fever is not always present, if it be, it is particularly at this stage that it is noticed. The lymph begins to get turbid, but it is none the less suitable for inoculation.
6thly. From the thirteenth day the crust, reduced to the size of a large lentil, gets still drier, and in drying becomes smaller. It falls off, as a rule, on the fifteenth to the eighteenth day. The scars, generally very superficial, are recognised rather by their reddish tint than by the depression which they leave on the skin. But after some months the skin returns to its natural colour, and the eye can hardly make out any traces of vaccination.	6thly. The vesicles, three to four lines in diameter and dried at the centre, present a circular, prominent, elevated ring; the transparency sufficiently indicates the state of the vaccine which it contains. This state continues until the fifteenth day, and sometimes longer. The areola is still very bright and extensive.
	7thly. From the fifteenth to the eighteenth day, the desiccation extends to the entire surface of the vesicle. The crust is flat, large, brown, and as if scorched. As to colour, I cannot do better than compare it to a burnt almond. At the same time the areola becomes pale, retires gradually, until completely effaced. The falling off of the crusts generally takes place from the twenty-fifth to the thirtieth day. The crusts are followed by large deep scars, which are traversed by a number of small lines, which give them a reticulated appearance. By examining with the finger, a cavity is felt, as if there had been loss of substance. It is not unusual for the crusts to leave behind them a suppurating sore—an ulcer—for the cicatrisation of which it is necessary to wait. I have seen vesicles hollow out the skin so deeply that they left regular holes.

are not constant; the areolæ do not always correspond exactly. Generally the areola of the old vaccine appears first, that of the new following one or two days afterwards; from which it is obvious that a moment must be reached when the inflammation subsides in one case while it is at its height in the other case.

In my first trials with the new virus, I made, according to my custom, three punctures on each arm. I soon had to give up this practice. The intensity of the inflammation was sometimes so great that it spread over the entire arm and as far as the glands of the axilla. M. Gasc cannot have forgotten a child whom he had vaccinated and had the kindness to show to me. The vesicles were enormous, the inflammation so violent that baths, poultices, fomentations, and complete antiphlogistic diet scarcely sufficed to reduce it. The crusts, when they fell off, left ulcerations which were very slow to undergo cicatrisation.

It was at this moment that I understood, for the first time, Jenner's anxieties. We know that he was so afraid of inflammation that he made only one puncture on each arm, and sometimes on only one arm, and he had hardly observed that slight onset of fever, which he believed to be necessary for complete infection, before he hastened to suppress the vesicle by all the means which art put in his power, even including cauterisation.

With regard to the progress of the vesicles, there is between the old and the new nearly the same difference as between Small Pox and Chicken Pox. Up to the seventh or eighth day everything is so exactly identical in these two eruptions, that it is difficult to distinguish them. But Chicken Pox has hardly passed this period when it stops, and desiccation commences. It is, I consider, nearly the same thing in the case of the old vaccine. Experience is necessary in order to distinguish it in the early stages from the new. The differentiation is not readily appreciable by everybody until towards the eighth day; it is then at its height; from this moment it only decreases. Observe, on the contrary, the new, follow it with the eye, and you will see that it develops, that it increases, and runs nearly twice as long a course as its rival.

[M. Bousquet then proceeds to discuss at length the advantage of the new lymph over the old, and concludes his paper with a reference to the disease in the cow.—E.M.C.]

* * * * * * *

In order not to interrupt the narrative, we have as yet said nothing of the cow which furnished the Cow Pox, the principal subject of this memoir. However, our first inoculation was hardly finished before we asked the favour of seeing the cow. Dame Fleury showed us a black cow, thin, and out of condition, about six or seven years old. She had calved six weeks when the eruption was first observed. We were informed that from this time she left off eating for two days, and the secretion of milk had considerably diminished. She appeared to suffer much when the attempt was made to milk her. She was only approached with difficulty. At our first visit there remained on the teats only the dry, reddish-brown crusts. Obliged to take things as we found them, we begged that these crusts should be kept for us. This was promised, but was not carried out. The crusts came off in pieces after the application of ointment (*vielle future*), and were lost in the litter. Bût though we had not seen the vesicles of the cow in their earlier stages, we had seen their scars; they appeared to us wrinkled and puckered like all scars. We expected them to be deeper.

ACCOUNT OF A SUPPLY

OF

FRESH VACCINE VIRUS

FROM

THE COW.

ESTLIN.

(Including a Report of the National Vaccine Establishment and Mr. Estlin's Reply.)

[*Reprinted from the Medical Gazette*, 1837—1838.]

MR. ESTLIN'S FIRST LETTER.

(New series, vol. ii., session 1837-38, p. 977.)

Account of a Supply of Fresh Vaccine Virus from the Cow.

To the Editor of *The Medical Gazette.*

SIR,

If you consider the following account of a successful effort to procure a supply of genuine vaccine lymph directly from the cow, as likely to prove acceptable to your readers, it will afford me satisfaction to have provided you with it.

Allow me, in the first place, to premise that, having been engaged in vaccinating (at one time rather extensively) for thirty years, I have watched with regret a decided decline in the activity of the virus; and for many years I have been endeavouring in vain to renew the lymph from its original source. To many agricultural and other friends I have repeatedly expressed my willingness to go twenty or thirty miles to see a cow with the vaccine disease; and though I have occasionally heard of cows thus disordered, and once took some matter from an ulceration upon the teat of one, I have never been able to succeed in reproducing the disease in the human subject, or to see, until within the last month, a decided instance of the complaint. Whether others have been more fortunate in similar attempts I know not.

The alterations in the vaccine affection which have appeared to me most marked are: the smallness of the vesicle and its attendant areola; its rapid course; the absence of constitutional disturbance, the small quantity of lymph yielded by the vesicle; and, especially, the diminished activity of its infecting quality. Twenty years ago it was a matter of comparative indifference how long the lymph taken was kept before it was used: after it had been preserved in a dried state for weeks, or even months, it almost certainly reproduced the disease. At the present time, virus a day or two old is very uncertain in its effects, and even fluid lymph often fails to communicate infection. On the diminished anti-variolous power of the present stock of vaccine matter I need make no remark; the public are too painfully aware of the fact.

Through the kindness of an acquaintance residing in Gloucestershire, who remembered my wish to procure some fresh vaccine virus from the cow whenever an opportunity offered, a small quantity was sent to me on the 18th of August upon a piece of glass, said to have been taken from a cow; and also some taken from the hand of a person who had contracted sores by milking the diseased cows. I lost no time in investigating the source of this unexpected supply, and on the morning of the 21st ult. visited a farmyard in which were about twenty-five cows, nearly all of which had been attacked with an eruption upon the teats during the four preceding weeks; the last of those thus affected had become so about a fortnight previous to my visit. Irregularly circular scabs existed upon the teats of many; in some the surfaces were raw from having been rubbed by recent milking: from none of the sores did any fluid exude, and most of them had been dressed with an ointment into the composition of which acetate of copper appeared to enter. The duration of the disease in the cows I ascertained to have been about a fortnight from the time that each had become affected. The hands of those who had been engaged in milking them presented sores in various stages; in one or two persons an eschar only remained, in others soreness still existed; in a boy of about thirteen years of age there was a large inflamed vesicle between the finger and thumb of the right hand, occupying all the space from the third joint of the finger to the second of the thumb. The skin was yellow at this part, as if a quantity of pus had been under it. Such, however, was not the case; for from a small opening through the thickened and yellow cuticle the boy squeezed out a perfectly limpid fluid, with which I charged some glasses. This vesicle had made its appearance six days before, at which time he had felt ill. The others before mentioned who had been engaged in milking (all of them females), reported that they had felt very ill before they discovered the "gathering" on their fingers; one represented herself as having been so much indisposed with headache, pain in the back and loins, and general weakness, as to be apprehensive she was going to have a serious fever; all described the sores as extremely painful, and as having occasioned enlargement and tenderness in the axillary glands. The course of the disease in them, as in the cows, was about a fortnight; and though it was known to them that the cows had something the matter with their teats, several days elapsed before the milkers suspected their malady to depend upon the disorder in the animals: never having witnessed the complaint before in the cows, they were ignorant of the nature of the existing disease.

All the persons I have now spoken of had been vaccinated in infancy, one of them by Dr. Jenner.

I next inspected three children who had been inoculated, by means of a needle, with lymph taken from one of those who had received the disease from the cows. One, a boy of fourteen years of age, who had gone through vaccination formerly, had four large, circular mahogany-coloured scabs upon his arm with the outer red line of an extensive areola still remaining. He was vaccinated about a fortnight before I saw him; the areola, I was informed, had appeared upon the eighth or ninth day, and he had been very unwell from the complaint. The next was a child who had been vaccinated from one of the milkers only three days before; scarcely any inflammation or prominence was observable about the punctures, and I have since learned that the inoculation produced no effect.

The third case was a little girl, Jane ——, about five years old, who had never had the cow-pox or small-pox. She had been vaccinated for the first time from the discharge taken from the hand of one of the milkers, during the activity of the complaint, on the 11th of August. I saw her, therefore, on the eleventh day of the disease. On one arm were three large, fine, prominent circular vesicles, flattened in the centre, and with some areola; on the other arm was one vesicle, much larger and less circular. I was informed that for three or four days after she was vaccinated it was difficult to decide if the infection had taken effect; and I have subsequently learned that the areola which I saw on the eleventh day continued to increase till the thirteenth day, and that the child had been "very poorly."

From this little girl I took a supply of lymph which was quite limpid and flowed very freely. I have not felt myself warranted in this account particularly to designate persons or places; but I am bound to acknowledge the great attention I met with from the inhabitants of the farm, and the facility afforded me of making every inquiry and investigation that I desired.

On my return to Bristol I employed, as soon as was practicable, the lymph with which I was furnished. In this proceeding I was kindly aided by Mr. Wilson and Mr. W. B. Carpenter, surgeons, of this city, who are much engaged in vaccinating. The matter I was possessed of was a little from the teat of a cow, which one of the milkers had placed on a piece of glass for me, before I had seen the cows; some which I took from the boy who had caught the complaint by milking; and that from the child Jane, now vaccinated for the first time.

The matter from the cow produced no effect, though tried on several children; nor did that from the boy's hand. Of those vaccinated with the lymph of Jane, two only out of many were infected. One of these patients had one well-formed vesicle, the other had two. In both the disease was late in coming on; in one of them no redness appeared at the base of the vesicle till the tenth day, and the areola was not fully formed till the thirteenth day. In this case, however, Sarah Owens, each vesicle was very perfect, rising abruptly from the arm, its upper part almost overhanging the base; its surface was much flattened, and it yielded freely limpid fluid when punctured before the areola appeared. On the thirteenth day the child's body and extremities were covered with a rash, in patches, much elevated from the skin, and she was constitutionally indisposed. On the fifteenth day the surface of the vesicle was becoming brown, and the areola, rash, and general indisposition, had disappeared.

From these two children many others were vaccinated; and now a second set has been inoculated from these last. In the majority of cases the vesicles have been inflamed round their base about the fourth or fifth day, and the areola has become extensive on the ninth. The areola usually continues for three or four days. In some cases it has been considerable on the eighth day. The vesicles are large, very well marked, and yield an abundant supply of clear lymph, and in every case there has been a good deal of constitutional disturbance. Some who have been vaccinated upon one arm with lymph taken on the eighth day from the other arm, have exhibited on the second vaccination a small vesicle surrounded with a miniature areola, appearing and subsiding with that upon the opposite arm. It appears clear to me that the new lymph is of a very active character; it so much resembles the original cow-pox in a more energetic form, that I feel no doubt of its anti-variolous properties: this, of course, must be decided by future experiments. I am happy thus far to be instrumental in propagating what I think promises to be a valuable renewal of genuine vaccine lymph. I have begun to re-vaccinate with this matter, some who had the cox-pox many years ago, and hope, ere long, to have the means of satisfactorily testing its protective character. Having sent some to Dr. Gregory, physician to the Small-Pox Hospital, I hope he will soon be able to make a favourable report of it; and if any gentleman attached to a public institution for gratuitous vaccination, is desirous of trying the new lymph, removed by so few degrees from its original source as it now is, it will afford me much pleasure to furnish him with a little of it. Should I become possessed of any additional facts that would be interesting either from my own observation or from that of others who have been employing lymph from the same source, I shall take the liberty of again addressing you.

I am, sir, your obedient servant,

J. B. Estlin.

Bristol, September 10th, 1838.

MR. ESTLIN'S SECOND LETTER.

(New series, vol. i., session 1838-39, p. 115.)

To the Editor of *The Medical Gazette*.

Sir,—

The letters I have received from various professional men, in consequence of my communication inserted in the *Gazette* of the 15th of September, convince me that my own anxiety to procure a supply of fresh vaccine virus from the cow, has not led me to overrate the interest of many of my brethren in the same object. The favourable light in which they are pleased to view the very moderate exertions I have had to make, cannot but be gratifying to me; and I feel it due to them to report the result of the farther experience I have had of the new lymph.

In my former letter I stated that the lymph brought to Bristol from the Gloucestershire farm, and successfully employed in inoculation, was removed from the cow only two degrees, having passed through one of the milkers, and the child Jane, inoculated from her. I have now (October 10th) under vaccination the sixth set of Bristol patients. A very few only have been unsusceptible of the disease, and there has, upon the whole, been much uniformity in those characters which appear to me to distinguish the new lymph from that commonly employed. I refer to a larger and longer-continued areola, more constitutional disturbances, and a much deeper indentation left on the arm. The depth in the cellular membrane to which the vesicle extends, is a marked feature in the new lymph. In some cases under my care, when during the third week the scab has been rubbed off, there have been deep, though not wide circular cavities, that would have contained the whole of a pea not of the smallest size.

The scab, if not rubbed, has seldom come away before the fourth week.

The period of teething being that during which children are most commonly brought for vaccination, it is not always easy to discriminate between the consequences of the inoculation and the irritation from the teeth; and the mothers certainly often attribute to the cow-pox symptoms which dentition produces; but I am satisfied I have in some instances seen vomiting occur at intervals, during the first week, in consequence of the vaccination. One child, vaccinated in four places, very near to the shoulder, had the vesicles so much disturbed by the dress as to represent rather deep circular ulcers on the fifth day; much inflammation accompanied the progress of the vesicles for about a fortnight, and two abscesses have formed in the axilla, one of them five weeks after the inoculation, and even after the cicatrization of the vaccinated spot. A scrofulous child, whom I vaccinated on one arm with lymph taken on the eighth day from the other arm, had an abscess produced on the spot of the second inoculation which I was obliged to open; it contained thick pus, had been twelve days in forming, and showed no trace of the inoculation. A similar abscess had formed under the child's chin previously to his being vaccinated. One or two more have had an abscess in the axilla.

More general cutaneous affection has been produced by this lymph than I believe to be often seen after the employment of the common matter. In some children a slight vesicular eruption has appeared during the first or second week; in others, rashes have come on at various periods, even after the third week. Though the parents have occasionally expressed uneasiness at these unusual cutaneous accompaniments, they have generally been pleased with the severity of the complaint, although so much greater than they have been accustomed to see, believing that more complete security against small-pox was thus ensured. I mention all these circumstances without any regard to the impression that they may convey respecting the value of the new virus; my only desire is, that others may have the same means of forming an opinion that I have, in order that its merits or demerits may be investigated. I must consider the evidence of its being even of equal value with the lymph previously in use, as incomplete, until it has been tested by small-pox inoculation. In consequence of the active inflammatory action which some children have had from three and four insertions of lymph, I now, for the most part, confine myself to two; and whenever the infection has taken in only one place, then the least local inconvenience has followed. My practice is, to insert the lymph by means of scratches made within a small space. Those vaccinations which have been least satisfactory were such as have been performed upon sickly children, or those that had eruptions. The re-vaccinations I. have practised tend to show the energy of the new virus. The following are the results in twenty cases:—In four no effect was produced beyond a little redness, or a small pimple, lasting two or three days. In eight persons, whose ages varied from three to sixteen years, there occurred irregular vesicles with more or less inflammation beginning on the third or fourth day, and continuing for eight or ten days. In four others there was rather severe inflammation, producing much uneasiness in the part, and pain in the axillary glands; (in one of them two sloughs formed where the virus had been inserted; the lady who was the subject of this vaccination was confined to the house for some days, and the ulcers had not healed at the end of five weeks). In two of the cases, ladies who had been vaccinated twenty and thirty years ago, flat and tolerably circular vesicles were formed, with a moderate areola; but the areola came on early, and continued for many days. These two cases, however, exhibited the nearest approach of any to a regular vaccine vesicle, but with neither should I have been sufficiently satisfied to have taken lymph for use, had they existed on persons not previously vaccinated. In the two remaining cases there were small vesicles, and slight areolæ for four or five days. In none, however, of these twenty instances did the vaccination run the same course that it has observed in children who had not previously been subjected to cow-pox infection. The cicatrices of the original vaccination in these individuals varied: some were well marked, others very faint, but there seemed no relation between the progress of the lymph and the extent of the original scar.

The new virus is now extensively employed in this city. Messrs. Wilson, Carpenter, Goodeve, Swayne, and several other surgeons of Bristol, are vaccinating with it, and are fully satisfied, as far as appearances go, of its superiority to the matter commonly in use.

Dr. Gregory, of the Small-Pox Hospital, in a letter (the words of which I am sure he will allow me to quote), after detailing the failure of a former trial, says, "The Bristol lymph is of very excellent quality. Had I any doubt of the good qualities of the lymph I have now in use I would forthwith have adopted it (the Bristol lymph), and I am sure I could fully have relied on it." Dr. Gregory was unable to continue the stock from accidental circumstances; but had he been able to do so, he must soon have relinquished it, from its not being in his power to keep up two different kinds of lymph during the winter.

It is too soon, probably, for me to become acquainted with the result of its use in other quarters; but as I have sent a supply to another medical gentleman in London, as well as to practitioners in Dublin, York, Bangor, Retford, Oxford, Bath, Falmouth Harbour, Gloucester, Swansea, Malvern, and many other places, and as the burthen of almost every letter I have received (with the exception of Dr. Gregory's) is dissatisfaction with the present stock of lymph, and unavailing efforts to procure a fresh supply from its original source, I have no doubt of its undergoing a sufficient trial.

One gentleman informs me that he has repeatedly inoculated cows with vaccine virus from the human subject without success. A more fortunate result attended a similar experiment in this neighbourhood. A friend having given me permission to vaccinate one of his cows, the experiment was conducted, during my unavoidable absence, by Mr. Wilson. Vesicles were produced on the cow's teat, running their course in about fourteen days. Children were inoculated with the lymph they furnished, and regular vesicles were reproduced upon their arms; but the lymph, after having thus passed through the cow, produced vesicles in no obvious character differing from those that it gave rise to before it was so treated; and after two or three weeks the stock was accidentally dropped.

The inquiries and correspondence I have been engaged in for the last two months have led me to the adoption of the following conclusions, though, I hope, with no undue confidence in their soundness:—

That the vaccine disease in the cow is not of very common occurrence, and that it is more prevalent in the south-west counties of England than in others; and that matter taken from the cow, and inserted into the human subject in the ordinary method with a lancet, seldom reproduces the disease; and that it is the greater exposure of the milker's hands to the morbid poison, sometimes probably with cutaneous abrasions, that renders them more liable to receive the infection than those who are comparatively slightly inoculated with it.

I still hope, with the aid of those friends who are also using the new lymph, to be able to furnish with it any medical gentleman connected with a public institution for gratuitous vaccination, who is anxious to give it a trial; but I would particularly urge, in order to secure a satisfactory beginning, that a healthy child be selected for vaccination, and one that is free from every kind of eruption.

I am, Sir, your obedient servant,

J. B. ESTLIN.

BRISTOL, October 10th, 1838.

P.S.—Oct. 11th.—After forwarding my letter of yesterday's date, I received from Mr. J. Soden, of Bath, the following report addressed to him by Mr. Gore, surgeon, of that city:—"I find the whole number vaccinated by myself or by deputy since September 15th, from Mr. Estlin's stock of matter, to be fourteen. It appears to be a very satisfactory kind; as regular in its progress as that we have been in the habit of using, but more severe as regards the extent and degree of the surrounding areola. I have watched it in three successive removes from the stock received from Mr. Estlin, and have not observed any modification or diminution of its intensity." "I am still keeping it up."

MR. ESTLIN'S THIRD LETTER.

(Vol. xxiii., 1838-39, p. 707.)

On the New Vaccine Virus.

To the Editor of *The Medical Gazette*.

SIR,—

As the recent supply of vaccine virus from the cow has excited the attention of many of your readers, and as the demand for it seems likely to increase, I think it may be satisfactory to those who are interested in the subject to be informed, that the new lymph has been sent for use to the National Vaccine Establishment, in order to facilitate its transmission to those members of the profession, who may desire to be furnished with it.

The following correspondence contains the communications I

have had with the respectable Registrar of that Board; and if not trespassing too much upon your pages, I shall be obliged by its early insertion, both as a matter of information to others, and for the purpose (whatever may be the future fate of the new virus) of placing upon record its history to the present period:—

"To the Registrar of the National Vaccine Establishment, Russell Place, Fitzroy Square, London.

"BRISTOL, *November 23rd*, 1838.

"Sir,—

"Being ignorant to what member of the National Vaccine Establishment I ought to address this application, I shall be obliged by your laying my letter before those who have the power of deciding upon the request it contains.

"This request is, that if it be not inconsistent with the regulations of the Institution, and not likely to be attended with inconvenience to those on whom the duty of vaccinating devolves, a stock of the vaccine virus, at present in my possession, which has been extensively used in this city, and circulated through England, may be employed at the National Vaccine Establishment, so that distant practitioners may receive supplies of it, on making the usual application.

"The grounds upon which I consider this virus as presenting claims to the notice of the Establishment, will be seen from the following account:—In August last I visited a farm in Gloucestershire (near Berkeley), where I saw cows and milkers, and the children who had been inoculated from the latter affected with cow-pox. I took some lymph from a very fine vesicle produced on the arm of a child, by inoculation with the virus from the hand of one of the milkers, and employed it for vaccination on my return to Bristol. The stock of new virus was thus fully established, and a succession of it is still kept up by many other practitioners in this city, beside myself.

"A statement of these facts is given in the numbers of the *London Medical Gazette* for September 15th and October 20th, and in consequence of these communications to the public, a strong desire has been evinced by medical gentlemen in various parts of the United Kingdom, to possess some of the new virus, and many have written to me for it. I have sent lymph (with a statement of the number of individuals through whom it has passed since it came from the cow) to the following places: Bath, Warminster, Swansea, Oxford, Retford, Bangor, Plymouth,

London (to four different quarters), Great Malvern, York, Dublin, Gloucester, H.M. ship *Pandora* (for the colonies); Langport, Madeira, Berwick-upon-Tweed, Liverpool, Chepstow, Bridgewater, Stafford, Somerton, Falmouth, South Petherton, Kidderminster, Cambridge (to two surgeons); Sussex, Newcastle-upon-Tyne, Stroud, Barbadoes, Plympton, Thirsk, Wincanton, Droitwich, and Sidmouth; to many places near Bristol, also to Paris, Switzerland, and America; and upon the application of the Consul General for Portugal, to Lisbon, and to the Portuguese physician of Madeira.

"Under these circumstances I think I am warranted in regarding the new virus as of sufficient interest in the estimation of the medical public, to entitle it to the notice of the National Vaccine Establishment, where more certain means will exist for keeping it up, and greater facilities will be given to its transmission to distant places. I have to acknowledge the polite attention of all who have written to me for it, in saving me from every avoidable expense, and it has been gratifying and instructive to me to communicate with so many intelligent practitioners. But if the demands for the matter continue, as it appears will probably be the case, it may not be in the power of an individual, engaged as I am in general practice, to supply them; and the means of keeping up the virus in this city may be lost. Having done all in my power to promote the interests of vaccination, I might upon personal grounds expect that the National Vaccine Establishment would now assist in relieving me of the duty I have hitherto cheerfully undertaken; but I would rather rest any claim for compliance with my request, upon the accommodation which will be thus afforded to a large number of my professional brethren.

"Should the Board be willing to introduce the new virus, I shall have pleasure in forwarding some which is recent, in any manner that may be desired; and I will send with it a correct statement of the progress of the lymph since it was taken from its original source.

"I ought to mention that the vesicle produced by the new virus has the well-marked characters of the vaccine disease; it is attended with more local and constitutional irritation, and, in the opinion of several elder practitioners, more resembles the vesicle which was met with twenty years ago, than that which is produced by the lymph in ordinary use.

"I am, Sir, your faithful servant,

"JOHN BISHOP ESTLIN."

To this letter I received the following satisfactory reply:—

"National Vaccine Establishment,
"*December* 11*th*, 1838.

"Sir,—I have the pleasure to acknowledge the receipt of your communication on the subject of a fresh supply of vaccine lymph. It was conveyed by Sir James Clark to this Board, and immediately taken into due consideration.

"I am instructed to inform you that the president and members fully participate with you in the zeal which you have manifested to promote vaccination. Their confidence in the genuineness of the lymph which they employ remains unshaken, after an experience of many years of its use; but they will gladly avail themselves of your kind offer to make trial of that which has been more recently obtained by yourself from the cow. If you will have the goodness to send us a supply in any form you please, it shall be used and tested with the greatest care, and I shall feel gratified in faithfully reporting to you the result.

"I remain, Sir,
"Your most obedient servant,
"C. HUE, M.D.,
"Registrar.

"JOHN BISHOP ESTLIN, ESQ."

Immediately upon the receipt of Dr. Hue's letter, I sent a supply of lymph from two healthy children to the National Vaccine Establishment, and I was in hopes that by this time the stock would have been sufficiently established to allow of its being forwarded to those who made applications for it; but from the following letter which I have received from Dr. Hue since I began writing this communication, I have reason to fear that either the lymph I sent has not been successfully propagated, or that the supply has been accidentally cut off.

"National Vaccine Establishment,
"*January* 23*rd*, 1839.

"Sir,—I am desired by the Board to request that you will favour us with an additional supply of the vaccine lymph which you have been in the habit of using. It is the wish of the Board to make a further trial of it, before they communicate to you their report.

"I remain, Sir,
"Your most obedient servant,
"C. HUE, M.D.,
"Registrar.

"J. B. ESTLIN, ESQ., BRISTOL."

In compliance, therefore, with this request, I have sent a second supply of lymph to the Board of the National Vaccine Establishment.

Since my second letter, inserted in your number for October 10th, I have continued to watch the progress of the virus. It has lost none of its activity at its present distance of about twenty removes from the cow. If any change have taken place, I would say that the vesicles are more firm and perfect, and less disposed to be broken during the first week, than was the case at an earlier period. Though I find the surest method of propagating the infection from dry matter is to rub it upon scratches of very small extent, the fluid lymph appears to me to answer best when inserted with a clean lancet into a minute puncture. A free insertion of lymph I find most liable to occasion excessive local irritation; and the vesicle produced upon scratches, from the injury done to the skin, is more inclined to break during the first week, than that which follows the introduction by puncture.

Mr. Humpage, surgeon of this city, informs me that since he has adopted the plan of having a piece of cotton wadding so stitched into the child's sleeve as to admit of the vesicle being completelv covered with it (the flocculent part being next the skin), he has seldom found a vesicle prematurely broken.

No cases of serious constitutional disorder attending the vaccinations in Bristol have come to my knowledge, though there have been instances of severe inflammation and ulceration in the arm.

From Langport, in Somersetshire, I have received a report, which shows that the new virus has exhibited a character of peculiar severity in that neighbourhood. The following is the result of the vaccinations practised on 68 children, by Messrs. Michell and Prankard, of Langport :—

In 52 cases the progress of the disease was regular.
1 Severe erysipelas.
4 Erythematous eruptions of a violent character.
2 Highly inflamed, ulcerated arms.
1 No effect after twice vaccinating.
8 Result unknown; supposed to have been favourable.
68

One of the patients with erythema, an unhealthy child, two months of age, died. It was vaccinated on the 29th of last December, and as no effect was produced, the inoculation was repeated on the 5th of January. On the 7th erythema attacked the back, and gradually extended to the feet, never affecting the arms, nor was there any appearance of vesicle. The child had much dyspnœa, with croupy cough, and died on the 21st ult. My correspondent observes :—"I do not attribute its death to vaccination, nor does the mother wholly, as she lost an infant previously with a similar affection of the air passages, but her neighbours set it down to vaccination entirely."

The case of erysipelas and the two others of erythema were serious ones. The attacks came on during the first week, two of them on the day following vaccination. One child had no vesicles.* It may be worthy of mentioning, that an uncle and aunt of the infant that suffered from erysipelas were similarly affected after cow-pox inoculation many years ago. The alarm occasioned by the violent symptoms which occurred in some of these children has induced Messrs. Michell and Prankard to suspend, for the present, the employment of this virus.

I have not yet had the power of inoculating with variolous matter any of the children recently vaccinated, but I have been favoured with a very satisfactory communication from Mr. Halton, house-surgeon to the Chorlton-upon-Medlock Dispensary, Manchester, in which he informs me, that in a family where there were four unvaccinated children, the three elder ones being seized with small-pox, he vaccinated the youngest, who took the cow-pox properly, and was preserved from the variolous infection. The interest felt by this gentleman and the other members of the profession in Manchester in the new virus may be inferred from the fact of his having at the date of his letter furnished seventy-one neighbouring practitioners with supplies of the matter.

And here I would remark that, as far as I have had an opportunity of collecting opinions from the extensive correspondence I have had on the subject, the confidence of the president and members of the National Vaccine Establishment in the "genuineness" of the lymph they employ and distribute, is not participated in by the profession generally, at least not by their provincial brethren. I am happy to perceive that the whole subject of vaccination is undergoing in this and in other countries some of that searching investigation which its importance demands. We are beginning to discover how much we have to learn respecting it. Careful observation of facts is more needed than theories and opinions. I am unable to feel any of that uncertainty with which some correspondents of the periodicals decide upon the precise time

* Having had the opportunity of seeing three of these cases referred to, I can testify to the severity of the inflammatory attacks.

when lymph ought, and ought not, to be taken; upon the necessity of re-vaccination, and even the period when it ought to be performed, and upon many other points of much intricacy. I know of nothing in the history of vaccination to warrant the assertion that lymph should be taken before the eighth day, to insure the successful propagation of the disease. I am in the habit of selecting those vesicles round which no areola has formed, for furnishing the lymph for future inoculation; but I am by no means certain that it would prove less effectual if used at a much later period. That the crust has been successfully employed for vaccinating is a well-known fact; nor is it conformable with my experience, that virus taken from a vesicle yielding but a small quantity of fluid is more active than when taken from one exuding lymph in greater abundance.

Most discordant are the opinions, and even the experiments, with regard to re-vaccination; and much patient and unprejudiced inquiry is required, to determine satisfactory results. From the extensive re-vaccinations practised in the Prussian army, when nearly one-half of the soldiers were affected with the regular disease, it has been concluded that the effect of the first vaccination decreases with advancing years, and that the risk of taking the small-pox is proportioned to the distance of time from the first inoculation of Cow Pox.

On the other hand, Dr. Neumann, a German physician (quoted in one of the numbers for the last year of the Belgian *Encyclographie des Sciences Médicales*), gives the results of 685 re-vaccinations, and comes to the conclusion, that those most liable to be attacked with small-pox after cow-pox are children who have been vaccinated but a few years.

Much discussion has also been taking place as to the proper period for re-vaccinating; but are we in possession of evidence adequate to prove that a second vaccination has more power to protect the constitution from an attack of small-pox than the first introduction of the cow-pox into the system? Two cases of small-pox after re-vaccination have lately come to my knowledge; one of them proved fatal, though the patient, a young gentleman of seventeen years of age, had gone through a satisfactory re-vaccination only four months before he died from the variolous attack.

To these, and to similar inquiries, as well as to the probable deterioration of the virus by passing through a great number of human beings, many of them probably affected with constitutional ailments, I trust an attentive consideration will now be [illegible] were ably [illegible] last meeting [illegible] cannot but [illegible] in that [illegible] in which it has been [illegible]

[illegible] servant,

[illegible]

INTRODUCTION OF THE NEW VACCINE VIRUS INTO AMERICA.

[illegible]

Sir,—

[illegible]

[illegible]

I am, Sir, your obedient servant,

[illegible]

[illegible]

some appearance of vesicles in five of the punctures,—on the seventh they had increased considerably, and the child became restless and feverish, and vomited several times. On the ninth day the vesicles were very distinct and full; the areola large and well defined. As soon as I became convinced that the virus you sent me had not lost its virtues (*i.e.*, on the fourth day after inserting some of it as above stated), I vaccinated two other children with the virus received from you, in both of whom it succeeded perfectly. From these three children I have taken virus and given some to the medical gentlemen of this city, who are using it with success and great satisfaction; I have transmitted some to medical friends in New York city, and to the vaccine institution of that place, and I shall exert myself to spread it over the country.

"Most sincerely do I thank you for this valuable present to myself and country. For several years, in common with other medical men of my acquaintance, I have noticed that our vaccine virus was less active than formerly; thus, frequently after very careful insertion no effect was produced, and at other times the vesicles were small, the areola indistinct, and the constitutional symptoms very slight, and often not observed.

"I have feared our vaccine virus had become less efficacious in preventing Small Pox than formerly, though I have no facts that positively prove this. The virus you have sent me is more active, produces a larger vesicle and more distinct areola, and more marked constitutional symptoms, than any I have used for ten years past.

"The history of vaccination in this country, briefly stated, is as follows:—

"In 1799, Dr. George Pearson, of London, sent at two different times, threads, imbued with vaccine matter, to Dr. Miller, of New York city; but this virus probably lost its virtues during the voyage, as experiments with it failed.

"In July, 1800, Dr. Waterhouse, of the University of Cambridge, Massachusetts, procured some good virus from England, and vaccinated his son: this was the first successful case in this country.

"From this source it was extended quite generally over the country; but this was not the only source.

"In 1801, it was obtained from the cow by Dr. Buel, of Massachusetts, and Drs. North and Trowbridge, of Connecticut. For a number of years vaccination was quite general throughout the country, but of late it has been much neglected.

"It is not in the hands of any particular class of medical men, but is practised by all physicians.

"Usually the physician who acts as accoucheur vaccinates the child when a few weeks old; but frequently, especially in the country when there is no alarm from the small-pox, medical men do not obtain the virus for a number of years: when a few cases of small-pox occur, then vaccination becomes general in that region.

"In some of the large cities are vaccine institutions, where the poor are vaccinated gratuitously. In some of the states, as in this, the law requires the town authority to adopt measures for the vaccination of the inhabitants twice a year, and those who refuse to have their children vaccinated are liable to be fined; but this law, I believe, is wholly inoperative, though the town authorities occasionally hire a physician to vaccinate all who wish it.

"Still we have had but very little small-pox among the civilized inhabitants, since the introduction of the vaccine disease. Cases out of the large commercial places are quite rare. During the last year it has prevailed to a frightful extent among the Indians in our western country. Several thousands perished in a short time, and no doubt many more would have done so, but for the prompt efforts of the army surgeons, who were despatched by our government to their relief with vaccine virus. In concluding this long letter I again wish to express to you for myself and my countrymen many thanks for the gift transmitted to me, and to assure you I shall endeavour to spread it over the country, believing it will be the means of doing great—very great good.

"With sentiments of great respect,

"I am your obliged servant,

"A. BRIGHAM.

"HARTFORD, STATE OF CONNECTICUT,

"*Jan. 16th*, 1839."

REPORT OF THE NATIONAL VACCINE ESTABLISHMENT

(WITH THEIR OPINION OF MR. ESTLIN'S COW POX).

(Vol. xxiii., 1838-39, p. 834.)

Report from the National Vaccine Establishment, February, 1839.

To the RIGHT HON. LORD JOHN RUSSELL, Secretary of State for the Home Department.

Feb. 11*th*, 1839.

MY LORD,—

The small-pox has prevailed epidemically, and with great severity, not only in England, but also in a considerable part of the continent of Europe, since our last report.

It seems, from the history of this disease, that it has recurred epidemically once in twelve or fourteen years, ever since its first introduction into these islands, and always with extraordinary violence and destruction of life; so that 45,000 persons are said to have died in one of these epidemic years, before inoculation was introduced, at the beginning of the last century.

Since that practice was brought here the loss of life by small-pox within the bills of mortality was 5,000 annually; but since vaccination has superseded inoculation, the number of deaths has decreased gradually, until it amounted to only 200 deaths in the ye 1837. In the course of the year which has lately terminated (during which small-pox prevailed epidemically) there have died 800 of this disease: not more, after all, than one-sixth of the number of those who died annually during the prevalence of inoculation, notwithstanding the increased population of the metropolis and its neighbourhood.—Surely this implies some generally protective influence, and our confidence in the efficacy of good vaccination remains unabated. We are indeed convinced that the indiscriminate vaccination which has been practised in this country, by ignorant and unqualified persons, with but little or no regard to the condition of body of the persons to be vaccinated, to the selection of the vaccine lymph, or to the progress and character of the vesicle to be formed, are to be regarded as amongst the main causes of the occasional failure of vaccination; and we are sorry to hear an anxiety expressed that a recurrence should often be made to the disease of the cow which first supplied the genuine protective matter: for, in the first place, it is not in the nature of any other communicable virus to degenerate and lose its influence; and, in the next, we have the opportunity of bearing our most ample testimony to the continuance of the efficiency of the original vaccine lymph introduced by Dr. Jenner through nearly a million of subjects successively, of whom many thousands have been exposed with entire impunity to small-pox in its most malignant form; and though we ourselves have taken a good opportunity more than once or twice of recruiting our stores with fresh genuine matter from the cow, yet we think it right to discourage an indiscriminate imprudent resort to this expedient; because the animal is subject to more than one eruptive disease, and a slight mistake might possibly be made in the selection of the proper pustule, by an inexperienced hand.

We have vaccinated, by our several appointed vaccinators, 18,659 persons this last year, and have sent out to various parts of the world 203,818 charges of lymph; the former amounting to 6,241 more than have been vaccinated in the metropolis and neighbourhood for any former year, and the latter exceeding distributions of lymph from the National Institution by 79,097 charges.

(Signed) HENRY HALFORD, President of the Royal College of Physicians, President of the Board.

HON. LEIGH THOMAS, President of the Royal College of Surgeons.

THOMAS WATSON, Senior Censor of the Royal College of Physicians.

CLEMENT HUE, M.D., Registrar.

MR. ESTLIN'S REPLY TO THE REPORT
OF THE
NATIONAL VACCINE ESTABLISHMENT.

(Vol. xxiii., 1838-39, p. 863.)

Vaccine Report.

To the Editor of *The Medical Gazette.*

SIR,—

It was not my intention to trouble you so soon with another communication; but as a report to the Government has just been published by the National Vaccine Establishment, bearing closely upon the subject respecting which I had before addressed you, I shall be obliged by your allowing me space for noticing two parts of that document. A very decided opinion has been given in that Report upon a most important point relating to vaccination, with all the *authority* certainly of the National Vaccine Board, but, as it appears to me, without that proof of its correctness by which such an opinion ought to be supported. In the present state of our experience, and of our *ignorance* with respect to vaccination—deficient as the virus in ordinary use has for several years been in reproducing a well-marked vesicle, attended by that extent of local and constitutional affection which characterised the disease twenty years ago—prone as the lymph has been, after being kept for only a few days, to lose its infecting properties, and painfully shaken as public confidence is known to be in every village and town throughout the kingdom, in the power now possessed by vaccination of affording protection against small-pox—I cannot but think that the attempt to renew our stock of virus occasionally, from the original source, is discouraged in this Report by a *dictum* little suited to the present age of philosophical investigation.

It is not my purpose to argue that the evils so seriously felt will be entirely, or even partially, removed by the introduction of fresh supplies of lymph into practice (though I hope soon to address you on this subject); but while so much uncertainty exists as to the cause of those evils, it appears to me that the National Vaccine Board was bound to adduce stronger arguments against the rational proceeding of occasionally procuring fresh virus from the cow than that "the animal is subject to more than one eruptive disease, and a mistake might possibly be made in the selection of the proper pustule by an inexperienced hand." The *mistakes* liable to arise from carelessness and inexperience are not peculiar to vaccination.

The other remark I have to make, refers to the number of individuals mentioned in that Report, through whose constitutions the virus now in use is said to have passed.

It is stated, that the lymph now employed at the National Vaccine Establishment, is some that has descended through an uninterrupted series of patients, from the original virus introduced by Dr. Jenner. Whether the records of the Establishment have been so accurately kept during forty years as to prove this satisfactorily, and to establish the fact that lymph, from some unknown source (perhaps from a cow more recently infected than those diseased in Dr. Jenner's day), has never superseded the older virus, I have no means of determining; but it is not difficult to perceive that much misapprehension will be the consequence of an implicit reliance on that document which is now presented to the Secretary of State, and circulated through this and other countries.

The Report, after expressing regret that a recurrence to the cow should be thought necessary, and after stating the opinion that "it is not in the nature of any other communicable virus to degenerate and lose its influence" (an opinion, however, contrary to that of many medical authorities), goes on to affirm, as a proof of the "efficiency of the original vaccine lymph, introduced at the Vaccine Establishment by Dr. Jenner," that it has "passed through nearly a million of subjects successively, of whom many thousands have been exposed, with entire impunity, to Small Pox in its most malignant form."

Now, it is only forty years since the introduction of vaccination, and, however numerous may be the subjects that have been vaccinated at one time from the same individual, the stock of matter at present employed at the National Vaccine Establishment can only have passed through 2,080 subjects, even supposing that lymph for subsequent vaccination had been taken every seven days from a fresh subject, without any interruption, from the time when Dr. Jenner first sent it to London. In order that it should pass through a million subjects, the lapse of 19,230 years and 10 months would be required.

In periods of general alarm, to what extent it may be justifiable to have recourse to the *pious fraud* of strong, and not very accurate statements, for the purpose of calming the public mind, I am not causist enough to determine; my preference, however, is for truth and correctness at all times; and I cannot but think it a matter of regret, on the present occasion, that an official document should have emanated from the National Vaccine Establishment of England, attested by the name of the learned President of the Royal College of Physicians, and destined to be circulated, not only throughout our own kingdom, but in countries where great attention is paid to the accuracy of medical statistics, so expressed as to refer the origin of vaccination to such a remote period as thirteen thousand years before the beginning of the world.

I am, Sir,
Your obedient servant,
J. B. ESTLIN.

BRISTOL, March 4th, 1839.

MR. ESTLIN'S FOURTH LETTER.

(Vol. xxiv., 1839, p. 151.)

On the New Vaccine Virus.

THIRD* LETTER.

To the Editor of *The Medical Gazette.*

SIR,—

As I have received an answer from the Registrar of the National Vaccine Establishment, in reply to my application for them to use the fresh vaccine lymph *for the purpose of distributing it* free of expense to those medical men who wished to have it, I shall be glad of permission to insert another communication in *The Medical Gazette.* My request is refused, and I am therefore preparing a letter of resignation of the office (rather an onerous one) of distributing lymph to all who apply for it. For the last six or seven months I have been constantly engaged in this business; and I cannot but hope that, eventually, I may be in some remote way instrumental towards procuring the permission to medical men of having vaccine lymph circulated *free of postage* from all quarters, as well as from the National Vaccine Establishment.

I know not what *your* sentiments are with respect to the proceedings of the National Vaccine Establishment; to me it appears a most *inefficient* institution, though provided with means,

[* *Vide*, p. 359.—E.M.C.]

and with abundant information, to be exceedingly useful in promoting a proper investigation into all the difficulties which surround vaccination. Under its present régime, with its meagre indefinite Annual Reports, it appears to me an *incubus* on the progress of vaccination in this country. I should be very glad, if it were in my power, to lend a helping hand in awakening this sleepy establishment, carefully, however, avoiding all allusions to, or reflections on *individuals*. I know there are those of much influence in our profession in town, who, though unwilling, from various circumstances connected with members of the Board, to take any ostensible part in finding fault, would be very glad to see a more efficient management pursued.

In the first volume of *The Medical Gazette* is an editorial article which quite accords with my views: if such be yours, would not the present be a suitable time to renew such observations?

I doubt if there be any one subject of communication to the *Gazette* that meets with attention from *so many* readers as vaccination, and therefore it is that I feel less reluctance in being so frequent a correspondent upon it as has been the case latterly.

I propose sending you a letter of four or five columns by the end of this week, or by Monday next, for insertion in the *Gazette* of Saturday week; and I have a communication from the Faculty of Medicine in Glasgow, in reference to the new virus, and containing some valuable observations on vaccination, which I think you would be glad to publish in the following week. I I must, however, write to Glasgow for permission to make this use of it, and hope to forward it to you for insertion in the number for next Saturday fortnight.

I am, Sir,

Your obedient servant,

J. B. ESTLIN.

BRISTOL, April 16th, 1839.

FOURTH* LETTER.

SIR,—

Having received a letter from the Registrar of the National Vaccine Establishment, in reply to my request that the stock of vaccine virus procured from the cow in August last might be kept at that Institution, in order to supply those professional gentlemen who wished to make a trial of it, I must trouble you with one communication more, probably a final one, in reference to this virus.

It will be in the remembrance of such of your readers as have

[* *Vide*, p. 359.—E.M.C.]

taken an interest in the subject, that in consequence of the numerous applications made to me for the new lymph, more numerous than probably I could continue to comply with, I wrote to the National Vaccine Board, requesting their aid in supplying the demands of the profession. My letter was dated November 23rd, 1838; and on the 14th December, by desire of the Registrar, I sent several charges of lymph to be employed in establishing the new supply. On the 23rd of January, 1839, an additional quantity was requested by the Board, which I also forwarded. On the third of this month (April) I received a communication from the Registrar, from which the following statement, being all that relates to this subject, is extracted :—

"I have the pleasure to inform you that we have duly tried the lymph which you were so kind as to send us, and that in four cases out of five we have succeeded in producing the true vaccine disease, and which in no respect appears to differ from that we daily witness from the employment of the lymph of this establishment. In two instances, however, the lymph taken from the above successful cases did not reproduce perfect vesicles; they were small, and without areolæ. I am instructed to add, that under the present circumstances the Board are not disposed to entertain any preference for your lymph, nor would feel justified in substituting it in lieu of that which they are in the constant habit of using, and of which, consequently, they have a most extensive and satisfactory experience."

The reference to the new lymph is concluded by the following extract from the letter of the Plymouth correspondent to the Board, dated March 9th, 1839:—

"Mr. Estlin's vaccine has been introduced here, and I have used it in two cases, but am not satisfied with it, and intend vaccinating with the true virus: many of the practitioners here have the same opinion of the Estlin vaccine." *

That the new lymph should supplant the stock previously in

* As the Registrar has seen fit to send me such an extract from the correspondence of the National Vaccine Board, perhaps I may be excused for giving a quotation from one of *my* correspondents—the surgeon of two extensive medical charities in one of our most populous towns, who vaccinated not *two*, but *two hundred* children, between January 28th and April 8th. He says: "Notwithstanding the *wise* letter of the Vaccine Board, with Sir H. Halford's signature attached to it, about twenty to thirty medical men have now received the new virus, and the old stock at the dispensary here is now obsolete. To-morrow the Hospital will receive the new matter, so that soon, all round this populous district, none but the new matter will be in existence; the hospital and dispensary being the only two places where vaccine inoculation is publicly done, from whence it is distributed to all the medical men around."

use, I neither asked nor wished; but considering how great the demand for it had been, and regarding the National Vaccine Establishment as one intended to promote, in all rational ways, investigation into the subject of vaccination, it appeared to me not unreasonable to hope—I thought, indeed, that the profession had a right to expect—that the Board would employ the facility it possesses for extensive vaccination, and the privilege accorded to it by government, of receiving letters and sending lymph free of postage, to meet the wish widely felt by medical men, and lend its aid to the experimental employment of a fresh supply of virus from the cow.

In this hope I have been disappointed; and if the grounds of the refusal are satisfactory to the profession generally, I have no right to complain.

I am, however, now desirous of considering myself released from the offer I made seven months ago, to furnish the new lymph to any professional man connected with an institution for gratuitous vaccination that applied for it.

That offer has been extensively embraced, and I have sent supplies to Bangor, Barbadoes, Bath, Berwick-upon-Tweed, Birmingham, Bridport, Bridgend, Bridgewater, Cambridge, Chepstow, Douglas, Droitwich, Dublin, Exeter, Falmouth, Glasgow, Gloucester, Hull, Ilfracombe, Ilminster, Kidderminster, Langport, Liverpool, London, Malvern, Manchester, Maxstock, Nevis, Newport, Oxford, Plymouth, Plympton, Retford, Sidmouth, South Petherton, Stroud, St. Vincent, Somerton, Swansea, Stafford, Thirsk, Warrington, Warminster, Wincanton, Winchester, Worcester, York, and to numerous other towns and villages; besides to America, France, Switzerland, Portugal, and Madeira.

Having thus testified my desire to promote the interests of vaccination, and being denied that aid from the New Vaccine Establishment which I thought I might calculate upon, I feel myself entitled to retire from an office which, though productive of much interesting correspondence, has not been unattended with trouble or expense. It is, I presume, unnecessary for me to add, that I have had no interest in the employment of the new lymph distinct from that of the profession and the public. I have declined all vaccinations but gratuitous ones (excepting in the families where I am the regular attendant), and I have freely given the matter to all who have applied for it.

In my former letters I have avoided giving any decided opinion with regard to the new lymph, and have withheld nothing that was unfavourable to it. I have been anxious to state the facts I had remarked, to induce others to make their own observations, and to have the experiments extensively made before any inference was drawn.

But having watched the virus through twenty-nine subjects successively (nearly one every week since the matter was procured from the cow), I have now no hesitation in stating that I consider it a valuable supply of virus, more energetic in its local and constitutional effects, and more inclined to produce vesicles, resembling what cow-pox was many years ago, than that employed by the National Vaccine Establishment.

It is so much estimated in this city, that I believe there is no other in use; and, as an institution has been established here, to be devoted solely to vaccination, we hope to be able to keep up the new stock.

What is the general opinion among the practitioners who have employed it in the numerous places to which it has been sent, I have had little means of ascertaining. I trust they will not withhold their views from the public. I presume, from the quotation sent me from the Plymouth correspondent of the National Vaccine Establishment, the Registrar considers the experience in the two cases referred to, and the opinion expressed by the writer, as evidence *against* the genuineness of the lymph: your readers must form their own judgment on this point. It is not impossible that even from Plymouth some opposing evidence may appear; and perhaps I may be allowed to adduce, as testimony of at least equal value, a published Report of the Chorlton-upon-Medlock Dispensary, Manchester, in which the decline in the activity of the former virus is spoken of as having "been long felt by the medical practitioner," and the new lymph is described as "a present of no ordinary value"; and, since writing the above, I have received a report from the committee of the Vaccine Institution connected with the Faculty of Medicine in Glasgow, especially made in reference to the new virus, minutely detailing its effects, and designating it as "a great boon to the public and that profession." This document contains some most judicious observations upon vaccination.

Whether it be dependent upon a more cautious mode of vaccinating (the introduction of only a very small quantity of lymph into never more than two points of insertion), or upon any alteration in the lymph, violent local irritation and cutaneous eruptions less frequently accompany the progress of the vesicle at present than was the case six months ago; but the character of the vesicle is most satisfactory. On the eighth day it may be compared in form to a minute coil of inflated intestine: it has a pearly hue, with scarcely a line's extent of redness at its base—often none at all: it is solid to the touch; freely yields pellucid lymph when punctured in the centre; and is so little affected by the escape of its fluid contents, that I have charged thirty points from a single vesicle without any perceptible change in its size or shape. On the ninth or tenth day the areola comes on. Sometimes the crust projects from the skin on the subsidence of the areola on the fourteenth or fifteenth day, and falls off in about a week more; in many cases, however, it becomes rather indented towards the fifteenth day, very like an eschar made with caustic potass, and accompanied by a secondary attack of surrounding inflammation, and of a more diffused character than the original areola; the crust is then separated, leaving a small but deep ulcer, that heals in a few days. And here I would express my surprise that in the report sent from the National Vaccine Establishment, the new lymph is spoken of as producing a disease "which in no respect appears to differ" from that which is daily witnessed from the use of the lymph usually employed there.

Most extraordinary, I am certain, will this statement appear to very many practitioners who have used the virus; and limited, indeed, must be the experiments made with it for such a conclusion to be formed. Perhaps, however, the opinion of the Board is founded upon no more than the seven cases referred to in the letter of the Registrar and the two cases from Plymouth. Very different is the experience with the new virus in this city. The only objection to it I hear of here is, its being much more active than the old lymph; and there are practitioners in other places, who from this cause, have thought it prudent to suspend the employment of it.

How far the introduction of a fresh stock of virus from the cow will have any influence in renewing the protecting power of cow-pox—which, of late years, it seems in some degree to have lost—I have not presumed to offer an opinion. It appears to me that one, and not an unimportant step is gained, if this recurrence to the original source have procured a virus more energetic in its course, capable of retaining its infecting properties for a longer time, and producing a vesicle more resembling that which was seen twenty years ago, than the lymph in common use.

That the new virus possesses these points of superiority I have no doubt, and though I have before commented upon the late Report of the National Vaccine Board, I cannot conclude this letter without repeating my regret that, in the present unsettled state of medical opinion upon vaccination, and under the failing confidence of the public in its protecting efficacy, the members of that establishment, with no better reason than an apprehension that the inexperienced might make mistakes, and with no evidence whatever to justify their opinion, should pronounce the recurrence to the cow for fresh lymph as an undesirable measure; and yet, while deprecating this application to the original source of the disease, and while extolling the purity of the lymph used at the Establishment, maintaining that it is a direct succession of that originally used by Dr. Jenner, the report declares that the stores of the establishment have been occasionally recruited "with fresh matter from the cow."

It is affirmed in this document, with the view of proving that cow-pox does not deteriorate, that "it is not in the nature of any other communicable virus to degenerate and lose its influence."

I would ask, is there any person long accustomed to vaccinate who cannot testify from his own experience that there is a constant tendency in the vaccine disease to degenerate? and that different constitutions so modify it, that, if care be not taken in the selection of the lymph for continued inoculations, it will become so weakened by passing through peculiar constitutions, as at length to be effete. The caution given in the Report is an implied admission of this fact.

Is it not also tolerably well ascertained, that, by a constant selection of the mildest cases for furnishing virus, inoculation for small-pox may be rendered comparatively safe? and that, at the time of the introduction of vaccination, this virulent morbid poison had been, in the opinion of some, so modified by successive inoculations, as to produce pustules for which the name of pearl pox was proposed?

The want of care and accuracy in statistical detail in the Report, which has given an age of nineteen thousand years to the lymph employed at the Establishment, has been commented upon by others as well as myself; * and, I have no doubt, will obtain much more notice when the document is perused by our continental neighbours.

Nor is it to the late Report alone that much may be objected. Considering the mass of information which the correspondence of the Board must have accumulated, it is impossible to read the reports of former years without being struck by their meagreness.

* See *Lancet*, March 9th, 1839.

[illegible] are given—no experiments detailed—no measures suggested either for the enforcement of vaccination or the prohibition of small-pox inoculation. It does not, indeed, require much reflection to perceive that however well intended the labours of that Establishment may be, we must look to other quarters for that amount of observation, that statistical accuracy, and that general energy, which, at the present [illegible] of the discovery of the [illegible], [illegible] the wants of the profession and public demand.

It is much to be desired that Government would allow the transmission of vaccine lymph from all quarters free of postage. Were this privilege extended only to the Small-pox Hospital, and the Royal Jennerian Institution in London, instead of being confined to the National Vaccine Establishment, the provinces would probably be often supplied with more efficient virus.

To those who prefer the new lymph, I would suggest, as there is no chance of their being supplied with it from London, that when a fine vesicle presents itself, two or three dozen of ivory points be thoroughly charged, and preserved in a dry, well-corked phial for future use. From the experience I have had, I have no hesitation in saying, that the virus will thus retain its infecting properties for several weeks.

I cannot conclude these letters without acknowledging the valuable information I have derived from the extensive correspondence in which I have been engaged, as well as the gratification I have felt at the favourable manner in which my humble efforts to serve the cause of vaccination have been appreciated: my professional brethren may be assured that I will not neglect any future opportunity that may occur of procuring information upon this subject that may be either useful or interesting, and with thanks for the promptitude with which you have been pleased to insert my communications.

I remain, Sir,

Your obedient servant,

J. B. Estlin.

Bristol, April 20th, 1839.

REPORT OF THE GLASGOW FACULTY OF MEDICINE ON THE NEW LYMPH.

(Vol. xxiv., 1839, p. 208.)

On the New Vaccine Virus.

To the Editor of *The Medical Gazette.*

SIR,—

I have pleasure in forwarding you a copy of the Report sent to me by the Glasgow Faculty of Medicine, which I am certain will be very interesting to many of the readers of the *Gazette.*

I am, Sir,

Your obedient servant,

J. B. ESTLIN.

BRISTOL, April 23rd, 1839.

REPORT OF THE COMMITTEE APPOINTED BY THE GLASGOW FACULTY OF MEDICINE TO SUPERINTEND THE EMPLOYMENT OF THE NEW VIRUS IN THE VACCINE INSTITUTION.

Before proceeding to the immediate object of this report, the Committee consider it their bounden duty to bear testimony to the prompt and courteous manner in which Mr. Estlin complied with the request of the Faculty of Medicine for a supply of the recent lymph, which he has been the honourable and praiseworthy means of introducing to the notice of the profession.

As the letter inclosing Mr. Estlin's vaccine points, stated that the use of this virus was occasionally followed by intense inflammation, and even abscesses, in the situation of the vaccine vesicle, your Committee, fearing lest the occurrence of such accidents might prove detrimental to the institution, and diminish their opportunities for observation, at first applied the virus to one case only, and then to a single puncture on one of the arms. On the eighth day this pock presented a most favourable appearance; and that your Committee might have a fair opportunity of judging of the course of the pock, it was left uninjured, and its progress observed from time to time by one of their number, who reported favourably of it throughout.

After this the virus was brought fairly into use; and since the 28th December, forty-three children have been inoculated with it, and upwards of a hundred and fifty charges have been distributed to members and other practitioners in town and country, so that this virus is now extensively diffused over this neighbourhood; and as your Committee have been at the pains to ascertain the results of the experience of many of the practitioners among their own private patients, they have embodied these results with what fell under their own observation at the Institution.

The first point in connexion with the new virus which your Committee would bring under notice, is the superior success attending its employment. Among these forty-three cases not a single instance is recorded in which it had failed; whereas, in the forty-three cases immediately preceding these on the record, ten instances of failure, and nine of spurious or imperfect vesicles, are noted. To this subject your Committee will again recur.

Secondly. As to the appearance of the vesicle on the eighth day, this has been in some degree modified by the size of the scratch, or scratches, made in vaccination; but at this period the vesicle has generally been in an immature rather than an advanced state, and the areola around it has been very slight, and in many cases entirely wanting. The centre of the vesicle has generally been much depressed, bearing the appearance of being firmly adherent to the substance beneath, and this appearance becomes still more marked as the pock becomes more matured. Indeed, the surface of the pock upon the eighth day has been rather flattened, and the quantity of virus contained has, in the majority of cases, been small; but this has always been perfectly pellucid, untinged by purulent admixture, and apparently in the most favourable state for the development of its peculiar properties.

Thirdly. The progress of the pock from the eighth day, or period of maturation, as this has been commonly considered, to the point of cicatrization, has generally occupied from ten to fourteen days; and although in none of the cases which have come under the observation of your Committee has the inflammation attending the pock run higher than they have repeatedly seen it in former cases, yet in a few instances they have about the fourteenth day observed in the site of the pock a deep cavity, resembling not a little that formed by caustic when the eschar has nearly dropped off. This deep and angry-looking sore has alarmed the friends of the child very much; but in none of the cases did the ulceration show any disposition to extend. Under the application of some mild absorbing powder, the sore has gradually filled up, taken on a scab, and become cicatrized; and in a few cases, when it has been examined, the cicatrix has been well marked.

Fourthly. The constitutional symptoms have been generally slight; but in some cases which have been closely under our observation they have come on early, been severe, and seemed to have no relation to the state of the local affection.

Before closing the report, your Committee feel called upon to make a few remarks upon the failures which occasionally occur in vaccination, and upon the probable causes to which this may be attributed; premising, that your Committee found these remarks chiefly upon the last volume of the Vaccine Record, which extends over a period of rather more than three years—viz., from August 1835 till December 1838—and embraces 2041 cases. During a portion of that time the appearance of each pock was minutely recorded, and during the whole period any deviation from the usual routine was noticed, and the state of the child's health, and especially the condition of the skin, accurately recorded.

From this record it appears, that at four different periods there occurred an entire degeneration of the lymph, and a consequent complete failure of the vaccination. The record further shows, that these failures have been preceded by certain circumstances which the Committee think worthy of being noted. In the first place a few isolated repetitions are recorded. In the second place, the pocks are remarked as being highly inflamed, or surrounded by a very diffuse areola. In the third place, many premature pocks are recorded; and finally, a vast succession of failures led to the renewal of the supply of matter from a new quarter.

The last of these entire degenerations occurred immediately before the introduction of Mr. Estlin's virus; and the whole of the children vaccinated upon the day week preceding, presented, instead of true vesicles, raw surfaces, resembling very closely spots that had been vesicated, and then denuded of the cuticle. Some of these surfaces were perfectly dry, and thinly scabbed over; others were pulpy-looking, and gave issue to a profuse discharge of serum. In fact, it appeared that in these cases the pock had run through its entire course in the time usually allotted to the mere development of the vesicle.

Your Committee, with these facts before them, are inclined to regard want of care in the selection of the pock to be vaccinated from, as one of the prime causes of the failures which have occurred, and even in that degeneration of the lymph which has been complained of; and they would earnestly recommend the selection of pocks for vaccination which are free from areola or much surrounding inflammation, as there is every reason to believe, that when a high degree of inflammation accompanies the vesicle on the eighth day, the pock is too mature to yield an active and pure virus.

Indeed, when the pocks, upon any given day, present the inflammatory character, your Committee would rather recommend the falling back upon the vaccine points than making use of matter from the arms of the children; and, that a good supply of these points may be always on hand, your Committee would further recommend that a number of them should be charged from time to time, from any decidedly characteristic pock which may come under observation. At all events, your Committee think it would be proper to renew the supply at intervals of two or three months, using the matter laid past at these intervals in preference to the recent lymph. In this manner, it will be obvious, that at the end of thirteen years, the matter will only be as many degrees removed from the original source as in the common routine it is in one. Your Committee would farther recommend that the appearance of each pock should be noted in the record.

In conclusion, with the conviction that the matter (in our institution at least), has shown a tendency to the production of premature vesicles, your Committee regard the introduction of Mr. Estlin's lymph as a great boon to the public and the profession; as it is very questionable whether these premature vesicles confer that immunity from the variolous disease which vaccination is calculated to bestow.

(Signed) J. P. Glen,
Convenor.

(Vol. xxiv., 1839, p. 222.)

MR. ESTLIN'S LETTERS ON VACCINATION.

The readers of the *Gazette* are aware that Mr. Estlin, of Bristol, has communicated the results of his interesting and important investigations connected with vaccination, through the medium of this Journal. We last week published our correspondent's "Fourth Letter," but by a mistake this was preceded by a communication intended to have been private, and which was headed "Mr. Estlin's Third Letter," whereas his *third* letter was published in February. The mistake is attributable to the temporary illness of the gentleman who supervises the press, and to his deputy not having perceived that the letter in question was intended to be private.

It was our intention to have referred to the circumstance this week, even had we not received the following note from Mr. Estlin:—

"To the Editor of *The Medical Gazette.*

"Sir,—

"On receiving, this morning, the last number of *The Medical Gazette*, I was concerned to find that a private note I addressed to you on the 16th instant, written solely to bespeak space for the insertion of my 'Fourth Letter on the New Vaccine Virus,' has been printed in the *Gazette*, and headed 'Mr. Estlin's Third Letter.'

"It is probable I may have omitted to write 'private' upon that note; but the nature of its contents, and the hasty manner in which it was obviously written, seemed to render such an explanation unnecessary.

"Many, I have no doubt, will perceive that the note could not be intended for the perusal of your readers, and will acquit me of the bad taste which writing such a one for publication would betray. To others the subsequent letter will show that whatever private opinion I might hold respecting the National Vaccine Establishment, I have been anxious to avoid any disrespectful expression in what was meant for the public eye.

"My 'Third Letter' on the New Virus was published in your number for February 9th, 1839. If the present error be not corrected, confusion will arise from any future reference to that letter.

"May I request that in the next number of the *Gazette* you will, as far as it is practicable, rectify the mistake which has occurred?

"I am, Sir,

"Your obedient servant,

"J. B. Estlin.

"Bristol, April 29th, 1839."

MR. ESTLIN'S PAPER AT THE MEDICAL SECTION, BRITISH ASSOCIATION.

(Vol. xxiv., 1839, p. 967.)

Mr. Estlin on the New Vaccine Virus.

[For the "London Medical Gazette."]

The following is an abstract of a paper which was read at the Medical Section of the British Association, during its late meeting in Birmingham.

ON THE NEW VACCINE VIRUS OF 1838.

BY J. B. ESTLIN, F.R.S.

The author stated that, as the history of this supply had been given to the public in various communications in the *Medical Gazette*, he should not enter into details respecting it, but merely describe the changes that had taken place in the effects produced by the lymph, during the twelve months he had watched its course.

He was induced to bring the subject forward, as in consequence of the dissatisfaction felt with the lymph furnished by the National Vaccine Establishment, he had been applied to for supplies of the new virus by practitioners in every part of England; and its employment in the charitable institutions of Liverpool, Manchester, Birmingham, and Bristol, was a sufficient proof of the extent to which it was used, and gave an importance to its past and present history.

The result of the author's observations was, that at first (during the three or four months following its inoculation from the cow) severe local and constitutional symptoms very frequently arose: so serious, indeed, did they appear to some medical practitioners, that they discontinued the use of the new lymph, and others were reproached by a few of the less intelligent class of their patients with having used spurious virus for inoculation.

The particular appearance of the vesicle at different periods was described, and it seems that a gradual change took place in the intensity of the lymph, though one that was hardly observable from week to week: at the present time, the lymph being forty-eight removes from the cow, the author stated that it had lost much of the activity it possessed when removed only fifteen degrees from its original source, while at the same time it retained all those appearances which Jenner describes as characteristic of a perfect specimen of the disease. The author observed that he was not aware that the course of one particular stock of vaccine virus, kept quite distinct from every other, had been often carefully watched in its progress from the cow during a considerable number of successive vaccinations, and he therefore thought the subject might not be uninteresting to the Section. He adverted to the statement made by the National Vaccine Establishment, in their last report, that the lymph supplied by them was of the stock originally introduced by Dr. Jenner, while in the same document it was declared that they had occasionally "recruited their stores" from the original source; and in a recent letter to the *Lancet* from Mr. Leese, a vaccinator at one of their stations, it is affirmed that the source of his supply was from cows which had the disease in 1836, from which he had furnished the parent institution with 27,183 charges.

The fact was noticed of the liability of the vaccine vesicle to become deteriorated in particular constitutions. A perfect vesicle, it was stated, will in some children produce a pock deficient in the characteristics of the genuine vaccine vesicle; matter taken from such a pock will reproduce other defective ones, and thus lymph of the best quality in two or three transmissions may become totally degenerated, and unfit for use. With this obvious fact in view, it was needless to theorize about the effects which frequent transmissions of virus have in "humanizing it": the practical suggestion is of more consequence, the careful selection of the best vesicles only for future inoculations, and a return to the original source, when satisfactory lymph cannot be procured.

At the conclusion of his memoir, the author adverted with high encomium to a series of experiments made by Mr. Ceely, of Aylesbury, and brought forward at the late meeting of the Provincial Medical Association at Liverpool, in which cows inoculated with small-pox had vesicles produced where the matter was inserted, with all the characters of the natural vaccine pock; lymph taken from these pocks, produced in children, through twenty-five successive inoculations, a most satisfactory and regular vaccine vesicle. The pathologist, it was stated, would feel great interest in this confirmation of Jenner's hypothesis of the identity of small-pox and cow-pox; and society at large would not too highly appreciate a discovery which furnishes an easy method of producing the vaccine disease at any time, so particularly important in countries where the ordinary supply of cow-pox could not be obtained when most required, on the breaking out of Small Pox. The author congratulated the profession at large, that under the want, so long felt in this country, of a National Institution with power and energy either to add to the stock of knowledge on the subject of Vaccination itself, or to encourage the pursuit of it in others, a Vaccination Section had been established in the Provincial Medical Association, which in so short a time had promulgated results of such importance.

The President (Dr. Yelloly) remarked that having received from Dr. Bright some of Mr. Estlin's lymph during the earlier period of its use, he employed it in his own family, and could testify to its activity.

Dr. Inglis stated he had lately received from a physician in Berlin, an account of the progress of vaccine virus, confirming Mr. Estlin's observations upon its diminished intensity when removed to a little distance from its original source.

OBSERVATIONS ON THE VARIOLÆ VACCINÆ.

. CEELY.

[*Reprinted from the "Transactions of the Provincial Medical and Surgical Association." Vol. VIII.*]

1840.

OBSERVATIONS ON THE VARIOLÆ VACCINÆ,

AS THEY OCCASIONALLY APPEAR IN

THE VALE OF AYLESBURY,

WITH AN ACCOUNT OF SOME RECENT EXPERIMENTS IN THE

VACCINATION, RETRO-VACCINATION, AND VARIOLATION OF COWS.

BY ROBERT CEELY, ESQ.,

Surgeon to the Buckinghamshire Infirmary.

"Que chacun dise ce qu'il sait, tout ce qu'il sait, et rien que ce qu'il sait."—MONTAIGNE.

ARDENTLY admiring the genius and philanthropy of Jenner, and entertaining a corresponding estimate of the value of the discovery which has rendered his name illustrious, and constituted him one of the greatest benefactors of the human race, I nevertheless could not divest myself of sundry doubts on certain points of extreme interest and very great importance connected with the natural history of the vaccine, and the theory and practice of vaccination. These doubts were not of easy solution. They required for this purpose not only time, but a concurrence of circumstances which I could scarcely hope to witness. Actuated, however, by the simple desire of observing, for my own personal satisfaction, the evidence upon which many of his fundamental conclusions were based, I sought, at an early period of my residence in this neighbourhood, to avail myself of those opportunities which the occasional occurrence of the natural and casual variolæ vaccinæ, and the existence of an ample field for vaccination, (if zealously cultivated), seemed capable of affording.

The events which have occurred, and the discussions which have arisen during that period, have greatly enhanced the interest, and materially augmented the necessity of such an enquiry. The active and judicious steps taken by this Association, prompted a more energetic and diligent pursuit; while the direct application of Mr. Dodd, one of the Secretaries of the Vaccination Section, on its first formation, for my humble co-operation in the investigation of the eruptive diseases of cows connected with vaccination and Small Pox, furnished an additional motive which I felt it both impossible and improper to resist. His *Queries and Suggestions on observing the Vaccine*, full of point and utility, have not been forgotten nor neglected during an active investigation of that and other contemporary and subsequent eruptive diseases which have prevailed in several dairies, during the last eighteen months, in the Vale of Aylesbury. The *Queries and Suggestions* of the same gentleman, relative to my intended experiments, induced me no longer to postpone the commencement of a series which I had long contemplated, and which nothing but an inability to procure suitable subjects had prevented me attempting during a previous variolous epidemic. The facts and arguments adduced and urged by the learned and able biographer of Jenner, in his late highly interesting work,* constrained me to persist in a course of experiments which my own observations had already taught me were difficult and troublesome of execution, and precarious in result. Biassed by no theory, but impelled by an earnest and anxious desire to discover truth, these observations and experiments were made and conducted amidst the fatigues and demands of active rural practice, and, though few and limited, under difficulties and sacrifices which it would be useless to enumerate or describe. To those who are practically acquainted with the subject, any detail of them would be superfluous; to others, a lengthened recital would be excessively tedious, if not altogether unprofitable. The manifold inherent and contingent difficulties to be subdued might well deter individual efforts, and defy private resources; but an unflinching interest has continued to urge, when other considerations ought perhaps to have restrained. The results of my humble but strenuous efforts, if they have no other effect than the corroboration and confirmation of the opinions and observations of others, will not, I trust, on so important and disputed a subject, be altogether without interest, or inappropriately placed in the *Transactions* of a Provincial Medical Association belonging to the country of Jenner, where, greatly to our discredit, less has been accomplished (if I am correctly informed), in some interesting branches of this comprehensive subject than has been effected elsewhere.

In the hope and with the expectation that our provincial brethren, at least, will see what is due to themselves, to the

* *Life and Correspondence of Dr. Jenner*, 2 vols., by Dr. Baron.

Association, and to the profession, (if other considerations could be disregarded),—that they will cultivate opportunities peculiarly their own, which more frequently occur than probably they are aware, I venture to offer the following hasty and imperfect sketch of still more imperfect labours. A subject which needed and obtained so much of the time and talents of Jenner, may, indeed, even for some of its less investigated parts, require the united and continued exertions of many. My own observations and researches, though commenced in scepticism, I have anxiously endeavoured to prosecute with all possible care and candour; and while I desire not to be considered as having pointed the way through a most intricate path, of which, in truth, I have but barely seen the entrance, it will be gratifying to me if a faithful record of them should arouse the enterprise or facilitate the progress of abler and more successful adventurers.—*Est quòdam prodire tenus, si non datur ultrà.*

TOPOGRAPHY.

The Vale of Aylesbury, which in natural fertility is considered scarcely inferior to Pevensey Level, or Romney Marsh, though for the most part composed of rich clays and loams, comprises within its limits most of the soils, variously intermingled, by which the county is characterized, viz., rich loams, strong clay, chalky mould, and loam upon gravel, in considerable variety. It extends from Thame in Oxfordshire on the south-west, to Leighton in Bedfordshire on the north-east, a distance of more than twenty miles. It is bounded on the south by a range of heights called the Chiltern Hills, which stretches across from the southern extremity of Bedfordshire to the southern part of Oxfordshire, being part of the great chain of chalk hills extending from Norfolk south-westward into Dorsetshire. On the west, at a distance of ten and twelve miles from the town of Aylesbury, which is situated nearly in the centre of the Vale, on a gentle eminence, it is bounded by a range of hills of the upper oolitic formation, constituting part of the chain which extends with interrupted continuity through Oxfordshire, Berkshire, and Wiltshire. The surface of the north and north-east border of the Vale, at a distance of six or seven miles, is diversified by a cluster of gradually rising insulated hills of nearly similar structure, taking the opposite direction, and blending in the distant prospect with the hills of Hertfordshire and the Chilterns. The Chiltern Hills consist of clay, upon chalk, of different qualities, with occasional beds of gravel and sand, and, in many places, an abundance of brick earth. The surface soil of the valleys between the hills consists of rich clays and clayey loam, which, upon the declivities, are in some places very thin, and form a clayey chalk; on some of the hills the surface is clayey, and on others it is composed in a great measure of chalk.

The highest of the insulated hills on the west and north-west verge of the Vale, and on which is situated the town of Brill, has, near the surface, broken strata of brick earth, limestone, grit, red sand, ochre, and rubble, a firmly consolidated bed of oyster shells, and, amongst the iron sand, large nodules of bright yellow, interspersed with lumps of pure white, in various forms, but chiefly cylindrical; these all rest on a basis of clay of unexplored depth, the ochrous beds being interspersed between the other strata in thin layers, imparting their colour and quality to the neighbouring springs. Purbeck, Portland, or Aylesbury limestone, and Kimmeridge clay rise from the river Thame on the south-west, and culminate on Brill Hill with a thin covering of iron sand, this being probably the highest point of these formations in England.

Fossils in great abundance are found here, furnishing a rich harvest for the collector. Large fossil wood, crustaceæ, and many vertebræ and bones of saurian reptiles; oysters and mussels, beautifully preserved; Ammonites giganteus, nearly two feet in diameter, and several other species; Trigonia clavellata, costata, nodosa; Pholadomya acutecostata, æqualis; Pecten; Helix obtusa; a species of Teredo; Trochus; Venus, two or three species; clams of Astacus, Ostrea, etc., etc.

The lower grounds consist of deep tenacious clay, intermixt with shells, loam, and sand, of various colours.

The highest of the north and north-east cluster of hills, at Quainton, is seven hundred and eighty-six feet above the level of the sea. The order of the strata near the summit to the depth of fifty-four feet is as follows:—Vegetable earth, gravelly small stones, ochrous (yellow) earth, white (like pipe) clay, sandy loam, with red, white, and blue sand, in small veins, under which are iron stone, fusible in a strong heat; loamy sand, beneath which is a thin layer of (sometimes interspersed) blue clay, resembling impure coal in colour, scarcely more than a foot thick; grey dirt and loam; hard blue solid stone; grey loamy sand and dirt, with a substratum of Pendril stone, formed like bricks; stone called building stone, in masses often exceeding two tons; limestone; brown or yellow sand; rubble stone, containing ammonites, ostrea, small screws, and other fossils; brown sand; and stone of a dark green colour, called bottom stone, not very hard. At the foot of the hills, on a basin of blue clay, prevalent throughout the Vale of Aylesbury, are strata of coarse sand of divers colours, hard grit stone, various loams, but little if any intermixture of water-worn pebbles. Fossils abound here: bivalves, ammonites, from the smallest to nearly two feet in diameter, with four or five volutes; belemnites in the sand and ploughed up from the clay, with sea shells in good preservation; and selenites in the clay to the north of the village, at the foot of the hills near the water courses.

The Thame, with many tributary streams, having their origin in the neighbouring hills, abundantly waters the Vale, which, in wet seasons, in many parts, is subject to copious and extensive inundations. Under draining has of late years been pretty generally and from necessity practised, and with manifest advantage.

ENDEMICS.

Here bronchocele has been from time immemorial an endemic. It is found in all parts of the Vale, but more particularly on or near the hills. It is chiefly observed in females, especially those with fair complexions and lax flabby fibres; occasionally in males under similar circumstances. It is often hereditary; not unfrequently of an enormous size;* and occasionally congenital, occurring in several successive births. It is remarkable, however, that when congenital it always spontaneously subsides within the first six months of infancy. The encysted form is very rare. Struma in all its varied forms and wretched complications is unhappily the lot of numbers of the ill-fed, indifferently clad, and badly lodged peasantry. Dyspepsia and neurotic disorders abound.

EPIDEMICS.

Fevers of the intermittent, remittent, and continued type, dysenteric and acute gastro-intestinal affections, are annually epidemic, one or other prevailing according to the season of the year and existing constitution of the atmosphere. They are often found co-existent in the same village and in the same family, and not unfrequently intercurrent in the same individual. In the remittent and continued (or continuous remittent) types, if of any duration or intensity, the intestinal mucous follicles are

* Although enlargement of the thyroid gland here seems in most instances to depend on the deposition of a glairy albuminous fluid in its cellular structure, yet now and then it appears to be composed of a compact and solid aggregation of calcareous particles, presenting to the touch a stony hardness.

invariably implicated. Originating palpably in malaria, it is nevertheless equally clear that they are under the contingent influence of contagion.*

Like most of this central part of the county, from the Chiltern Hills northward to the Watling Street, the greater part of the Vale of Aylesbury is devoted to grazing and the dairy. An immense number of sheep, cows, and oxen are kept on these extensive pastures. The dairy farms are in general large, and in number and extent greatly predominate. The cows and grazing stock are for the most part bought in. The short-horned Yorkshire breed of cows is used principally for the dairy; Hereford, Devon, and Welch for grazing.

EPIZOOTICS AND ENZOOTICS.

In common with many other parts of the kingdom, this neighbourhood suffered much from the contagious epizootic which prevailed so fatally among horned cattle from the years 1745 to 1780. The places of interment of many of its victims are yet pointed out, and the dismal tales of its ravages are remembered by many with whom I have conversed.

In wet seasons the sheep suffer extensively with the "Liver Rot," a disease which at the same time assails hares and rabbits.

Lately the disease which has for the last twelve months prevailed so extensively on the Continent, the aphtha epizootica,† has appeared among us, but not very extensively. I have seen it rapidly pass through one large dairy. Its mode of attack is not uniform in the same situation. Some have the characteristic vesicles on the membrane of the mouth, lips, and tongue, on the teats at their apices, and also on the heels; while others have only the mouth and tongue affected, others only the heel, and most with different degrees of severity.

---

* In the observation of the rise, progress, variation, and decline of these kindred epidemics, it is impossible to forget the graphic descriptions of Sydenham, of those occurring in and near London in his time; or the later and very interesting accounts of the Gottingen mucous fever, by Rœderer and Wagler. Distressing as these visitations are to the unhappy poor, and harassing as they prove to the country practitioner, yet he cannot fail to derive some compensation in the interest these cases excite. Having obtained from experience and reflection correct principles of treatment, he may, with safety, pleasure, and advantage, often recur to the consideration of the theories and precepts of Clutterbuck, Armstrong, Broussais, Louis, Smith, Maculloch, and others.

† For information on this recent epizootic, I must refer to the *Veterinarian* for September last,—a very able periodical, in which medical men may often find very interesting papers and remarks; and to an elaborate and very excellent article in the *Dublin Journal of the Medical Sciences* for the same month, translated from the French of M. Rayer.

From the general richness and luxuriance of the pasturage, and especially in wet seasons like the past, dry cows,* and even young heifers, are attacked with inflammation and induration of the udder, called the "Garget," a disease which has been more than usually prevalent throughout the past summer.

Besides the true Cow Pock, the variolæ vaccinæ, the milch cows here appear to be very subject to the following eruptive diseases and spurious pocks :—Inflammation and induration, sometimes suppuration of the cutaneous follicles at the base of the teats: small hard knots, cutaneous or sub-cutaneous in the same locality, about the size of a vetch, a pea, or even larger, which often remain indolent for a time, at length become red, vesicate, enlarge, suppurate, and burst after attaining not unfrequently the size of a walnut or more, occasionally affecting the hands of the milkers, and often the other cows milked in the same shed by the same hands : an eczematous eruption, with intertrigo on the udder and near the roots of the teats: warty growths of two kinds ; one consisting of long, narrow, pendulous, and linear-shaped prolongations, easily removed, and often detached ; the other of short, thick, compact, broad elevations, lighter in colour generally than the ground from which they rise, of various sizes, from that of a pea to that of a horse-bean, frequently very numerous on the teats, where they are often found bleeding and partially detached: *the Yellow Pock;* a pustular eruption resembling ecthyma on the teats and udders, succeeded by thin, dirty brown, or black irregular crusts: *the Bluish or Black Pock;* bluish, or black, or livid vesications on the teats and udders, followed by thin, dirty brown, or black irregular crusts, and some degree of impetigo on the interstices, near the basis of the teats: *the White Pock;* a highly contagious disease among milch cows and to the milkers, quickly causing vesications and deep ulcerations ; often or almost always confounded by them with the true vaccine, and certainly not readily distinguishable in all its stages by better informed persons than milkers.

Before entering into a detailed description of these eruptive diseases or spurious pocks, I shall proceed to the consideration of the variolæ vaccinæ as they appear:—1st, naturally, or are produced casually on the teats and udders of cows by the manipulations of the milkers; 2ndly, by vaccination; 3rdly, by retro-vaccination; 4thly, by variolation.

---

* Cows not in milk.

GENERAL OBSERVATIONS.

The *variolæ vaccinæ* seem to have been long known in the Vale and neighbourhood. They have been noticed at irregular intervals, most commonly appearing about the beginning or end of spring, rarely during the height of summer; but I have seen them at all periods from August to May, and the beginning of June. By some it is presumed that cold and moisture favour their development; by others that the harsh winds of spring, after a wet winter, are supposed to have the same influence. I have, however, seen the disease in the autumn and middle of winter after a dry summer. The disease is occasionally epizootic, or prevalent at the same time in several farms at no great distance, more commonly sporadic or nearly solitary. It may be seen sometimes at several contiguous farms; at other times one or two farms, apparently under like circumstances of soil, situation, etc., amidst the prevailing disease entirely escape its visitation. Many years may elapse before it recurs at a given farm or vicinity, although all the animals may have been changed in the meantime; I have known it occur twice in five years in a particular vicinity, and at two contiguous farms, while at a third adjoining dairy, in all respects similar in local and other circumstances, it had not been known to exist for forty years. It is sometimes introduced into a dairy by recently purchased cows. I have twice known it so introduced by milch heifers. It is considered that the disease is peculiar to the milch cow,—that it occurs primarily while the animal is in that condition,—and that it is casually propagated to others by the hands of the milkers. But considering the general mildness of the disease, the fact of its being at times in some individuals entirely overlooked, and that its topical severity depends almost wholly on the rude tractions of the milkers, it would perhaps be going too far to assert its invariable and exclusive origin under the circumstances just mentioned; yet I have frequently witnessed the fact that sturks, dry heifers, dry cows, and milch cows milked by other hands, grazing in the same pastures, feeding in the same sheds and in contiguous stalls, remain exempt from the disease. Many intelligent dairymen believe that it occurs more frequently as a primary disease among milch heifers; but I have not been able to confirm this remark by my own observation. It does not appear to be less frequent on the hills than in the Vale. It has been seen primarily on the stall-fed as well as on the grazing animal.

Origin of the Disease.—I have met with several intelligent dairymen whose relatives had seen good reason to ascribe its occurrence to the contagion of the equine vesicle, communicated by the hands of the attendant of both animals; but very little of that disease has been noticed of late years, though I know of several farriers who have been affected from the horse, and resisted subsequent variolation or vaccination, and have seen a few who distinguish between the equine vesicle and the grease, a recurrent disease—eczema impetiginodes—as it appears to me. For many years past, however, the spontaneous origin of the variolæ vaccinæ in the cow has not been doubted here. In all the cases that I have noticed, I never could discover the probability of any other source.

There is much difficulty in determining with precision, at all times, whether the disease arises primarily in one or more individuals in the same dairy; most commonly, however, it appears to be solitary. The milkers pretend in general to point out the infecting individual; but as I have more than once detected the disease in a late stage on an animal not suspected of having it, I am not very prone to confide in their representations, unless my own inspection confirms or renders them probable.*

In some animals the disease being mild, and their tempers good, little notice is taken of tenderness in milking, which is of frequent occurrence; whereas an ill-tempered animal, with not more of the disease, being very troublesome to milk, is sure to be considered the infecting source. Moreover, in the same dairy, at the same time, with the true disease, some one or other of the spurious forms may occur in some individuals, causing difficulty in milking, and producing deep sores on the milkers' fingers, thus complicating the investigation and deceiving the indiscriminating milkers. The very frequent occurrence of inflamed, tender, and chapped nipples, in connexion with the time and mode of milking in closely arranged stalls, and in comparative darkness, renders these men in general

* An early conviction of the necessity of almost entire self-dependence in these dairy investigations soon led to the adoption of the following rules:

1st.—Not to be too fastidious in my footsteps.

2nd.—To be on the best possible terms with the milkers.

3rd.—To obtain all possible information from them, and believe nothing important which could not be confirmed.

4th.—To enquire into the temper and habits of every animal to be inspected.

5th.—To inspect with gentleness and caution, remembering that there was danger from behind as well as before.

6th.—Never to be without a small pocket lanthorn, glazed with a thick plano-convex lens, wax candles, and the means of ignition, either to explore in the absence of daylight, or to obtain a perlustration of parts on which daylight can rarely impinge.

manifestations of any specific disease till it has made pretty extensive progress through the herd. Their general incompetency to distinguish between the true and the false eruptive diseases, added to the above disadvantages, often creates insuperable difficulties in obtaining very important information, and frequently precludes implicit reliance on it when obtained. Hence another source of the numerous inherent difficulties which attend these investigations, and hence the cause of late intelligence precluding successful enquiries, and not unfrequently the loss of all knowledge of the fact of the existence of the disease; hence also the multitude of vexations, perplexities, and disappointments which too often await the enquirer after facts, and the searcher after lymph. For the acquisition of a very moderate amount of real knowledge on this subject, much time and many sacrifices are required, since actual personal observation is indispensable; and even then it is only after extreme vigilance, quickened by repeated disappointments, with much inconvenience and considerable labour, that some of the objects sought can be obtained. The remote causes appear to be entirely unknown.

Condition of the Animal Primarily Affected.—Here, again, the difficulties above mentioned often thwart enquiry, and the preliminary signs of the disorder are rarely noticed. Yet it must be admitted that this fact, though negative, justifies the presumption of the absence, in many instances at least, of any appreciable or very notable constitutional derangement. In the majority of instances I could not learn that food was refused, or any palpable febrile indications were noticed. In August, 1838, three cows were affected with the disease: the first was attacked two months after calving, and seven weeks after weaning. This animal was considered in good health, but to me appeared out of condition: it had heat and tenderness of teats and udder as the first noticed signs. The other two were affected in about ten days. In December, 1838, in a large dairy, a milch cow slipt her calf, had heat and induration of the udder and teats with vaccine eruption, and subsequent leucorrhœa and greatly impaired health; the whole of the dairy, consisting of forty cows, became subsequently affected, and some of the milkers. In another dairy, at the same time, it first appeared in a heifer soon after weaning, and in about ten or twelve days extended to five other heifers and one cow milked in the same shed, affecting the milkers. In another dairy, at the same time, thirty cows were severely affected, and also one of the milkers. It appeared to arise in a cow two months after calving. The only symptoms noticed were that the udder and teats were tumid, tender, and hot, just before the disease appeared.

Condition of the Animals Casually Affected.—There is rarely any manifestation of fever or constitutional disturbance. In some seasons it appears milder than at other seasons. In some animals it is less severe than in others, depending on the state and condition of the skin of the parts affected, and the constitution and habit of the animal. It is sometimes observed to diminish the secretion of milk, and in most cases commonly does actually affect the amount artificially obtained, beyond which, and the temporary trouble, plague, and accidents to the milk and the milkers, little else is observed : the animal continues to feed and graze, apparently as well as before.

The topical effects vary much in different individuals, whether primarily or secondarily affected, the mildness or severity being greatly influenced by the temperament and condition of the animal, and especially by the state of the teats and udder, and the texture and vascularity of the skin of the parts affected. Where the udder is short, compact, and hairy, and the skin of the teats thick, smooth, tense, and entire, or scarcely at all cracked, chapped, or fissured, the animal may and often does escape with a mild affection, sometimes only a single vesicle. But where the udder is voluminous, flabby, pendulous, and naked, and the teats long and loose, and the skin corrugated, thin, fissured, rough, and unequal, then the animal scarcely ever escapes a copious eruption. Hence, in general, heifers suffer least and cows most from the milkers' vaccinations and manipulations. Dark red and red-spotted animals are often seen more affected than those of a lighter colour, as might be expected, from the occurrence in them of the respective conditions above mentioned.

Progress of the Disease.—The variolæ vaccinæ once arising or introduced, and the necessary precautions not being adopted in time, appear in ten or twelve days on many more in succession, so that amongst twenty-five cows, perhaps by the third week nearly all may be affected ; but five or six weeks or more are required to see the whole number perfectly free from the disease on the teats at least.

The facility with which the disease may be and often is propagated by the milkers, is very remarkable. In December, 1838, on a large dairy farm where there were three milking sheds, the variolæ vaccinæ first appeared in the home or lower shed. The cows in this shed being troublesome, the milker from the upper shed, *after milking his own cows*, came to assist in this for several days, morning and evening, when in about a week some of his own cows began to exhibit the disease. It appears that having chapped hands, he neglected washing them for three or four days at a time, and thus seemed to convey the disease from one shed to another. During the progress of the disease through this shed, one of the affected cows, which had been assailed by its fellows, was removed to the middle shed, where all the animals were perfectly well. This cow being in an advanced stage of the disease, and of course difficult to milk, and dangerous to the milk pail, was milked first in order by the juvenile milker, for three or four days only, when, becoming unmanageable by him, its former milker was called in to attend exclusively to it. In less than a week all the animals in this shed showed symptoms of the disease, though in a much milder degree than it had appeared in the other sheds, fewer manipulations having been performed by an infected hand.

The progress of the disease, however, is not always so readily or so satisfactorily traced; and I have felt nduced to think sometimes that more than one animal has had the natural form in different parts of the same dairy. Nor is the disease necessarily communicated to all the animals milked by the same hand: not only do some older animals escape, but I have seen several times young milch heifers, exposed to all the circumstances favouring contagion amidst the rest of the herd, entirely escape.

Topical Symptoms of the Natural Disease.—For these we are almost always, in the early stage, by reason of the circumstances above mentioned, compelled to depend on the observation and statements of the milkers. They state that for three or four days, without any apparent indisposition, they notice heat and tenderness of the teats and udder, which are followed by irregularity and pimply hardness of these parts, especially about the bases of the teats and adjoining vicinity of the udder; that these pimples, on skins not very dark, are of a red colour, and generally as large as a vetch or a pea, and quite hard; that in three or four days, many of these having increased to the size of a horse bean, milking is generally very painful to the animal, the tumours rapidly increase in size and tenderness, and some appear to run into vesications on the teats, and are soon broken by their hands; milking now becomes a troublesome and occasionally a dangerous process. It is very seldom that any person competent to judge of the nature of the ailment has access to the animal before the appearance of the disease on others of the herd, when the cow first affected presents on the teats acuminated, oval, or globular vesications, some entire, others broken, not unfrequently two or three interfluent. Those broken, have evidently a central depression with marginal induration ; those entire, being punctured, effuse a more or less viscid amber-coloured fluid, collapse, and at once indicate the same kind of central and marginal character. They appear of various sizes, from that of a pin's head, evidently of later date, either acuminated or depressed, to that of an almond, or a filbert, or even larger ; dark brown or black, solid, uniform crusts, especially on the udder, near the base of the teats, are visible at the same time ; some, much larger, are observed on the teats ; these, however, are less regular in form, and less perfect ; some are nearly detached, others quite removed, exhibiting a raw surface, with a slight central slough. The forms of the crusts on the udder are either circular or ovoid, slightly acuminated or depressed, and the crusts seem imbedded in or surrounded with more or less indurated integument. On the teats the crusts are circular, oval, oblong, or irregular ; some flatter, others elevated and unguiform, several irregular, some thin and more translucent, being obviously secondary. The appearance of the disease in different stages, or at least the formation of a few vesicles at different periods, seems very evident. The swollen, raw, and encrusted teats seem to produce uneasiness to the animal only while subjected to the tractions of the milkers, which it would appear are often nearly as effective as usual.

Most commonly, however, the observer, instead of seeing the above phenomena, does not arrive at the dairy until the cicatrices are nearly healed on the animal first affected, when he commonly finds the greater part of the animals in the same house in different stages of the disease. When he is fortunate enough to have an opportunity of watching the disease in its progress through the different parts of a dairy, and can carefully and diligently inspect all the animals in succession, he may observe the

Topical Symptoms of the Casual Variolæ Vaccinæ.—It is very rarely that any indications of contagion, after undoubted exposure, are manifested before the sixth or seventh, sometimes not till the eighth or ninth, day ; but a vigilant observation of thin-skinned animals, with chaps and cracks on the teats, will exhibit small red, rather tender papulæ near the udder and on the body of the teats about the fifth day. On the sixth and seventh days, in cows with white clear skins, on the lower parts of the udder are observed circumscribed indurations, generally of a reddish colour, and of a circular, ovoid, or lozenge shape, as large as a vetch or a pea ; a few are still larger, six lines or more in diameter, and have

have a slight depression on the apex; they may be found from the size of a pin's head to that of a pea. But generally, the majority of the tumours are more or less abraded or otherwise injured, either by the animal while recumbent, or by the merciless manipulations of the milkers; hence is seen lymph exuding from the centres, with cuticle loose or partially detached, raw surfaces, brown or black crusts, either primary or secondary, and here and there the cuticle entire raised from the centre of the tumour, forming a vesicle of a conoidal shape, often slightly depressed at its apex with a dark central spot, and distended with pellucid lymph, around which there is generally some appreciable intumescence and induration. Many tumours are found coalescent and several vesicles interfluent. In very dark-skinned animals, instead of a bluish tint of the centre of the tumours, a leaden-coloured or metallic glistening hue is apparent there and over the intumescent margin. In those less dark, with thin skins, a yellowish or dirty yellowish white, sometimes pustular appearance is observed in the centre and on the margin, and instead of a well-defined surrounding areola there is in some perhaps a reddish brown or tawny hue; but in all, heat and circumscribed induration, especially where the skin is thick, corresponding to the limit of the areola in others.

Between the tenth and eleventh days the disease in general reaches its acmé. On the udders the tumours are often from eight to ten lines in their largest diameter, and in white skins the centres and central edges of the intumescent margin are of a deeper blue or slate colour, and the areola, which is usually of a pale rose colour, is seldom more than four or five lines in extent, under which the integuments are deeply indurated. Lymph, which two days before was difficult to procure from beneath the cuticle of the central depression of some tumours, is now so copious that it raises the cuticle, forming a globular or conoidal vesicle, or freely flows out from its rupture. Other tumours have a greatly extended brown or black central crust, either slightly acuminated or depressed, encroaching on the marginal intumescence; others have become flatter, entirely encrusted, and perfectly passive. On the teats, the few which remain unbroken undergo similar changes, but appear to have less extent of areola, and less circumferential induration; the skin here being loose and extensile, the coalescent tumours are more or less abraded, and have acquired primary brown or secondary black crusts, or a combination of both; the interfluent vesicles are more or less covered with brown or black, oblong, irregular, solid or unguiform, strong, compact crusts, or, denuded of cuticle, are raw, swollen with elevated margins, discharging blood, lymph, and pus. On and after the twelfth day, on the udder nearly all is passive; the central brown or black crusts have rapidly increased, and the marginal induration and intumescence have proportionately subsided: the few remaining unbroken vesicles gradually acquire a brown or blackish hue, shrink, and desiccate within their subsiding induration. The central crusts above alluded to, if undisturbed, though they may become thicker and darker and more compact, seldom increase in breadth after the thirteenth or fourteenth day. The marginal indurations within which the central and vesicular crusts are always enclosed, though they now and then, for a day or two, seem irregularly to renew their former elevation, gradually subside, and have nearly disappeared on the spontaneous separation of the crusts, which takes place on the twentieth or twenty-third day; but even then some traces of induration are left surrounding the cicatrix or pit, which is shallow, smooth, oval, or circular, of a pale rose, white, or whitish colour, according to the contrast of the surrounding pigment.

On the teats about this period—the twelfth day and onwards—around their base, the tumours and vesicles which are left entire, exhibit the like appearance; central crusts of various sizes, brown or black, imbedded in less indurated marginal elevations; vesicles in various degrees of advancement towards desiccation; some with flaccid, flattened cuticle, of the colour of the surrounding pigment; others, more advanced, with yellowish light brown, and others desiccated into dark brown and blackish, slightly acuminated or centrally depressed, oval or circular uniform compact crusts. On other parts of the teats, out of the way of the milkers, and where the tumours or vesicles have been small, few, or solitary, the same may be observed: but most commonly, and always where these have been large, numerous, and coalescent or interfluent, the skin thin, loose, and vascular, and the animal inordinately irritable, a very different state of things is observed. Large black solid crusts, often more than an inch or two in length, are to be seen in different parts of these organs; some firmly adherent to a hard and elevated base; others partially detached from a raw, red, and bleeding surface; many denuded, florid red, ulcerated surfaces, with small central sloughs, secreting pus and exuding blood; the teats excessively tender, hot, and swollen.* Not unfrequently one or more teats form a tumid

* Compare this description with Plate X., Vol. I.—E.M.C.

mass of black crusts and naked red sores, secreting a discharge which imparts to the finger that touches it an odour strongly resembling that which emanates from a patient in the last stage of Small Pox. In some animals, under some circumstances, this state continues little altered till the third or fourth week, rendering the process of milking painful to the animal, and difficult and dangerous to the milker. In many, however, little uneasiness seems to exist; the parts gradually heal; the crusts, though often partially or entirely removed and renewed, ultimately separate, leaving apparently but few deep, irregular cicatrices, some communicating with the tubuli lactiferi, the greater part being regular, smoothly depressed, circular, or oval. Occasionally warty or fungous growths succeed some of the deeper ulcerations. It not unfrequently happens that the central deeper part of the depressed cicatrix, even when not very large, continues to retain a thin flimsy irregular incrustation (secondary or tertiary), as late as the end of the fifth week, or even longer.

Varieties, Anomalies, and Analogies.—Although the medical observer, practically acquainted with the varieties and anomalies of the vaccine disease in man, will neither be much surprised nor long perplexed at less obvious though strictly analogous occurrences in the cow; yet there are some particulars connected with this part of the subject which appear to me not unworthy of remark.

The normal course of the natural and casual disease is completed in about twenty or twenty-three days, viz., four days, in the natural form, from the probable period of invasion (in the casual, three or four from the presumed period of incubation,) to the appearance of the eruption; six or seven from this period to the full development and perfect maturation of the vesicle; five or six from its decline to perfect desiccation; five or six from this period to the spontaneous separation of the crust, and the formation of the cicatrix. Irregularities however, both real and apparent, are observed. In the natural disease the first two stages often seem materially abridged. In the casual, the first seems prolonged, and the second proportionately abridged; or the first is prolonged, and the second and subsequent stages are normal. In both forms the third stage seems often abridged, sometimes prolonged. Lastly, the eruption is not always simultaneously developed. All these irregularities do occur, some more frequently than others; but some of them are very often merely apparent anomalies.

It would frequently appear, from the representations of the

milkers, that the eruption in both forms of the disease reaches its acmé in four days; and this would be perfectly correct if we could admit that the period of detection was coeval with the period of eruption; but in very few instances, on their parts, does this appear to be the case. It has been already stated that these men rarely, if ever, detect any precursory fever; they often disregard the first occurrence of topical heat, and as seldom notice the first period of papulation. Nor is this in the least to be wondered at: it is, in truth, very difficult for an experienced observer at all times to escape error in this latter particular, and oversights will occur to the most vigilant from various causes, especially from peculiarity of colour, vascularity, and texture of skin, as well as temperament of the individual. It is indeed surprising, at times, to observe with what suddeness and rapidity the second stage appears to be completed, seeming scarcely to occupy more than three or four days. In this, of course, we see nothing more than what is occasionally observed in man from various causes. Greater difficulty in detecting the commencement of papulation in the cow, however, is the fruitful source of apparent anomalies of this kind; but vigilant observation, I am persuaded, by leading to the earlier detection of the obscure indications of this stage, will materially diminish their number, Topical heat, slight discolouration, slight tenderness, some induration, will often exist three or four days before any well-defined circumscribed tumefaction is perceptible. When the corium and epidermis are thin and vascular, the pigment not very dark, and the examinations are carefully and repeatedly made in a good light, the respective stages are better observed, and fewer irregularities are apparent. Although the exact period of incubation of the casual disease cannot always be positively determined, yet there seems good reason to believe that it is occasionally prolonged from five to eight days, the subsequent stages being perfectly regular.

The abridgment of the third stage, or the too early appearance of turbidity in the lymph, or the premature occurrence of vesicular desiccation, and the circumstances upon which these and other real and apparent anomalies depend, are well deserving of consideration. In order that they may be more correctly appreciated and better understood, it seems necessary to furnish an analysis of the principal phenomena of the eruption in connection with some of the varied circumstances under which they arise; and this I shall proceed to attempt, although it must necessarily involve some repetition, which to many, I fear, will prove tedious, and be deemed surperfluous. The eruption commences in papulæ, which have their seat in the corium. They are not always simultaneously developed, either in the natural or casual form. In size and colour the papulæ differ according to their age, the thickness and colour of the skin. In thin, fair, and vascular skins, at a very early period, they resemble flea or bug bites, and are of a deep rose red; they become in a day or two as large as a pea, and have frequently a dark damask or even livid hue, which gradually diminishes as they acquire their vesicular character. In very dark skins of this texture, at this period, some degree of redness, a coppery-reddish brown, or a tawny hue, is observable. In thick skins, though fair, the colour is much paler, and is, of course, sooner lost. In dark thick skins, and even in flesh-coloured skins if very thick, the red colour is often entirely wanting, or is scarcely appreciable. Here, therefore, the papulæ are seldom noticed till they have acquired the size of a vetch or a pea. They feel hard, raised, more or less round, are hot and tender. Many of these varieties may occur at the same time in different parts of the same animal.

In three or four days from their first appearance, the papulæ acquire their vesicular character, and have more or less of central depression, continuing gradually to increase; in three or four days more they arrive at their fullest degree of development, and sometimes are surrounded with an areola, and always embedded in a circumscribed induration of the adjacent skin and subjacent cellular tissue. The first change in the pimple is indicated by the appearance at its apex of a dull or dusky yellowish point; the circumference gradually increases in substance and extent, and the centre becomes wider and deeper; at length a flattened vesicle is formed, with a dimpled or depressed centre. The degree of central depression differs not only in different stages of the vesicle, but also in different animals, and in different parts of the same animal at the same time. It is in general more considerable about the fifth or sixth day of its formation. In very fair skins, (especially on the udder,) just before the appearance of the areola, and in very dark skins of a slate, blue, or black colour, where no areola appears, the depression is better felt than seen; but in the former a dirty ochre or dusty spot in the centre is rarely ever absent to aid the eye. The depression is sometimes wanting in some small vesicles on the teats at their early stage; but it appears in the middle or termination of their course, and is again entirely lost. An anatomical examination of the structure of the vesicle just before it attains maturity shows that its colour, indurated margin, and central depression, depend on the existence of an adventitious membrane formed in the corium and secreted by the papillæ. It is raised in the form of a zone, and is intimately connected with the epidermis. It has a cellular structure, in which is secreted and contained a clear viscid lymph. The cells appear to be arranged in two concentric rows, and are separated from each other by whitish radiating partitions, which, at their converging extremities, are united by a central membranous band. The dusky central spot which marked the first change of the pimple into the vesicle, and which has now become darker and more distinct, seems to be caused by a greater or less degree of separation and desiccation of the epidermis, stretched over a crypt-like recess, which contains a small quantity of semi-concrete lymph-like matter, occasionally a turbid opaque fluid. This cellular, adventitious, membranous conformation, though differing in texture and amount in different vesicles, is invariably present, and is not less essential than diagnostic. About the fourth or fifth day of the eruption, or two days before the decline of the vesicle, there often appears at its base a red circle, which gradually increases in extent till that event occurs. During this period the lymph within the cells, having become more abundant and less viscid, and somewhat opaque, bursts and breaks up the cells and their connecting band, separates the epidermis from its attachment to the subjacent adventitious membrane, and the vesicle, losing its central depression, becomes more or less acuminate, presenting a conoidal or semi-globular form. The lymph soon acquires a pale straw-colour or light amber hue, and speedily becomes more serous, turbid, and opaque. Acumination of the vesicle, however, is not always confined to this period. It takes place earlier, later, or never occurs. It is earliest in small, comparatively superficial vesicles, which seem to resemble the supernumerary vesicles in children; is later in thick skins, not very vascular, being postponed till the tenth, eleventh, or twelfth day of the disease. It is earlier on the teats where the cellular tissue is more lax, than on the udder where it is more compact. There are different degrees of acumination: in some vesicles it is barely visible, especially on the udder; but on the teats it is very often strongly marked.

The quantity and quality of the lymph varies, not only at different stages, but also in different parts of the same subject. It is generally more abundant and less viscid on the teats than on the udder; more copious commonly in the cow than the heifer In the early stage of some vesicles, chiefly those which are comparatively superficial, and often others which have been irritated, the lymph is occasionally turbid, and even bloody, without any impairment of its efficiency. In these vesicles, too, are often observed pustular or vesicated margins, analogous to those seen in the puffed irregular vesicles of adults, or the vesicles of irritable habits, either with or without local irritation. They are more apt to occur on the teats, but happen in thin skins, on the udder, from the slightest irritation. Here the cuticle appears sodden and rumpled, and is soon removed. A premature decadence of the vesicle sometimes occurs from an accidental escape of its contents; it is then covered with concrete lymph. An irregular escape of lymph will give rise to alternate decline and revival. When the escape is slight and progressive, it constitutes another form of vesicle—the vesicle with a central crust, which being liable to be mistaken for a desiccated vesicle, deserves notice. This vesicle or "vesicular tumour" assumes its characteristic form at various periods, most commonly at an early stage. It depends generally on a deep fissure in the epidermis and corium, through which the lymph slowly oozes, and concreting, exhibits a central crust. The fissure may not have completely closed before the formation of lymph: it may have re-opened during any part of that process, therefore the characteristic form may be acquired at different periods. When it exists at an early period, the dusky yellowish spot of the centre of the vesicle is absent, its place is occupied by concrete lymph, and the vesicle commonly has more central depression, and more elevation and induration of the margin.

The crust gradually changes from an amber to a yellowish brown or black; sometimes, from an admixture of blood, it is black at an early stage. It partakes of the form of the vesicle, though sometimes it is irregular. As the vesicle enlarges, the central crust in the same ratio increases in breadth and thickness, advancing towards the circumference, and resting *upon* the epidermis until the tenth or eleventh day, when the elevated margin beginning to decline, the central crust having become darker, thicker, and larger, in all directions, often reaches its inner circle, occasionally partially overtops it, about the thirteenth or fourteenth day. The epidermis around and beneath this crust, if punctured at any part except the immediate centre, yields nothing but blood. It often has a rumpled and pustular appearance. These vesicles, and a few others scantily supplied with lymph, never acuminate.

The areola differs in colour and extent, and is often entirely absent. In thick white skins, at its acmé, it is of a pale rose-colour, and seldom, when the vesicles are distinct, more than three or four lines in diameter. In dark skins it is entirely absent, except when they are very thin: in that case it will appear as a circular line of a dull vermilion, a reddish brown, a tawny, or a coppery hue. When absent, the erythematous inflammation of the superficial, surrounding, and subjacent tissues, of which it is one of the signs, is still indicated by others, viz., heat, tenderness, and circumscribed induration. This induration is greater where the tissues are thick and compact, though more circumscribed and better defined. Where they are thin and lax, it is less regular and more diffuse. The former is the case on the udder, the latter on the teats.

Seat of the Vesicles.—The vesicles are found principally on the teats, but are often seen on the udder, especially on the lower and naked part. They are very frequent around the base and neck of the teat, and also on the body, now and then on the apex. The number varies considerably—occasionally one or two; not unfrequently twenty, thirty, or even sixty dispersed about the teats and udder.

Size and Form of the Vesicles.—Perfect vesicles may be seen scarcely much larger than a pin's head, and not unfrequently as large as a sixpence, sometimes even larger. On the same animal they often appear as large as a vetch, a pea, a horse-bean; the latter is a common size. In general the more numerous they are, the smaller they are. The form of the vesicles is circular or oval; now and then, in some parts, somewhat irregular; almost invariably circular around the base and neck of the teats. The oval form is to be found on the udder, but principally on the body of the teats. Its axis seems to be determined, as well as its form, by a fissure or furrow in the skin. Where the skin is thin, vascular, and much furrowed and corrugated, which is often the case on the teats of red cows, the form is irregular, more especially when the vesicles are coalescent.

The Colour of the Vesicles.—This varies according to the age of the vesicle, and is again modified by the colour and texture of the skin. At an early period, from the first to the third day, where the skin is thin and vascular and the colour fair, that of the vesicles varies from a florid red to a deep damask or purple. At a corresponding period, in thick skins of a light colour, that of the vesicles is less intense, but often bluish. In thin skins, very dark, a degree of redness is still visible, often a light damask or bright rose; but when the skin is thick and dark, the colour is more obscure. In general the vesicle is lighter in colour than the surrounding pigment; but in all cases there is presented a striking metallic glistening aspect. As the vesicles advance, the depth of their colour proportionately diminishes. It is, however, always darker at the base than on the surface, especially on the elevated border, where it is also more glistening. In the fairer skins, the glistening lustre resembles that of silver or pearl; and some vesicles, where the skin appears diaphanous, have a bluish white or pale slate colour, particularly towards their centre. In very dark thin skins, the colour of the vesicles is occasionally reddish at their base, and they have their surface much lighter than their ground, glistening with the lustre of mica or of lead. When fully developed on the light-coloured skins, the vesicles vary from a bright to a pale rose or flesh colour, which is deeper at the base, and blends softly with the varying tint of the areola, when present, or terminates in a narrow rose-coloured ring when that is absent. At this period, even in the dark reddish brown skins, the raised and tense margins of the vesicles have a rosy hue, which increases towards the base, where it terminates, except in very thin skins, insensibly in a deep tawny hue. The bluish, bluish white, grey, or slate-coloured tint of the depressed surfaces of some vesicles is most apparent, and the metallic lustre is most conspicuous in all. But these are not all the variations of colour met with; there are others, some of which are not unfrequent. On white skins, when very thick, and at the same time much corrugated, the vesicles have a dull white or cream colour. This will also appear when some vesicles have been injured and a portion of their contents has escaped, diminishing their tension, and plumpness. A recovery of tension restores their former warmth of colour and glistening aspect. On light brown thin skins, especially when the vesicles are not deeply seated, the depressed centre is of a dirty yellowish white. These and other superficial vesicles, which resemble more the human vaccine vesicle, have a tendency to become pustular on their surface, and, at their margin, often vesicate.

After the tenth day the vesicle loses its plumpness, its warmth of colour, its glistening aspect, its areola, and its indurated base and in general, when undisturbed, rapidly subsides. Those which early exhibit the central crust, in a day or two after this period, have their centres completely occupied with its oval, or circular, or irregular form and scabrous substance. By the thirteenth or fourteenth day this crust is at its greatest magnitude, is of a brownish black colour, and adheres more or less tenaciously to the epidermis and skin beneath, and is bounded almost always by some traces of indurated margin, even at the twentieth or twenty-third day, when it separates and leaves a smooth cicatrix,

[illegible]

[illegible] Some of the masses are sufficiently [illegible] produced that, by pressure [illegible] self-[illegible] may occur; but a more frequent and more efficient cause are the [illegible] manipulations of the millers. These men, night and morning, [illegible] another task, [illegible] perform on an extensive scale a very important process—a series of [illegible], not from the infecting and infected animals. Hence many of the apparent anomalies and incongruities above alluded to. Some papulæ, appearing late, never pass into the other stages; others, of earlier date, possess some of the vesicular attributes; others, still earlier, exhibit them all, and hasten on with rapid but unequal steps to the final stage of desiccation.

A due consideration of all these phenomena and their associated circumstances would make it appear, therefore, that the disease in the cow has few if any anomalies by which it may be distinguished from the disease observed in man. The phenomena in man called supernumerary vesicles, and those produced by what has been called Bryce's test, seem as strictly analogous to those appertaining to the cow as can well be desired. It is in the supernumerary vesicles alone of man, whether eruptive or not, that we are able to trace the corresponding changes from the papular to the vesicular state.* The inoculated vesicle in him, of course, will not suffice for that purpose any more than the casual vesicle in the cow, palpably induced by the manual application of lymph to a visibly abraded or fissured surface. The two kinds of vesicle in the cow, it has been seen, exhibit some striking differences from the supernumerary and inoculated vesicle in man. In the

* Eruptive supernumerary vesicles of course are not seen every day; but vesicles which exhibit their peculiar features may often be successfully sought for by those who will spare the time and trouble for the purpose of observing the phenomena alluded to. Use active liquid lymph in great abundance to every puncture, made so as to draw blood rather freely; wipe the lancet over the puncture, leaving it covered all around with lymph; take care, by attention to position, etc., that the blood shall dry over and around the wound, and thus cover the lymph. It will often happen, in young and favourable skins, that one or two supernumerary vesicles will appear at a greater or less distance from the punctures, which, in time, nearly or completely coalesce. Sometimes they will appear even two or three inches distant from the puncture, when the blood, mixed with lymph, has trickled down and dried there. Nearly the same thing may be produced by direct vaccination: insert a point, well charged only at its extremity, cautiously and deeply into a puncture, running obliquely along the skin, and let no portion of the lymph come in contact with the lips of the wound. In general the vesicle will form at a distance from the puncture and exhibit, like those just mentioned, a resemblance in miniature to the natural vaccine. These and the really eruptive supernumerary vaccine vesicles alone afford us an opportunity of observing the striking resemblance which subsists between the vaccine and human variola. Here we may see the granular elevated pimple, its ash-coloured summit, its early and obvious central depression, the gradual loss of that, and the final acumination, precisely like casual variola, from which, in anatomical structure, from the fourth to the fifth or sixth day, as shown by M. Gendrin (*Histoire Anatomique des Inflammations*, tome i.), the vaccine vesicle does not essentially differ. The subjects of these experiments, however, must be inspected daily from the third to the eleventh day, between which periods these and other supernumerary vesicles appear. By adopting this step in one hundred and fifty cases, I have succeeded in watching the progress of fifty such vesicles.

supernumerary vesicle, though the tendency suddenly to acuminate does exist, as in the cow, yet it always possesses more obvious indications of the vesicular character on its surface and at its margin than is ever seen before acumination in that animal, where an indurated and more or less elevated solid substantial margin alone appears. This remark applies also to the vesicular tumour, or the vesicle with a central crust; its margin is solid, indurated, tense, and shining, but the epidermis is not raised by distended cells giving an obvious vesicular appearance as in man. The central crust of this vesicle, of course, has its analogy in man, and in him depends on a corresponding though artificial cause. It is always progressive and more obvious in the cow. The lymph in man has not that tendency to escape, in the form of a crust, from a deep puncture or accidental fissure; the containing cells, readily distending, elevate the yielding and thinner cuticle; whereas, in the cow, the lymph is slowly and scantily secreted for a time, the cuticle is thick and resisting, and an epidermic fissure affords the readiest outlet. A near approach to this tumour-like form sometimes, it is true, is found in children in particular states of the health, or in those of phlegmatic habits, otherwise healthy, with thick skins, where the vesicle, of a rose or damask hue, rises boldly and in a solid form above the level of the skin, covered with an ash-coloured or bluish epidermis, which being punctured, like that on the cow, yields scarcely anything but blood, even till the tenth day. In form, size, colour, etc., the analogies, exceptions, and their causes, are too obvious to need particular description.* In the irregular appearance of the eruption, hitherto, I have seen nothing essentially different from what occasionally occurs or may be induced in man, as above alluded to; and as I have never yet succeeded, after numerous attempts, to revaccinate the cow, subsequently to the development of the areola or its attendant phenomena, I should look with suspicion and some distrust on vesicles apparently evolved after the twelfth day.

The cow, like children, and the young of other animals,

* In the smooth, really beautiful, and white or flesh-coloured skins of some cows, so closely resembling the plump, tense, velvet-like surface of a fine healthy infant's arm, there is often an obvious approach to similarity of colour in an advanced stage of the vesicle. The prominent circular or oval form, now and then varied by some irregularity, is evidently often connected, in the casual disease (as in man), with a pointed or linear opening in the epidermis. Folds, furrows, and fissures of the skin, cause irregularity in form, and stand, to a certain extent, in the place of those irregular punctures accidentally or designedly made by the vaccinator, which produce, till the ninth or tenth day, crescentic, reniform, and other fantastic shapes.

particularly high-bred dogs, is subject to a purely vesicular eruption, consequent upon vaccine fever, which often bears a striking resemblance to vesicular varicella. This commonly occurs about the ninth or tenth day of the vaccine, in the form of erythemato-papular elevations of different sizes, solitary or in groups, evidently of sub-epidermic origin, which, within twenty-four hours, contain a pellucid serous fluid, raising the epidermis. This fluid, being more or less imbibed by the cuticle, gives, in the white skins, an early appearance of opacity to the vesicle; in the darker skin's, a yellowish brown or dirty yellowish white colour is soon apparent. On the second day the fluid is straw-coloured, and becomes speedily turbid; the cuticle collapses or bursts, turns yellowish brown, and before the fifth day the vesicles desiccate with brown and black, thin, flimsy, brittle crusts, which speedily fall. They vary in size from a mere point to that of a vetch or small pea, or are even larger, may occur on any part, but most commonly appear on parts void of hair; sometimes they arise later, and not unfrequently continue to form and desiccate for three or four weeks.

Besides this vesicular and other occasional co-existent eczematous and ecthymatous eruptions, less likely to be mistaken, it must be borne in mind that the state of the teats and udder, during and after the specific eruption, is very favourable for the generation and reception of other contagious eruptions, which are sometimes seen to occur in the same dairy. Hence it is no uncommon thing for cows which have recently passed through the former to become the subjects of the spurious pocks. In the winter of 1838-9, I witnessed this phenomenon most satisfactorily. In a dairy farm, containing several sheds, the animals in one shed, scarcely recovered from the true disease, became affected with the white vesicle (to be hereafter figured and described*), from the introduction of an affected cow from another shed, and several of them continued under its influence for two or three weeks longer. The character of the eruption of genuine vaccine, its seat, its cellular structure, its hard and knotty feel, its glistening aspect, its tardy and progressive change to the vesicular form, its central depression, its late acumination, afford in general broad and palpable grounds of distinction. Difficulties in the way of prompt and accurate discrimination, especially in solitary vesicles, will be better indicated and more appropriately discussed in a special account of the spurious pocks.

* The original drawing is preserved in the Museum of the Royal College of Surgeons, London. The promise of publication was not fulfilled.—E.M.C.

Recurrence of the Disease.—At what period the disease may recur in the cow, and with what amount of modification, I have had no opportunity of personally observing. Here the animal is rarely kept for dairy purposes after the fourth or fifth period of calving, often not so long; and as it is not very common to notice the disease in the same dairy more than once within that time, recurrent or modified cases are not likely to be met with.

CASUAL COW POX IN MAN.

If reliance could be placed on the judgment of persons concerned in the management of milch cows, we should be induced to believe that the Cow Pox is of very frequent occurrence in this neighbourhood; but as such persons in general decide on the existence of this disease mainly on the grounds of severity and communicability, it is impossible for others, acquainted with the eruptive diseases of cows, and therefore aware of the fallacy of such a diagnosis, without collateral evidence or personal observation, to form an accurate estimate of its absolute or relative frequency.

From my own observation, and the testimony of persons competent to judge, the disease would appear to be of more frequent occurrence here, especially in the central and northern parts of the Vale, than in many other districts; but it is, doubtless, considerably more rare than other eruptive diseases of the animal, although I am aware that the fact of its occurrence may not always transpire, unless a milker need surgical assistance, or the medical enquirer be perpetually on the watch. My own observations do not extend beyond a period of nineteen years, during which time vaccination has made great progress among the peasantry, and, consequently, diminished the number of individuals likely to be the subjects of the casual disease in so severe a form as to require medical attention; yet I am inclined to believe, from all the information I have been able to procure, that the Cow Pox is not so often met with here as it was forty or fifty years ago. But upon this point of course I speak with much hesitation, especially when it is seen that so much uncertainty attends all general enquiries into the subject. The lack of discrimination amongst those persons from whom we seek information is not only a formidable obstacle to successful investigation, but has been the source of serious and often fatal consequences to themselves. Contagious eruptions on the teats and udders of the milch cow, communicated to the hands of the milkers, producing considerable local irritation, and much constitutional disturbance, often interrupting their avocations, and occasionally confining them to bed, have not only proved the source of much misinformation, but have imparted to many a confident assurance of safety from Small Pox, which subsequent attacks of that disease, by leading to particular enquiries, have proved entirely unfounded. I have met with several instances of this kind, where, upon investigation, no doubt could be entertained of the delusion under which these individuals had been labouring for several years. Often, too, I have had the good fortune, by a careful enquiry, to discover many who were unconsciously exposed to the like danger, and who, by a successful and perfect vaccination, have been saved from a like fate.

Although the casual Cow Pox in man is mostly found on those who have not previously gone through variola or the vaccine, it is by no means rare to meet with it on persons who have passed through the latter, and a few who have had the former, disease. It is no novelty to see individuals who have taken the casual disease more than once, at various intervals, but not severely · and now we often see cases after vaccination, at periods of frcm two to fifteen years, of different degrees of severity, not always, but often proportioned to the time elapsed, many declaring their symptoms to be more distressing than those which they remembered of the previous vaccination.* On the other hand, we now and then meet with persons who, without any protection, have used every endeavour to acquire the disease by milking, but have failed amidst their more fortunate fellow labourers.

As in the cow, so in man, it does not appear always necessary that the skin should be visibly fissured or abraded to ensure infection,† although very often we find those conditions in existence. A thin and vascular skin seems capable of absorbing lymph if copiously applied and long enough retained.

The parts upon which the disease is commonly observed are

* In estimating the degree of comparative severity in the symptoms of such cases, we ought not to overlook the influence of age. I may here also add that I have several times succeeded, with ordinary *humanized* lymph, in producing modified vesicles, with smart constitutional symptoms, on persons who, from seven to thirty years before, had had the casual Cow Pox severely.

† One of my medical acquaintances in the neighbourhood, who had been engaged, four or five years ago, all the morning in vaccinating, and had wiped the lancet on his pocket handkerchief, on his return home unconsciously vaccinated his infant son on the right ala nasi, by the application of the handkerchief to this part. The child suffered severely, and bears now a large deep scar in testimony of the event.

the back of the hands, particularly between the thumb and fore finger, about the flexures of the joints, and on the palmar, dorsal, and lateral aspects of the fingers. The forehead, eyebrows, nose, lips, ears, and beard, are often implicated from incautious rubbing with the hands during, or soon after, milking. In women, the wrists and lower parts of the naked forearm, coming in contact with the teats, are apt to be affected. If the skin of the hands be very thin and florid, especially if chaps and fissures abound, the individual often suffers severely, having, soon after the decline of the disease, abscesses and sinuses of the subcutaneous cellular tissue, and often considerable swelling and inflammation of the absorbents and the axillary glands.

The inflamed spots or papulæ which announce the disease are more circumscribed, better defined, harder, deeper, and more acuminate than the papulæ produced by some of the other contagious eruptions of the cow. They vary in colour from a deep rose to a dark damask or purple hue, according to the vascularity and texture of the parts affected. If the papulæ be small, there is often no perceptible central depression in the early period of their change to the vesicular state; but they exhibit an ash-coloured or bluish rather acuminated apex, which gradually becomes relatively flatter as the base enlarges and elevates, when the central depression is more obvious, and exhibits a yellowish tinge. Vesicles of this size become more or less elevated in their centre on the development of the areola, retaining their yellowish tinge. Larger vesicles, especially on the back of the hand and sides of the fingers, have a well-marked central depression in the early stage, and often a livid or irregularly ecchymosed appearance, similar to what is frequently observed on the cow; when fully developed, they present a bluish or slate-coloured hue, which increases in depth, and is more conspicuous towards their decline.* This bluish colour, though very common, is often absent, even in some of the vesicles on the same hand. It evidently depends upon and is influenced by the vascularity of the part, the greater or less translucency of the epidermis, the quantity of lymph, the depth and extent of the vesicle. When the epidermis is stripped off from such vesicles, the zone-like adventitious membrane appears diaphanous, and has a bluish or livid hue, derived, doubtless, from the highly congested state of its vessels; here and there are often seen spots of actual

* The plate of the casual Cow Pox on the hand of Sarah Nelmes, (Jenner's *Inquiry*, 1798) is a beautiful and faithful delineation of the disease on a fair skin.

ecchymosis.* Where the epidermis is thick, the vesicles are generally well defined, circular or oval, if the parts will admit, and have only a light slate-coloured tint in the centre; but more frequently this colour is superseded by an opaque white or a dusky yellowish hue. Where the skin is loose, thin, dark, or dusky, the vesicles are jagged, irregular, and puffed at their margins, and, saving the central depression, very much resemble a scald. In size they vary from that of a vetch to a fourpenny piece, sometimes larger, especially when depending on a wound or extensive fissure. The vesicles are frequently broken, or, when the epidermis is thin, spontaneously burst, causing deep sloughing of the skin and cellular tissue, and ulcerations, which slowly heal. There is often, consequently, much attendant local irritation, and considerable symptomatic fever.

Although there can be no doubt of the greater severity of the local and constitutional symptoms attending the casual Cow Pox on the hands, etc., it is equally clear that these symptoms are greatly aggravated by the rupture of the vesicles on parts so vascular, tense, and sensitive, and subject to motion. There is the same variety in the period of their occurrence in this, as in the inoculated form of the disease with ordinary lymph. In some, long before much vesication is apparent, the constitutional symptoms are well marked—three or four days before the appearance of the areola; in others, they are not complained of till the areola is well developed. There is a corresponding variety also in the intensity of the symptoms which often distinguishes different ages and temperaments under ordinary vaccination. Instances are occasionally met with (arising probably from an insufficient application of lymph, or a local or constitutional indisposition to receive the disease in the usual way), where the vesicles are imperfectly developed, and there is little or no obvious constitutional disturbance, exhibiting a marked contrast to the local or general effects on other individuals affected at the same time from the same source. I have seen such cases followed by distinct though mild Small Pox. From these occurrences, and others presently to be related, I have been accustomed to consider milkers liable to Small Pox, contrary to their own expectations: first, from having been the subjects merely of the spurious diseases; secondly,

* This hue and some of these appearances are often seen in other vesicles:—eczematous vesicles, produced by various irritants, especially tartarized antimony; the vesicles of herpes zoster, etc., at their acmé or towards their decline; aphthous and other vesicles on the hands of the milkers; but in these last vesicles this colour is generally confined to the base and outer margin.

from imperfect vaccination, at a late period of the disease, with *deteriorated* and purulent virus, or even with *perfect* lymph, of which they had not at the time been sufficiently susceptible.*

In general there is no great difficulty in distinguishing the casual vaccine on the hands, etc., from other eruptions caught from the cow; but I have seen many mistakes committed by those who ought to have known better, from a hasty inspection, and a neglect in ascertaining the period of the disease. The white vesicle will, on some hands, approach very nearly to the form and appearance of the vaccine vesicle in its declining stage. On very thick skins, about the sixth or seventh day of its existence, it sometimes appears as a raised, circular, well-defined, firm vesicle, with a small violet or pink areola, and a slight central depression, with a light brown discolouration. But, on examination with the lancet, it is found neither cellular nor possessed of fluid contents; it is in a state of desiccation, and has retained this appearance and its integrity so long on account of the thickness of the epidermis.

Papular, vesicular, and bullous eruptions, are occasionally seen attendant on casual Cow Pox, especially in young persons of sanguine temperament and florid complexion, at the height or after the decline of the disease. They are generally of the same character as those known to attend the inoculated disease; but now and then we are told by the patients that these eruptions, either solitary or in clusters, resemble the vaccine vesicles. They seldom meet the eye of the practitioner; but occasional scars, in the situation pointed out, would induce the belief that such do sometimes occur as secondary vesicles.

PRIMARY LYMPH.

It has already been stated that to procure primary liquid lymph, in a condition fit for use, is a task of no ordinary difficulty; the most vigilant and active endeavours too frequently proving unavailing. Acuminated vesicles, containing a thin, serous, and straw-coloured fluid, and of course of little value, more commonly vesicles broken and nearly destroyed before that period has arrived, are often all that remains. Often, too, there are no crusts present or in prospect that can be depended upon. Unless the disease arises in a large dairy, and a consequent succession of cases occurs, it will seldom happen that vesicles are found capable of yielding that which is sought for. More frequently than would be suspected, the practitioner will have the mortification to find on his

* See section below, "Primary Lymph."

arrival, that, from the lateness of his information, a whole dairy of cows has passed through the disease, and he can scarcely find even a useful crust. The hands which have damaged the vesicles have also prematurely removed the crusts. Still a careful inspection of all the subjects should never be omitted; *primary* crusts should be sought for on the lower part of the udder and around the base of the teats. During this search it is not improbable that small vesicles of later formation may be found yielding efficient lymph.* A recollection of the real and apparent anomalies of the eruption, and a little experience, will detect other resources which might be overlooked or disregarded.

The best lymph is to be obtained from perfect vesicles before the period of acumination; after this period it is less to be depended on, particularly if very abundant, thin, or discoloured. Taken immediately before acumination, it is quite as active as that of an earlier date. In the earlier period, from the fifth to the ninth days, it is often scarcely possible to obtain it in any quantity except the skin of the part be very thin and lax. Lymph from a vesicle which has not acuminated, even if turbid, should not be rejected; it will often succeed when limpid lymph from an acuminated vesicle will fail. Acuminated vesicles which have been broken are rarely to be relied on; and vesicles which have been broken at an earlier period are not much better, and, on account of their liability to afford more than the specific secretion, may prove highly objectionable to some individuals. Entire unacuminated vesicles, or vesicles with central crusts, should be sought for where they are least exposed to injury, viz., on the lower and naked parts of the udder, and the adjoining bases of the teats; but as there is some difficulty in obtaining lymph in sufficient quantity from these sources, the greatest care and circumspection is necessary. It is impossible to exercise too much delicacy in the proceeding. It is scantily secreted, as before stated; the exudation of blood will obscure, and the sensitiveness of the animal under a rough manipulation sometimes altogether prevent, the process. The puncture should be made with a sharp lancet as near the centre of the vesicle as possible, and the epidermis be gently raised to a moderate extent around the discoloured or most

* Vesicles which appear either between the commencement of the areola and its full development (from the ninth to the eleventh day), and which, in many instances, as in man, would appear to depend on the scanty or imperfect application of lymph to the mouths of the absorbents; or, still more rarely, and needing a careful inspection, vesicles of secondary formation arising after the twelfth day, and during the period of strictly vesicular desiccation. Vide page 390.

depressed part. Slight pressure, either with the blade of the instrument or between the thumb and finger, if done with tenderness, will enable the operator, after some time, to charge a few points with the slowly exuding lymph. Patience and a treble charging of the points are always to be recommended. From what has been stated in another place, it will be understood that the puncture at the elevated and indurated margin of the vesicle will be perfectly useless, as it yields only blood ; it may be pernicious by irritating the animal.

Vesicles with central crusts will be found perhaps most convenient, and nearly as productive as those just mentioned, particularly if the crust be small, and the margin of the vesicle tender, hot, and tumid. The crust may be wholly removed or pressed on one side, the epidermis underneath may then be carefully raised if the lymph does not soon exude, and a perfectly limpid fluid, in small quantity, can thus be procured.*

When we are, as too often happens, deprived of the above advantages, we may yet succeed in procuring useful substitutes for liquid lymph in—first, amorphous masses of concrete lymph; secondly, central irregular crusts; thirdly, vesicular crusts or desiccated vesicles. The first are often found upon or in close proximity to broken vesicles; and are either colourless, like crystals of white sugar candy, or of a light amber colour, resembling fragments of barley sugar, according to the period of their escape, and the length of time they have been exposed to the air. With a few drops of cold water they may be reduced again to the liquid state, and employed with a probability of success. The central rough and irregular crusts, often more or less conical, occasionally contain an admixture of blood or some discolouring secretion or other adventitious superficial coating : the more transparent and the nearer a dark brown the better. Desiccated vesicles should be carefully abstracted by the milker before they are casually removed or spontaneously fall, and those only of primary formation, the model of a vesicle, dark brown and somewhat translucent, should be retained.† Secondary and tertiary crusts are of scarcely any value : these are more or less thin, ill-defined, or irregular in form, of a dirty yellow, or yellowish brown, more transparent though not unfrequently more dusky and opaque, containing a large admixture of concrete blood and pus.

Good crusts, treated in the manner first suggested by Mr. Bryce

* Small superficial vesicles are often more yielding than contiguous larger vesicles more deeply seated.

† See page 338.

for human vaccine crusts,* may as frequently be depended on, in suitable subjects, as liquid lymph, and more frequently than much of that which is commonly met with. After all, however, where there is often so little choice, we must not be too fastidious as collectors, nor rely too confidently, as experience proves, on the precepts deduced and the expectations formed from the use of the humanized vaccine. It will frequently happen that much of the lymph taken in confident assurance of success, will, from causes presently to be alluded to, prove utterly unavailing in propagating the disease in man; and, on the other hand, some that is taken from necessity, and in despair, will be followed by unexpected and complete success. With the exception before mentioned, in reference to broken or irritated vesicles, disappointment from failure is all that results from the use of late lymph; and the best lymph, it will shortly appear, will not always avert such an occurrence.

VACCINATION OF MAN WITH PRIMARY LYMPH.

The rarity of the natural Cow Pox, the difficulty of obtaining information of its existence, even in the very neighbourhood where it arises, the mischief so often done to the vesicles by the milkers, and the advanced stage of the disease before inspection, preclude the frequent *practice* of vaccination with primary lymph, if it were necessary or desirable. But there are also formidable obstacles to the *success* of the process, even when primary lymph is obtained in all its purity. These impediments to successful vaccination seem to arise from two causes: first, the natural difficulty with which animals of one class receive a morbid poison generated in animals of another class; and secondly, deficiency or imperfection in the mode of communication. Although it is admitted that man more readily receives some of the morbid poisons of the lower animals than they receive his, yet it would appear that even in him there are various degrees of susceptibility, and that some individuals seem altogether insusceptible under ordinary circumstances. This certainly may be asserted with respect to primary and imperfectly assimilated vaccine lymph, at least by the usual mode of transmission. The following facts, which have often fallen under my own observation, and which have been repeatedly witnessed by many of my medical acquaintance, seem to me to justify these conclusions.

1. More than half my attempts to vaccinate with primary

* *Practical Observations on the Inoculation of the Cow Pox*, by James Bryce, F.R.S., etc. Edinburgh, 1809.

lymph, taken from vesicles at a proper stage, and possessing all the characteristics of perfection, have entirely failed. The same individuals have immediately afterwards been successfully vaccinated with dry or liquid lymph which had been long current in man.

2. A small number, vaccinated from the same primary sources, afforded results in various degrees of imperfection. In general, the seventh or eighth day has elapsed before any indications of infection have appeared: a dark red pimple has slowly advanced, and gradually assumed a tubercular or tuberculo-vesicular form,* being either perfectly lymphless, or a dark red tubercle on the thirteenth or fourteenth day with a scanty supply of lymph on its acuminated summit, with a moderate areola, slowly subsiding, attended by very trifling or scarcely appreciable constitutional symptoms. Nearly all these subjects have been successfully re-vaccinated with ordinary lymph, from periods of nine to eleven months, in different degrees of modification, but always with a nearer approach to perfection.

3. A still smaller number, vaccinated from the same primary stocks, have furnished vesicles in the highest degree of beauty and perfection. But even in many of these there has been more or less delay in the full development of the vesicles; and in nearly all, the number of the vesicles has seldom equalled one-half of the punctures.

4. Precisely similar phenomena of entire failure, imperfect, or complete vaccination, with all their attendant circumstances, have followed the use of lymph from perfect casual vesicles on the hands of the milkers; and the like results have frequently attended the early removes of lymph from the most perfect primary vaccinations.

5. The whole of these phenomena—abortive punctures, tubercles, tubercular vesicles, imperfectly developed, and perfectly normal vesicles—may be frequently seen co-existent on the same individuals, either from primary lymph, casual lymph, or the early removes of both from any given vesicle.

6. Although, with the few exceptions previously stated,† the copious, repeated, and long-continued casual application of Cow Pock lymph to a highly sensitive, vascular, mobile, and extended surface, with or without abrasions, chaps, or fissures of the cuticle during the process of milking, proves a more perfect and successful

* Similar to those of earlier formation and more rapid progress, which often follow re-vaccination.

† Pages 393 and 395.

mode of communicating the disease, yet it is abundantly obvious that even this superior mode is in general more prompt and certain in infecting the cow than the milker.* Other facts, which will presently appear, and some that will be related in the next section, might here be adduced if it were necessary, but it is expedient to pass on to the consideration of the particular phenomena of primary vaccination.

Whether vaccination with primary lymph—lymph direct from the cow—be successful or not, I have always observed that the puncture which receives it exhibits on the next day a remarkable and unusual degree of redness, more or less intense and diffused according to the habit of body and the condition of skin of the recipient. It resembles the prompt inflammatory blush often attendant on re-vaccination, the vivid redness which marks the haste of spurious vesicles, or still more nearly that early indication of effect so well known as the unwelcome harbinger of what has been called the "irritable vesicle," which ordinary lymph will often produce in strumous or erysipelatous habits, with light and fair complexions, thin and florid irritable skins, and a flimsy cuticle incapable of concealing the network of plethoric capillaries beneath, and where the smallest puncture produces a torrent of blood, and the mildest lymph proves a destructive poison. This early and vivid blush, which follows the insertion of primary lymph, gradually declines on the third or fourth day, and, where the vaccination fails, soon entirely disappears. When successful, and the vesicle is normal or nearly so in its progress, the redness becomes more and more concentrated, and at length blends with the red elevation of the vaccine pimple.

But there is often an interval of longer or shorter duration between the decline of the blush and the commencement of the first stage of the disease, papulation being sometimes postponed to the sixth, seventh, eighth, ninth, or even tenth day. Hence there is much irregularity in the period of full development of the vesicles, and the areola is frequently not complete till the eleventh, twelfth, thirteenth, fourteenth, or even sixteenth day. About this stage of the areola, especially on children, small supernumerary vaccine vesicles in miniature often appear within its limits, sometimes on the shoulder, and still more rarely on the face and body. The well-known papular, vesicular, and bullous eruptions occurring in such subjects are frequently observed. The colour and extent of the areola vary of course in different subjects, being very florid and

* Vide Casual Cow Pox and Vaccination of the Cow.

extensive in the sanguine and irritable, pale and limited in the leucophlegmatic and apathetic; but at its height, and about the decline, there is considerable induration of the surrounding integuments in all, influenced by the same circumstances certainly, but manifestly existing to a greater degree than is observed in corresponding temperaments from ordinary lymph. The areola, under these circumstances, *declines and revives*, continuing to exhibit a brick-red or purplish hue while the hardness remains indicative of deep seated inflammation in the corium and subjacent cellular tissue.

The process of desiccation, even in perfectly normal vesicles, is generally protracted. Although not quite so late in the thick clear skins of infants and some young children, even here it will be seen for some days confined to the centre, while the circular margin remains of a dull or dirty yellowish white or pale horn colour, retaining a fluid to the sixteenth or eighteenth day. When the regular vesicle is neither ruptured nor spontaneously bursts, the crust is often retained to the end of the fourth or fifth week, bringing away with it a circle of the corium, often the whole depth of it, and some of the subjacent cellular tissue, leaving a deep foveolated red cicatrix, or a yellow foul excavation, which ultimately furnishes the pink, shining, puckered aspect of a Small Pox scar. But it too often happens, especially in subjects with thin and vascular skins, that the vesicles burst or are easily broken during the height or about the decline of the areola; and if the subject be of a strumous or erysipelatous diathesis, of full habit, and possess an irritable skin, secondary inflammation is set up and becomes more diffused and deeper seated, the corium is destroyed completely, and a slough of the subjacent tissue is soon manifest, the surrounding integuments are deeply indurated, often a multitude of ecthymatous pustules are formed on the enlarged papillæ and on other parts of the skin, and abscesses in the cellular membrane and axillary glands ensue, causing proportionate constitutional irritation. When the slough separates, the wound often has the appearance of a caustic issue, seeming capable of receiving a small marble. All this mischief, however, generally soon subsides: the ulcers speedily clean, throw up luxuriant granulations, needing repression; the surrounding irregularly and superficially denuded skin soon heals, and an unexpectedly small circular or oval, red, shining, puckered, elevated, and uneven cicatrix succeeds.

Character of the Vesicles, and Other Effects of the Lymph.—Vesicles produced by primary lymph, like those from good ordinary lymph are not only subject to all the well-known modifying contingencies of temperament, habit of body, quality and condition of skin, form and extent of puncture; but their character, as might be expected from what has been stated, is subject to still further variety from special qualities in the lymph itself. These qualities are not equally manifest in all subjects. The vesicles very often exhibit a bluish, ecchymosed, or livid appearance, not only at their commencement in thin skins with an active circulation, but are more than usually blue towards their decline where such conditions are absent. Yet this effect cannot be produced in all cases. Although the vesicles are often remarkably large and finely developed, yet they are commonly not more so than others produced by ordinary lymph, and could not be distinguished from them but by the circumstances above stated, when describing the extent and depth of skin affected. They are not unfrequently less fine and much less developed than other vesicles, but they admit of very remarkable improvement by transmission of the lymph through a series of well selected subjects. By this process, also, in a very short time most of the defects and some of the evils connected with the use of primary lymph may be dissipated, and the lymph rendered milder and more suited to general purposes.

In attempting this, it will be recollected that it is quite possible to lose the stock unless a large number of suitable subjects are at hand. Children are the best certainly for the purpose, and such should be selected as possess a thick, smooth, clear skin, and have a dark complexion, and are not too florid; but still plump, active, and healthy. Infants of this description are decidedly the best; their vesicles, we know, are almost always better defined, less liable to burst or be broken, have less areola, and, in fact, if between four and nine months old, are capable of furnishing with this lymph all that can be desired, with the least amount of risk. By a steady and judicious selection of these and similar subjects, in a few (even three or four) removes, the severity of the local mischief becomes manifestly materially diminished, the vesicles acquire a magnitude and beauty often greatly superior to what is daily witnessed, and, in a short time, the lymph may be transferred with safety to others, even more sanguine and robust, where, it is well known, lymph, if good for any thing, will produce the finest and most perfect vesicles.

Three or four punctures, according to the size, age, and habit of the patient, when the lymph is thus thoroughly assimilated, will in general be amply sufficient; a less number will be safer for some subjects.

Too much care, however, cannot be taken at all times to avoid rupture of the vesicles, or what might and does otherwise pass off with moderate inflammation and the erosion of about half the texture of the corium, leaving a magnificent well-excavated scar behind, will most certainly lead to great inconvenience, and probably to all the mischief formerly described as resulting from the first remove. As we advance we find the necessity of preparing the most objectionable subjects, and the advantage of subjecting many of them to the same preliminary treatment which the best and most expert inoculators of Small Pox formerly so successfully adopted for their patients ; for it is a long time before some individuals can be safely vaccinated with this active lymph, even though taken from the mildest vesicle.*

In the succeeding removes, among a diversity of subjects, there is of course endless variety in the character of the vesicles. They are meagre, ordinary, or equally fine as before, some bold and elevated, with rounded margins, turgid with lymph, or, having narrow acute margins and broad centres, yielding as abundantly, thick and fleshy, or flat and level with the skin, affording scarcely any lymph on the eighth day,† without the least abatement of any needful activity ; while every now and then we have all the characters of the earlier removes, and all the inconvenience of primary lymph. It is quite allowable to admire, and perfectly right to endeavour to produce, beautiful vesicles ; but we must admit our failures in such attempts while relying on lymph alone : the soil is of as much importance as the seed. Lymph from the smallest vesicles, if normal, will, in a good subject, furnish in its turn the finest vesicles, and *vice versâ.* We are constantly reminded, too, that the finest vesicles often exist where there are the least indications of constitutional disturbance, and that remarkable intensity of symptoms is seen where the vesicles are strikingly small.

In using primary lymph and its early removes, however we may be disposed to attribute to it the power of aggravating the constitutional symptoms in certain temperaments well known to be obnoxious to them, yet we are also forcibly reminded that the very same lymph will appear to produce scarcely any appreciable

* I have seen too much evil result from a neglect of such salutary precautions, and have several times positively refused to vaccinate, with very active lymph, certain subjects with the obnoxious characteristics, mistaken for health, till they have been reduced to propriety. There are a few such who for a long time must be avoided—*cane et pejus angue.*

† But in these and other vesicles the lymph is abundant on the tenth and eleventh days, perfectly limpid and quite efficient.

symptom in others. Roseola, lichen, etc., with vomiting, diarrhœa, delirium, &c., arise in some, while in others mere acceleration of pulse is observed without complaint. In many instances the symptoms appear as early as the fifth day, on the sixth and seventh very often, with morning remissions and evening exacerbations, terminating on the ninth, or augmenting till the height of the areola. In other instances they are not manifest till the eighth or ninth day, sometimes later; occasionally they are scarcely observable. In some subjects a single vesicle will be attended with earlier, more severe, and longer protracted symptoms than four or six will produce in others.

Although the greater part of my experiments with primary lymph and its early removes have exhibited the above as its qualities and accidents, I think it not improbable that primary lymph may vary in these respects, and be modified by seasons and other circumstances, both individual and local. In passing through a large number of cows, it has appeared to me generally milder in the latest than in the first subjects, and I have certainly succeeded in effecting a mitigation by artificial means while in the prosecution of experiments with another view. As I shall have to recur to this subject, and to a detail of the effects of other kinds of lymph, I think it better to proceed at once to a narrative of the experiments themselves.

VACCINATION OF THE COW WITH PRIMARY LYMPH.

Never having observed or heard of the occurrence of Cow Pox, in this neighbourhood, in any other than milch cows, I was desirous of ascertaining the degree of susceptibility of the sturk (or young heifer) to the disease, and its attendant phenomena, when artificially induced by primary lymph. I commenced, therefore, by vaccinating some of these animals, about ten months old, in the inside of the ear, on the teats, and in the soft and vascular structure on and near the vulva, with lymph taken from milch cows in the winter of 1838—9, while the disease was prevalent in many of our dairies. Punctures were made in the ordinary way with lancets well charged and with points thoroughly imbued with good lymph; two or three of the latter were broken off short, and allowed to remain in each wound. Although I could not boast of the almost unvarying success which attends the casual vaccination of the milkers,* yet I found much less difficulty in succeeding

* These men, without knowing it, are unquestionably the most successful vaccinators with primary lymph, and the most careful too, for they never

than I had supposed, or than is experienced in vaccinating these animals with lymph taken from man. Though the punctures in general were early inflamed—on the second day—the papular stage was not well marked, and appeared postponed; the vesicles were normal, but declining on the eleventh day. On the teats there was much tumefaction of the integuments until the thirteenth day. On the parts near the vulva the vesicles, though declining on the eleventh, occasionally revived and declined for two or three days, as they often do in the natural and casual forms. When the crusts fell spontaneously at the proper time, a moderately deep smooth scar was observed; but if prematurely removed, a deep erosion of the skin ensued. On the inside of the ear the vesicles appeared less developed, though the lymph was reproductive. No indisposition in the animals was noticed beyond a slight acceleration of the pulse. The lymph used in the above experiments was from the same source and of the same date as some which had been applied to children and adults. On these last, however, it either failed altogether, produced more or less imperfect vesicles, or perfect vesicles with the areola not fully developed till the twelfth, thirteenth, or fourteenth, and fifteenth or sixteenth days. The lymph resulting from these vaccinations of the cow, taken on the tenth day, and transferred to man, differed in no respect from that which has been described,[1] except that the inflammation and induration at the base of the vesicles were certainly less considerable, and the subsequent scars rather less deep, but remarkably well defined, and even now appear to have extended through two-thirds of the substance of the corium. I could not spare subjects to carry on this lymph.

VACCINATION OF THE COW WITH HUMANIZED LYMPH, OR RETRO-VACCINATION.

My experiments in retro-vaccination were almost entirely confined to the sturk under twelve months old; and the parts selected for the operation were those in close proximity to the vulva. These animals were easily procured, while milch cows in any number, at least here, are difficult to obtain for such a purpose. The parts chosen are most easy of access, and in every respect, I think, most

neglect Bryce's test. We cannot fail to be vexed at their destructive proceedings, and impatient of their general lack of discrimination; but we must stop to admire the splendid success of their performances, which it would be well if we could imitate. They may indeed smile at our puny efforts!

[1] Page 400.

desirable.* The operation was performed either with a lancet or a sharp straight bistoury. The lymph was either dry, or liquid in capillary tubes. No other precautions were taken than excluding the animals from wet and cold immediately after the operation for a few hours or perhaps a night. Those of a light colour and with thin skins were generally preferred, but often without avail, scarcely one-half of the operations succeeding. Tubercles, nearly or completely lymphless, were often produced: but sometimes every puncture succeeded. In the majority of instances the vesicles ran the normal course, declining on the eleventh day. Four kinds of lymph were at different periods employed, each having been current in man for a longer or shorter period. But a detail of some of these experiments will best explain some interesting particulars elicited in their progress.

Retro-vaccination with Lymph which had been Several Years in Use.—It appeared sufficiently active, and from arm to arm was attended with satisfactory results. *Subject:* a small ill-conditioned sturk, strawberry coloured, thin skin. Seven punctures were made near the vulva, and eight points inserted recently charged with *fifth-day* lymph from a fine child on February 1st, 1839.

Second Day.—Nothing remarkable.

Fourth Day.—Some of the lower punctures rather red.

Fifth Day.—Scarcely any traces of punctures left.

Sixth Day.—Punctures appear perfectly passive.

Seventh Day.—Two punctures rather elevated and inflamed.

Ninth Day.—All the punctures raised in the normal form, but in different degrees, the vaccine tumours being of different sizes; tried to procure lymph, but failed, both on the surface of the tumid margins, which yielded only blood, and in the centres, where there is a slight crust.

Tenth Day.—There are four fine large and three small vesicles, from two of which were charged one hundred points, abundantly, with clear adhesive lymph, some of which was used on the same and subsequent days. The punctures made yesterday had given rise to the exudation of lymph which is now visible in the form of light-amber-coloured concretions on the parts.

Eleventh Day.—The vesicles appear diminishing, and amber-coloured lymphatic concretions are formed in their centres. *Vespere:* Crusts enlarging: vesicles subsiding.

Twelfth Day.—Upper vesicles have a pustular appearance in places; others have a yellowish brown crust; others flattening.

Thirteenth Day.—All subsiding; crusts larger.

Fourteenth Day.—Subsiding.

Fifteenth Day.—Crusts more elevated; margins flatter.

Sixteenth Day.—Declining.

Seventeenth Day.—Intumescent ring nearly disappeared; black crusts alone remaining.

* The scrotum of the male sturk (young bull) would answer very well indeed, on the continent, I learn that it is very often thus appropriated.

Eighteenth Day.—Every thing diminishing.

Nineteenth Day.—Small elevations in the site of the vesicles, still lighter than the ground.

Twentieth and *Twenty-second Days.*—Some crusts prematurely removed by accident; others spontaneously fell on the *twenty-second* and *twenty-third* days, leaving small pale rose-coloured smooth scars, slightly depressed in the centre.

February 26th.—Inoculated with liquid Small Pox lymph (variola discreta, *seventh day*), in five punctures, from capillary tubes, on right side of labium pudendi, the wounds being at the same time deluged with fluid.

Third Day.—Slight tumidity around the punctures.

Fourth Day.—A shining glassy tumidity around the punctures, which are larger.

Fifth Day.—*In statu quo.*

Seventh Day.—All subsiding; no result.

March 12th.—Re-inoculated with dry *sixth-day* confluent Small Pox lymph, inside and outside the left labium pudendi, with several points; four punctures. Re-vaccinated with *seventh-day* "variola vaccine lymph,"* two removes, inside and outside of the right labium pudendi; several points; four punctures. No result from either.

Experiment second (June 6th, 1839).—Retro-vaccination with lymph which had been in use at the Small Pox and Vaccination Hospital since March, 1837. It was then introduced by Mr. Marson, the resident surgeon, from casual vaccine vesicles on the hands and arms of a dairy woman, to the ultimate exclusion of the old lymph, whose declining activity Dr. Gregory had long noticed, and has clearly pointed out.† *Subject:* a young sturk, colour strawberry, skin thick; lymph used from points and tubes; punctures four, deep, near the anus and vulva.

Third Day.—All the punctures closed with a plug of adhesive or "modelling" lymph, but all tender.

Fifth Day.—Three of the punctures tumid and tender, filled with a black plug.

Seventh Day.—One very fine vesicle near the anus, on a dark fleshy ground, with a thin central crust; two smaller vesicles below. Charged twelve points with great difficulty; used some the same day, and sent others to the Small Pox and Vaccination Hospital.

Eighth Day.—Large vesicle glistening, but a little flattened from the loss of lymph; centre filled with a hard crust, which was removed; appearance bloody and raw, and no more lymph could be procured. The smaller elevations do not appear to increase.

Ninth Day.—Large vesicle increased in size, is plump and glistening, hot and tender; centre depressed and filled with dark central crust, which has everted edges. The other two scarcely altered.

Tenth Day.—Vesicle arrived at its maximum of development, and remarkably fine. The smaller ones are abortive, or lymphless tubercles.

Eleventh Day.—Evidently flatter; black central crust has its centre depressed; tubercles flatter.

* Vide Variolation of the Cow.

† *Medical Gazette*, February 24th, 1838.

Twelfth Day.—Vesicle much flatter, with projecting crust.

Fourteenth Day.—Intumescence nearly gone, crust remaining; very small crusts in the two smaller supposed tubercles, proving that they did furnish some lymph.

Twentieth Day.—A small crust still remaining on the site of the large vesicle; nothing visible on the others.

Twenty-third Day.—A very small smooth scar visible on a dark ground, from the large vesicle only.

Twenty-sixth Day.—*Re-vaccinated* in four punctures, eight points, and two tubes charged with *eight-day* retro-vaccine lymph.

Fifth Day.—slight tumefaction of the edges of the punctures; three wounds, raw; one closed. Failed.

Experiment third (July 9th, 1839).—Retro-vaccination with points charged with "variola-vaccine" lymph, nineteenth remove. *Subject:* a young sturk, colour red and white, skin dusky and thin; punctures four, very superficial, and not deeper than was necessary to hold the points, as in ordinary vaccination, inserted near the vulva.

Second Day.—Inserted four more points of the same lymph in the four wounds of yesterday.

Third Day.—Punctures closed with plugs, rather inflamed.

Fifth Day.—Punctures rather tumid; three plugs removed; four small vesicles resembling the vaccine in man, three reddish, flesh-coloured, and glistening, on a dusky ground; centres depressed.

Sixth Day.—The four vesicles rather more enlarged, more distinctly vesicular, of a bluish colour, two upper more elevated, two lower flatter, but all glistening with a bluish tint blended with a pale rose near the base.

Seventh Day.—Vesicles contain more fluid, look bluer, have a pale lead colour, irregularly blistered, very little raised, centre slightly depressed, base reddish flesh colour; charged three points with turbid opaque fluid.

Eighth Day.—All four vesicles broken, have been slightly rubbed, and the blue cuticle rather rumpled; no hardness of the base; no elevation; no fluid to-day; no central crust.

Ninth and *Tenth Day.*—No induration at the base; no central crust.

Eleventh Day.—Vesicles have a thin brownish crust, and fragments of lead-coloured cuticle, but no marginal induration.

August 1st.—Re-vaccinated in four punctures with "variola-vaccine" lymph, twenty-one removes. Slight scars of the previous vaccination visible. No result.

Experiment fourth (July 13th, 1839).—Retro-vaccination with retro-vaccine lymph, obtained from the second experiment, and from that, the fifth remove. *Subject:* a young sturk; skin dark, not very thick; colour red and white; punctures four, very superficial, as the last, near the vulva.

Fourth Day.—No apparent effect; re-vaccinated by opening the closed punctures and inserting four more points charged with the same lymph.

Tenth Day (July 22nd).—Four vesicles at their acmé, with slight central depression, and slight annular red areola; no central crusts; colour of the vesicles, dirty yellowish white. Charged eight points with a turbid fluid.

Fifteenth Day.—Nothing apparent but four small crusts the size of [illegible] in their centres; slight [illegible]

[illegible] Re-vaccinated carefully [illegible]

[illegible] first experiment had been in [illegible] the effects of my [illegible] had become visible, [illegible] warbles, [illegible] the integuments on [illegible] change in the [illegible] to state the [illegible] experiment, I have [illegible] current for several [illegible] active, and could [illegible] constitutional [illegible] a vesicle for [illegible] or *sixth day*, [illegible] was then pursuing [illegible] was used at that [illegible] slight aberration of the [illegible] health was noticed. [illegible] were unequivocally [illegible]

[illegible] it will often happen, [illegible] appear suddenly to [illegible] without passing through a [illegible] as if they had [illegible] thus to be disappointed of by the [illegible] are noticed [illegible] and casual disease. Analogous [illegible] take place in man, [illegible] re-vaccine, and unassimilated [illegible] lymph till the tenth day, [illegible] not uncommon when the vesicle [illegible] but tenth-day lymph from such [illegible] as good as that of an earlier date; [illegible] as well, sometimes better, the points being more fully charged. Though the vesicle appeared so late, it still commences to decline on the evening of the eleventh day: the lymph instead of raising the cuticle, as in man, at the margin of the vesicle especially, or accumulating in the centre, as it often does in the natural and casual disease under different topical circumstances, was slowly discharged upon the epidermis through fissures made in vaccinating and abstracting, and thus formed a central crust.* Slight pustulation is sometimes observed on the margins of vaccine vesicles, even without accidental irritation.

The lymph, taken on points thoroughly and trebly charged, and immediately used, produced perfect vesicles. The papular stage, however, was late—the sixth or seventh day; but the areola was complete on the tenth, and declined on the evening of the eleventh or twelfth day. It was employed on subjects of different ages, and, with this exception, and some vesicles being rather smaller, the local and constitutional effects did not differ materially from those resulting from its former use. The slight change which it had undergone in its transit through the cow was not apparent after the third remove, when it appeared to possess no more than its former qualities. The object of the subsequent variolation and vaccination is sufficiently manifest: both entirely failed.

The subject of the second experiment possessed a much thicker and darker skin than that of No. 1. Similar experiments with this lymph on subjects apparently more eligible had failed, and even in this case, although liquid lymph from tubes, as well as points recently charged, was used, but one good vesicle arose out of four punctures, yielding a very small quantity of lymph; the other vesicles were ill-developed, and presented only, on their decline, slight and ambiguous traces of lymphatic exudation.

In man, the lymph employed for this experiment was prompt and effective, possessing the desired "maximum of vaccine intensity," as those who have used it or seen its effects at the Hospital can testify. In this subject, too, the papular stage was short, but lymph was obtained much earlier than in the former experiment, though the quantity was very small, and none could be readily procured after the seventh day. This lymph, transferred to eligible subjects, produced vesicles in various degrees of perfection. The areola was not at the height till the twelfth or thirteenth day, papulation not appearing till the fifth or sixth day; but by the third remove it acquired its former power, and its use was followed by vesicles of the greatest perfection and beauty. The same results attended the employment of the charged points forwarded to the Small Pox and Vaccination Hospital; and when I observed there the vesicles of many subsequent removes, I was incapable of distinguishing them and their effects from those produced by the parent lymph. The lymph

* See Natural and Casual Cow Pox.

had gained nothing by the transit; it could not be improved. Imperfectly developed vesicles, such as appeared in this retro-vaccination, are not unfrequently observed; the presence, though late, of concrete lymph in the centre is the only means of judging of their character; tumours, tender, circumscribed, and glistening, are frequently produced, and slowly subside without this indubitable sign. The course of the vesicle here was perfectly normal, and it affords a good specimen of a vaccine vesicle on a thick dark skin, yielding, as usual, very little lymph. This animal was not only re-vaccinated, on the subsidence of the disease, without effect, but was tested on the seventh day with its own lymph, and also with Small Pox lymph, but with doubtful results in both cases, there being merely glistening, well-defined, but equivocal lymphless tubercles in both sets of punctures.

In the subject of the third experiment the skin was very thin and of a singularly dusky colour. The punctures were designedly made as superficial as in ordinary vaccination with points, for the purpose of producing a variety in the character of the vesicle. The lymph was little more than four months old, but had failed in previous attempts at retro-vaccination on other subjects apparently equally favourable. The punctures were again opened on the second day by the thumb and finger, in near imitation of the re-infecting process of the milker. The first operation it appears was successful. Lymph, in very small quantity, was obtained on the sixth day immediately under the epidermis, which, however, was not raised. There was never much secreted, and the vesicles did not exhibit the induration and marginal elevation, etc., which other vesicles do when implanted deeply in the corium. The lymph was not used, but would have been available, though a little turbid. Very minute crusts subsequently adhered to the centres of the vesicles; the scars were slight, smooth, and superficial. This animal was re-vaccinated with liquid lymph, and inoculated with Small Pox lymph twice before the eighth day, with the production only of tender and reddish elevations around the punctures, but not affording unequivocal appearances of the formation of lymph. Re-vaccination after the decline of the disease had no result.

In the fourth experiment the skin was thicker than in the preceding subject; the lymph scarcely more than one month old. The punctures were made as in that case, with the same object, and with the same result,—the production of a vesicle more nearly approaching in character the human vaccine. The effects

were as prompt and as regular as in the former case, and on the tenth day a scanty supply of rather turbid lymph was obtained. In the first removes the vesicles were postponed a day or two, or diminished, but on the third had acquired their former perfection. This animal, also, was inoculated and re-vaccinated before the sixth and seventh days without any satisfactory result from either set of punctures.

GENERAL OBSERVATIONS.

These experiments are neither intended nor calculated to illustrate the best mode of vaccinating or retro-vaccinating the cow. The method here used was adopted, as before stated, more for its convenience than from any belief in its superiority. Other plans of procedure, doubtless, there are, better calculated to ensure a greater measure of success. Nevertheless, it does appear that many individuals are affected with difficulty, or are altogether insusceptible by the ordinary known modes of vaccination. Even those persons who profess to have "discovered, after a long series of experiments, a mode of perpetuating the natural Cow Pox at will,"* confess that a selection of subjects must be made. Probably much of the difficulty attending the operation, and impeding or preventing its success, depends upon the condition of the tissues as natural to the subject, or as induced by season or circumstances. Whether with points or with tubes, some subjects are promptly affected; while others, in every respect, to all appearance, not less eligible, require a repetition of the process, and then yield but a small number of vesicles for a large number of punctures. The difficulty and uncertainty of the operation, by our usual defective means, are still further manifest by the apparent failure and doubtful effects of Bryce's test, employed in two of these experiments, as well as in others. I have made incisions into the cellular tissue and inserted crusts of natural Cow Pox; the wound has healed without any result. The above experiments, however, will serve to show the greater difficulty of vaccinating the cow with humanized than with primary lymph, and that, when successful, a much milder disease is the result. Take an abundance of humanized lymph from one of the finest and most productive vesicles ever seen, and if you succeed in retro-vaccinating the cow, you may perhaps be able to charge scantily only a very few points from

* Vide *Lancet*, June 29th, 1839.

a vesicle which excites but trifling topical inconvenience. Vaccine lymph, it is obvious, therefore, in passing from the cow to man, undergoes a change, which renders it less acceptable and less energetic, on being returned, to many individuals of the class producing it; some refuse it altogether. But this reluctance or absolute refusal, this difficult imbibition or total insusceptibility, does not exist to the same extent as observed in the converse of this experiment, viz., in passing primary lymph from the cow to man by the same means. Here we have considerable difficulty; but when we succeed, a severer disease is induced. These experiments clearly show that the *age* of humanized lymph does not seem to influence its reception by the cow. Provided that the lymph be of ordinary activity, and possess the normal qualities, it is as likely to succeed in its operation on the animal whether it may have been current in man a few weeks or many years, and will excite equally perfect and productive vesicles. The effects of retro-vaccine lymph on man, as compared with primary and current lymph, are worthy of notice. Lymph which had passed from arm to arm with the greatest promptness and facility, and produced the finest effects, in its first removes from the costive vesicle of the retro-vaccinated cow, is not so readily absorbed by many individuals. It rarely fails; but papulation is retarded, and though the vesicle may attain maturity at the normal average period, the completion of that stage is frequently postponed. The vesicles are often smaller, and the disease really not so well developed, as by the stock from which it was derived. But these changes do not appear after the second or third remove. The lymph is restored to its former qualities, and produces its [illegible] effects. Some of the retro-vaccine lymph of the second experiment, transmitted to the Small Pox and Vaccination [illegible], from whence it was originally derived, was passed through a long series of subjects, under the inspection of Dr. [illegible] and Mr. Marson, who, though better able to make the comparison, were unable to detect any sensible difference in its local or constitutional effects after the second remove. On the [illegible] remove it became "very fine," as it was before its transit through the cow.*

[illegible] the practice of retro-vaccination of any real value as a means of renovating humanized vaccine? I confess that from my limited experience (these few observations and experiments), I am unable to discover its advantages, or to admit more than its questionable utility, from one transit through the cow. What humanized vaccine might acquire by repeated and indefinite transmissions, I am not prepared to say. From what has been observed above, I have no doubt that primary vaccine, passed by artificial means through a series of cows, would lose much of its acrimony, and produce on man a milder but abundantly active and characteristic disease; but that humanized vaccine, by a similar process, should ever acquire all the attributes of primary vaccine, or become so much more *brutalized* as to deserve the epithet of "renewed," is more than many are prepared to expect. Few persons, I apprehend, are likely to succeed in conducting such experiments; and being of doubtful utility, in the estimation of many, the difficulty, trouble, and expense necessarily attending them, will, in all probability, long operate to the exclusion of positive proof. But it has been stated by those who doubt the advantage of a single transmission through the cow of lymph which had passed through many individuals, who may be variously affected with the germs of scrofula, etc.,* that where primary Cow Pock is not met with, and the vaccine hitherto in use shows a falling off in its essential properties, "retro-vaccination is advisable." But if vaccine lymph, at any time, and under any circumstances, shall have lost its *essential properties*, surely the chances of a successful, much less a useful, retro-vaccination of the cow are very few. It is highly probable that by a proper selection of the animal, and an experienced choice of topical and other advantages, pretty uniform success may be obtained with the use of ordinary lymph; but when we see the effects of the very best and most recently humanized lymph on parts of the animal not ill adapted to the operation, it seems reasonable to fear that lymph deprived of its "essential properties" is not likely to prove a very manageable agent. This, in fact, is practically admitted by the best and most successful retro-vaccinators, who select the lymph for their operations from "well-developed vaccine vesicles."† But, from facts which will shortly appear, although the practicability of the operation may not be disproved, its utility may be still further questioned.

Before quitting this subject, I may be permitted to make a few

* *British and Foreign Medical Review;* Dr. Prinz; January, 1840, p. 85.

† *British and Foreign Medical Review*, January, 1840, p. 85.

brief remarks on the following question. Is vaccine lymph, in passing through many individuals with all due care and selection, susceptible, in process of time, of actual degeneration or essential diminution of intensity? Without speculating on the asserted immutability, under ordinary circumstances, of the essential properties of any known morbid poison, which seems to me not quite so easily maintained, or entering into a discussion as to the safety or propriety of implicit reliance on the analogy instituted between a virus of human and one of brute origin, I shall content myself with a reference to facts. In warm climates it is well known that actual and speedy degeneration does take place. In India, at Silhet, we are told by Mr. Brown, in a highly interesting paper on the regeneration of the vaccine,* "that in the course of three or four months the lymph gradually changes to a thin purulent-looking fluid, of a dirty white colour at first, and afterwards more resembling thin pus of an unhealthy character. Vaccination from such sources puts on the appearance of the pustular variety of imperfect and irregular vaccine noticed by Bateman—premature formation with much itching: the constitutional influence about the eighth day is rather less in this than the regular vaccine, and it is necessary of course to discontinue the practice from such degenerate virus." In other places these changes occur at different periods. Now is it unreasonable to enquire whether, in other climates, under the influence of occasional intemperature of season, slight changes may not take place, from time to time, which may ultimately lead to actual though less palpable alteration in some of the qualities and properties of vaccine lymph? Without presuming to assert that this is the *cause*, it seems impossible to deny the *occurrence* of the fact in temperate climates. M. Bousquet, whose zeal, ability, and experience in the practice of vaccination are well known and justly appreciated, in a very interesting and satisfactory memoir on the subject,† in comparing the vaccine of 1836 with that from which it was derived in 1800, by the aid of a coloured engraving, clearly shows a positive diminution of intensity, and explicitly states that the course is changed:—"*Aujourd' hui la pustule vaccinale n'est jamais plus belle, plus apparente qu au septième jour, mais cet état ne dure pas; à peine est-elle entrée dans le huitième jour, qu'elle jaunit et le vaccin se trouble dès le lendemain, la desiccation commence au centre et elle marche si rapidement que la croûte, réduite à la grosseur d'une lentille, tombe*

* *Quarterly Journal of the Calcutta Medical and Physical Society.* April 19th, 1837, No. ii.

† *Notice sur le Cow Pox decouvert à Passy, &c. &c.*, 1836.

du quinzième au dix-huitième jour." An accompanying engraving illustrates this perspicuous description, and contrasts the character and stages of the lymph in question with some new vaccine, found at Passy that year, which had then passed through scarcely twenty-five removes, and which M. Bousquet considers threatened with the like fate. Dr. Gregory* had observed that the vaccine lymph which had been in use at the hospital for a long period was of "diminished intensity—eight or ten punctures produced not more irritation than the three to which he had been accustomed fifteen years before." New lymph from a different source was introduced by Mr. Marson, and was found to be far more intense and active than the old. Three or four punctures were now amply sufficient; and Dr. Gregory, assured of the superior quality of the new lymph, discontinued, eventually, the old, and concludes his report by the expression of a belief that vaccine lymph, passed through the bodies of many persons, loses, in process of time, some essential portion of its activity. It is worthy of remark that the conclusions both of M. Bousquet† and Dr. Gregory are contrary to former belief.‡ Mr. Estlin, whose success in obtaining, and whose kindness and laudable diligence in diffusing, a new and active lymph are well known, and properly estimated,§ states that in his opinion the alterations in the vaccine affection consist in—first, the smallness of the vesicle and its attendant areola; secondly, its rapid course; thirdly, the absence of constitutional disturbance; fourthly, the small quantity of lymph yielded by the vesicle; and, fifthly, especially the diminished activity of its infecting quality. At the Vaccine Institution at Glasgow, and by many competent persons in this country and on the continent, similar opinions are entertained; though all do not, therefore, conclude that the vaccine, *pro tanto*, has lost its protecting property. On the other hand, persons of high authority and large experience can see no diminution of the needful activity of the present vaccine, and assert that it possesses all the exterior qualities and characters which new lymph exhibits. In a description of the variolous epidemic of 1829, in Turin, Griva‖ gives an

* Report on Small Pox, etc., etc., *Medical Gazette*, February 24th, 1838, p. 860, No. xxii.

† *Traité de la Vaccine*. Par M. J. B. Bousquet. Paris, 1833; p. 217.

‡ *Cyclopædia of Practical Medicine*: Article "Vaccination," p. 413.

§ *Medical Gazette*, September 15th, 1833, No. li.

‖ *In tutti questi sperimenti era impossibile rintracciare una qualche differenza dal corso del vaccino cosi detto umanizzato.—Epidemia Vajuolosa del* 1829, *in Torino; aggiuntivi I. Lavori Vaccinici.* Per T. D. Griva. Torino, 1831.

account of a few of his own experiments with primary lymph, and analogous observations of many distinguished persons who had favoured him with a detail of theirs, and asserts that he could see no difference, at that time, in the course and operation of the ordinary humanized and the primary vaccine. That the vaccine has undergone no essential change in its protective property is maintained in the report of the National Vaccine Establishment,* and the fact stated that lymph thirty-eight years old, obtained from Dr. Jenner, had manifested its peculiar influence in all the numerous subjects, in descent, through which it had passed. Many others contend that Jenner was correct in his belief of the improbability of future supplies from the cow becoming necessary. Jenner remarks, "Whether the nature of the virus will undergo any change from being further removed from its original source in passing successively from one person to another, *time alone can determine.* That which I am now employing has been in use nearly eight months, and not the least change is perceptible in its mode of action, either locally or constitutionally. There is, therefore, every reason to expect that its effect will remain unaltered, and that we shall not be under the necessity of seeking fresh supplies from the cow." †

Let us enquire, therefore, of Jenner himself, what was *then* the local and constitutional action of the vaccine. "The constitutional symptoms," says he, "which appear during the presence of the sore, while it assumes the character of a pustule (vesicle) only, are felt but in a very trifling degree." ‡ Two cases, in illustration, are detailed,—one vaccinated with primary lymph, the other from the second remove,—perfectly characteristic of the mildness of the constitutional *primary* symptoms, and not less so of the severity of the *secondary*, derived from the local, wide and deep spreading ulceration. The latter he was solicitous to prevent by local applications, caustic, etc.,§ remarking, emphatically, that the indisposition which was most sensibly felt "*does not arise primarily from the action of the virus on the constitution, but that it often comes on, if the pustule (vesicle) is left to chance, as a secondary disease.*" Analogy, Jenner's constant guide, here directed his judgment and

* *Medical Gazette*, May 19th. 1838, p. 348.

† *Continuation of Facts and Observations on the Variolæ Vaccinæ*, 1800, p. 258.

‡ *Further Enquiry*, p. 171.

§ M. Bousquet (*Traité de la Vaccine*) has gone much farther, and shown that the vesicle may be destroyed with caustic, at an earlier period, without interrupting the constitutional influence.

determined his practice.* Further observations convinced him of the correctness of this conclusion; and that a single vesicle was adequate to the production of the anti-variolous effect. Repeated vaccinations also taught him that his solicitude concerning the local irritation was unnecessary, and that, ultimately, the mildest remedies were rarely required, the acrimony of the virus having been subdued.† Jenner's description of the constitutional and local effects of the vaccine, with the accompanying illustrations, may therefore be confidently appealed to as a standard by which we may and ought to compare those of the present day. He rarely failed in communicating the disease from arm to arm; and dried lymph, he asserts, would prove effective at the end of three months.

From an early period, struck with the fidelity of Jenner's description, and always having recognized his distinction of the primary and secondary symptoms, I have looked upon the local affection, which is so much under the influence of temperament, tissue, etc., as of inferior importance, provided it did not materially differ from the average mild and normal character indicated by him. Where symptoms of constitutional affection are so mild, and often scarcely to be recognized, as in the vaccine,‡ of course it is necessary to have exterior local indications of the desired influence. It behoves us, therefore, to adhere as nearly as possible to the model furnished and recommended by the great discoverer of the vaccine and the inventor of vaccination. My own repeated applications to the cow have been chiefly for the purpose of experiment, for the satisfaction of patients, or the accommodation of friends, not from any belief in its superior protective efficacy over active humanized lymph. But when lymph is found uniformly deficient in infecting property, vesicles abnormally rapid in their course, at their greatest development on the seventh day, yellowish in appearance on the eighth with turbid lymph, central desiccation on the ninth, and a miserably small crust falling on the fifteenth or eighteenth day, common prudence dictates its discontinuance, and urges the adoption of a new supply, although constitutional symptoms may not be absent, for *weak* lymph may not be better than *late* lymph.

* He remarks that confluent Small Pox did not more effectually prevent a recurrence than the mildest Small Pox.—*Further Enquiry*, p. 180.

† *Continuation of Facts*, p. 264. 1800.

‡ Where no complaint is made, or is otherwise indicated by the patient, I have very frequently found an acceleration of the pulse mark the silent but sure progress of the disease.

There surely, in so delicate and important an affair, must be more satisfaction in using that which will affect promptly and certainly, produce a vesicle in its greatest beauty on the tenth or eleventh day,* which will then and even later contain a limpid and often an effective lymph, and desiccate not completely till the fourteenth or fifteenth† day. Such we know was the vaccine of 1800.

AFFINITY OF COW POX AND SMALL POX.

Neither the protective nor the modifying power of the vaccine, its co-existence with variola in the same individual, the striking resemblance in the form and structure of the two vesicles at a given period, nor its occasional occurrence as a secondary eruption,‡ had satisfied me of their common origin. So marvel lous a modification of so disgusting, malignant, and contagious a disease as variola, by the medium of the cow, and its conversion into a beautiful, benignant, and non-contagious affection, which it preserved when transmitted to man, did appear to me to require positive proof to be admitted with satisfaction. The announcement of Dr. Sonderland's experiments interested and astonished me, I confess, and I regretted the existence of impediments in the way of their repetition, but cherished the hope that other trials would be made to corroborate the fact. I was particularly struck with his seventh aphorism:§ "It is now clear why, in recent times, Cow Pox has been seldom or never seen in the cow; for the Cow Pox of the cow arises merely from infection by the variolous exhalations from men recently affected with Small Pox, and coming in contact with the cow. As epidemics of Small Pox have been rare during the last thirty years, cows could seldom be exposed to infection, and have, therefore, seldom exhibited the disease." I resolved, therefore, to enquire into the validity of the two propositions contained in this aphorism, viz., the origin of Cow Pox from man, and the rarity of the disease of late years,

* As in the acuminated natural or casual vaccine vesicle.

† Very active lymph will require sixteen or seventeen days for complete desiccation. See p. 402.

‡ *Medical and Physical Journal*, vol. ii., p. 402 (the Rev. Mr. Holt's cases); and vol ix., p. 309 (Dr. Adams's cases); also Dr. Adams on *Vaccine Inoculation*. A young lady, a member of a family resident here, was vaccinated in infancy, fourteen years ago. During the desiccation of the vesicles a secondary eruption of perfect vaccine vesicles appeared on the face and trunk, about twenty in number, and went through the regular course, leaving characteristic scars. Four or five on the face, which I saw a few days since, attest the fact. A few similar cases will be presently related.

§ *Medical Gazette*, November 9th, 1831, vol. i., No. 5, p. 162.

doubting the correctness of the former from my own previous observations. The result of careful and extensive enquiry induced the belief that the asserted comparative rarity of the disease was true as regarded this neighbourhood. From similar enquiries, made on every suitable opportunity, among the proprietors of cattle, of individuals who had had the casual Cow Pox, and from my own personal observations when the disease has arisen, I have collected the following facts :—

The Cow Pox has occurred: First, during epidemic Small Pox, but when no cases of variola have been known in the neighbourhood; secondly, when variola has been prevalent in neighbouring towns; thirdly, when variola has been in contiguous villages; fourthly, when in the same village (perhaps a solitary case) in which the affected farm was situate; but, fifthly, I have never succeeded in tracing positive or probable intercourse of convalescents from Small Pox, their friends or attendants, with a dairy or its occupants, except in one instance, in the autumn of 1838, during which time, and the early part of the following year, Cow Pox was prevalent, and in this case it can scarcely be supposed to have had any influence; the milker had carried a child some miles labouring under modified Small Pox (I merely relate these facts,* leaving others to draw their own conclusions, adding, what I have before stated, that although occasionally I have suspected the occurrence of Cow Pox in more than one individual in a dairy at a time, it is generally observed to appear first on a single cow, and spread by contact): and

* In the course of my enquiries I have heard many strange and unaccountable tales. I cannot forbear relating the following :—A resident in this town has repeatedly assured me that when a lad, more than forty years ago, he with several others, assisted in holding a milch cow while the late Mr. Allsop, of Watlington, Oxon., inoculated it with Small Pox matter in the teats and udder, at a farm called Standals, about seven miles from that place. That the whole herd subsequently had the Cow Pox thus produced. He caught it from them, as well as other milkers, and great numbers of people around were vaccinated on the occasion, the Small Pox being then prevalent and fatal. He understood the operation on the cow was done to render the Small Pox milder; and assures me that a copious but small vesicular eruption on the body followed his casual vaccination on the hands. The matter was taken, for the cow's inoculation, on the point of a lancet out of a small bottle. Mr. Allsop is dead, and I am unable to procure further particulars. I vaccinated this man: he had one *modified* vesicle, which left no permanent scar. A milker, detailing the particulars of the outbreak of Cow Pox in a herd, when he caught it, more than thirty years ago, assured me that his employer had men to sit up and watch nightly during a fortnight to detect, if possible, the approach of the d——d doctor (in search of lymph), whom he suspected of having inoculated the cows with Small Pox! his suspicions arising out of the facts that the disease was on no other farm, and the Small Pox was very bad in the adjoining towns.

lastly, that it is often seen in a single animal, but not unfrequently in several at the same period.*

[illegible] OF THE COW.

Nothing but direct experiments seemed available in determining the point at issue; but unfortunately there were many difficulties in the way of performing them satisfactorily. I obtained only negative results, and these [illegible] for me not to attempt any experiments except under a concurrence of the most favourable circumstances. These were not to be met with at any time; and arrangements for the purpose, made in the spring of 1838, were set aside for want of a sufficient number of eligible subjects. Under a more satisfactory concurrence of events in August 1838, I commenced some experiments with a view to ascertain the possibility of infecting the cow with variola after the manner of Dr. Sunderland.† I [illegible] two milch cows and one heifer, all in calf, with the sheets and blankets of a Small Pox patient. The sheets and blankets had been used for a deceased patient, and were removed from the same bed where lay another patient under confluent Small Pox of the twelfth day. The two milch cows were shut up in their shed for three days and nights, and afterwards for three days more, but not at night. During their confinement they perspired freely from the warmth of the covering. The heifer was placed under an open shed during a week. I could detect no indisposition, nor find any eruption on any part of them. A fortnight after this all these animals were inoculated with Small Pox virus of the [illegible] day, [illegible] by the lancet and by setons in the ear, the udder, and the teat, but without any apparent result. On examining the setons inserted into the udder [illegible] afterwards they were found [illegible] and as [illegible].

This fact afforded a [illegible] of what might be expected from the tissues of such animals, but they were subsequently [illegible] with points, setons, and the lancet, on the teats, udder, and the back, with [illegible] eighth-day lymph. No result.

One was subsequently re-vaccinated with [illegible] lymph of the seventh day, [illegible] had furnished it. No result.

* [illegible]
† [illegible] November [illegible] No. [illegible]

One of these animals was, some time subsequently, *re-invested* with blankets from the bed of a Small Pox patient of the ninth day. No result.

Such inconclusive results could not be otherwise than unsatisfactory. This, to me, at least, did not appear to be a land of promise, but a *terra incognita*, enveloped in clouds and abounding in mists, and where retreat was as difficult as advance was discouraging. Reflecting, however, on the experiments of M. Viborg, of Copenhagen,* on other animals, the statements of Dr. Sonderland, and the varied results of similar experiments by Dr. Numann, of Utrecht,† and those said to have been performed in Egypt;‡ but considering more especially the strong presumptive evidence advanced by Dr. Baron,§ that variola had been common to men and brutes, and the not unfrequent occurrence of malignant vaccine, if not of actual varioloid disease, in the cows of Bengal,‖ I resolved to persevere; and accordingly subjected several sturks (young heifers) to variolous inoculation. The following are the details of one of the series of experiments, and their results:—

February 1*st*, 1839: Inoculated three sturks with Small Pox virus (variola discreta), seventh or eighth day, on large points—the teeth of a comb—charged twelve hours previously. Sturks about ten months old.

Experiment first.—Red and white sturk, thin skin, gentle, well bred:—Made seven punctures, and introduced fourteen points, charged half their length, near the left side of the vulva and below it. Inserted two setons, charged with Small Pox virus from the same subject, at the same time.

Fifth Day.—Two or three of the punctures tumid, all closed with brown plugs; setons tumid.

Sixth Day.—Some punctures tumid.

Seventh Day.—Less tumid.

Eighth Day.—Still less so; setons passive, dry, adherent.

Ninth Day.—No material alteration, and therefore *vaccinated* on the *right side* of the vulva, in seven punctures, with fifth, sixth, and seventh day lymph, on fourteen points, from a young child; and *below* the vulva, in four punctures, with eight points.

Tenth day of variolation, *second* of vaccination: Some of the variolated punctures hard and elevated; but *one*, near the margin of the

* *Medical and Physical Journal*, vol. viii., p. 271.

† *Johnson's Medico-Chirurgical Review*, January 1834, p. 208.

‡ *London Medical Gazette*, vol. i., p. 673.

§ *Life and Correspondence of Jenner*, vol. i.

‖ *Ibid.*, vols. i. and ii.; also *Quarterly Journal of the Calcutta Medical and Physical Society*, No. 2, April 19th, 1837.

under fold of the labium of that side, with fourteen points, charged, as in the Experiment No. 1, from the same source; and with two setons, charged in like manner, near and below the vulva.

Third Day.—Incisions tumid, encrusted.

Fourth Day.—Less tumidity, less crust.

Fifth Day.—Incisions appear healed; two or three more tumid than the rest.

Sixth Day.—Some incisions more tumid.

Seventh Day.—Less tumidity.

Eighth Day.—Still tumid, but not advancing.

Tenth Day.—Seem lymphless tubercles.

Eleventh Day.—Tubercles less elevated; setons passive.

February 15th.—Re-inoculated with Small Pox virus of the seventh and eighth day (variola discreta) on the left side of the vulva and under fold thereof, as before, and near the verge of the anus. Virus liquid, some pellucid, some opaque and puriform, in capillary tubes, was forced into eight punctures, which were deluged with it; the punctures being afterwards irritated with points deeply charged with the same, which was suffered to remain in the punctures.

Third Day.—Nothing remarkable.

Fifth Day.—Four upper punctures near the verge of the anus, enlarged and elevated; four on the under fold of the labium, elevated and red, but less enlarged.

Sixth Day.—All present the appearance of the vaccine vesicle. The four upper are larger, but seem only tubercular; four lower, on the under fold of the labium, have a deep damask hue, and appear like oval or circular solid elevated rings, with central depressions: from one of these took clear lymph with much difficulty, and scantily charged thirty-nine points.

Seventh Day.—Upper tubercles seem diminishing, lower vesicles seem flatter, but broader.

Eighth Day.—Four upper appear still tubercular, of a slighter colour than their ground; four lower vesicles rather augmented, have a light damask hue. Took lymph again from one of them; the other three, not readily yielding lymph on a careful puncturing, were not further disturbed, from a desire to witness their progress; slight central crusts.

Ninth Day.—The four vesicles enlarging; again opened the inner margin under the daily increasing central crust of the vesicle first opened, and charged twenty points; tubercles diminishing.

Tenth Day.—One of the tubercles rather larger; four lower vesicles increasing. Charged twenty-seven points. Vesicles have a bluish, reddish, glistening appearance; two of them rather red at the base; one or two rather raw on each side.

Eleventh Day.—Brown crusts cover the centre of the vesicles, which appear declining.

Twelfth Day.—Declining, with increasing crusts of a blackish brown colour, within a slightly elevated margin. *Vaccinated* in several punctures on the margin of the right labium with many points, well charged with sixth-day retro-vaccine lymph; two removes. Punctures slighty tumid for a day or two, but quickly subsided. No result.

March 12th.—Four scars, as large as peas, in the situation of the four vesicles, depressed, pale rose colour. *Re-inoculated* with Small

Pox virus (confluent), fifth day, in four punctures, on inside of left labium. *Re-vaccinated* in three punctures, many points, of fifth and seventh-day lymph from a child. No result.

Experiment third.—February 1st.—Sturk, dark red and white; thick coarse skin. Inoculated in seven punctures, fourteen points, on the right side of the vulva, and beneath it, in the same manner and from the same source as No. 2. Two setons, charged with Small Pox virus, inserted still lower.

Third Day.—Punctures tumid.

Fourth Day.—Incisions closed with dark brown plug.

Fifth Day.—Tumid.

Sixth Day.—Several punctures tumid.

Seventh Day.—Less so.

Eighth Day.—Appear subsiding.

Ninth Day.—Only one or two small tubercles, and they are perfectly lymphless.

Tenth Day.—Diminishing in all respects; setons passive.

February 15th.—Re-inoculated with Small Pox virus of the seventh and eighth day (variola discreta), on the left side and under part of labium and verge of anus, with liquid virus, some pellucid, some opaque and puriform, from capillary tubes, and with points deeply charged with the same, taken twelve hours previously, in eight punctures, which were deluged with the variolous fluid, and afterwards irritated with the points which were allowed, when shortened, to remain in the wounds.

Third Day.—Two or three punctures a little tumid.

Fourth Day.—Some rather hard and elevated.

Seventh Day.—One puncture rather more tumid, about the size of a vetch.

Eighth Day.—Three or four tubercles rather larger.

Ninth Day.—One (the largest) tubercle seems pustular, the others appear subsiding.

I considered this a failure, and of course did not use the pustular product of the tubercle.

This animal was vaccinated in December last, with two other sturks, with primary lymph, but without any other result than that just described. The vaccination of the others succeeded.

Remarks.—In the experiments for the purpose of infecting the cow, those animals were selected which, from their age and the appearance of their teats, had not, in all *probability*, been the subjects of the vaccine disease; they were all under four years. I could not detect any eruption by a careful inspection of those parts of the body where it was most likely to have appeared; yet I cannot affirm that none existed in parts thickly covered with hair. All I can say is, that eruptions, consequent upon fever, are most commonly observed on parts of the animal void of or thinly covered with hair, viz., the teats and udder, as in the vaccine, the apices, chiefly, of the teats, the interdigital membrane, the skin over the coronet, of the feet, the mucous membrane of the mouth, gums, and tongue, as in the aphtha epizootica,* except in the malignant exanthemata, where any part of the surface may be affected, when the hair of course falls off on recovery. I have seen, on one occasion, both haunches of a milch cow covered with a multitude of the white blisters, which are apt to form on the teats and udder; but such an occurrence, at least in this neighbourhood, is exceedingly rare. It appears to me, therefore, from the absence of any fever in the animals in question, and the freedom of the parts above mentioned from any eruption, that we may fairly suppose that none occurred. I took no precaution to shave any hair from the back, which it appears was done in one, at least, of M. Numann's cases,† the reason for which I cannot understand. On the contrary, I took every precaution to prevent the infected blankets from coming in contact with the naked or thinly covered skin, my object being to *infect*. Hence portions of the blankets were suspended round the necks of the animals, and hung up near them, so that the variolous effluvium had every chance of being inspired. The uncertainty of these experiments, therefore, seems manifest; and the same may be said of the others, for I failed to succeed in *vaccinating* the same animals—a circumstance which at once prohibits our drawing any other inference.

The experiments by inoculation, from their importance, need a few remarks. The animals employed for the purpose were not those which I should have chosen if circumstances had permitted proper selection; but the difficulty of obtaining a *number* of milch cows upon which to operate, and *conveniently* inspect, is almost insuperable in a neighbourhood where these animals are so valuable. Few persons will permit operations which have a tendency to make milch cows irritable, much less such operations as these; and the importance of the operation requires careful and daily inspection. I decided, therefore, that there was no alternative but to subject the best I could obtain to the process of inoculation, in that manner and on those parts which I had ascertained would sometimes favour vaccination. There was an inducement also, of no trifling importance to the employing of these animals, that I was able to keep them on my own premises, and an advantage in selecting the parts, in their superior acces-

* Since the writing of this paper commenced this disease has been very prevalent here; and from the kindness of many of my friends, and especially of Mr. Lepper, our active, intelligent, and zealous veterinary surgeon, I have had numerous opportunities of watching the disease in all its interesting forms.

† *Johnson's Medico-Chirurgical Review*, January 1834, p. 209.

sibility to operation, facility of daily inspection, and tolerable freedom from injury. Yet I was fully aware of the loss of those advantages which the teats and udders of milch cows were capable of affording. The animals were much out of condition when they came under my care, but were beginning to improve when subjected to experiment.

The uncertainty attending similar experiments, and the importance of their results, were sufficient inducements to the adoption of every precaution calculated to avoid error and remove all possible doubt and misgiving; accordingly I took the Small Pox virus myself, in the presence of my assistant, Mr. Taylor, on points that never could have been used before, for they were the teeth of a large comb cut for the purpose, and charged new capillary tubes for the second experiment. The performance and progress of these experiments, as well as others of a similar nature, were witnessed by Mr. William Vores, house surgeon of the Bucks Infirmary; Mr. Charles Vores, his pupil; Mr. Henry Lepper, veterinary surgeon, and his assistant; my colleagues at the Infirmary, Mr. Henry Hayward, and Mr. James Henry Ceely; and my assistant, Mr. Taylor, who aided me in taking the virus.* The subjects from which the virus was taken were healthy young men, the pocks were remarkably fine, large, plump, and numerous; but at no time were either of the patients considered in danger. In using the points just described, I thought I obtained another advantage in having them large and capable of holding much virus, for they were doubly charged above half their length, cut in two, and allowed to remain where they were inserted, the punctures being made with a straight bistoury or a large lancet.

In the first experiment, during the first five or six days, there seemed some chance of a result in the tumefaction of the punctures; but on the ninth day, as this result seemed very unlikely, I decided on an endeavour to ascertain the susceptibility of the subject to the vaccine, and, therefore, inserted the vaccine points. The next day, to my great surprise, that which I considered an inert tubercle had assumed the form of a vaccine vesicle, and some of the other tubercular elevations had increased in size; the vaccine punctures, too, all looked red. The lymph obtained from the vesicle was perfectly limpid, and it so slowly exuded

* To all these gentlemen I am much indebted for valuable assistance, on many occasions, in the conduct of these and other experiments, especially to Mr. W. Vores, who has for a long time been my most zealous and untiring assistant in these pursuits.

that much time was spent in charging a few points. On the following day it appeared that the abstraction of lymph had diminished the energy of the vesicle; it looked flatter, duller, and smaller in size, as if declining, yet the vaccine punctures were evidently advancing. On the next day, twelfth of variolation, the vesicle had acquired more than its former size, and looked in a most vigorous condition, with all its characters augmented; there seemed some promise, too, of some of the other variolous punctures advancing; two below the vulva were certainly larger. The vaccine punctures (fourth day of vaccination,) were evidently forming, almost vesicular. On the thirteenth day nothing could exceed the interest of the scene. The highly vigorous state of the variolous vesicle—tense, florid, and glistening with a silvery hue from the tension of the epidermis, and the palpably vesicular state of the vaccine punctures, were, I need not say, very gratifying. Having before seen the temporary injury done to the variolous vesicle by the abstraction of lymph, I had not the courage to touch it again, being desirous to avoid interrupting its progress; besides, I had already enough lymph, and had inserted it into the arms of some children, whom I was daily watching with much anxiety. I took however, some lymph from the vaccine vesicles (their fifth day). Here was Bryce's test on the cow! Variola on one side in vigour, tested by vaccine on the other, hastening to declare the fact of constitutional affection. The variolous tubercles made no advance. On the fourteenth day all the vesicles seem diminished in activity and plumpness, owing to an escape of lymph, partly from injury, partly from the use of the lancet to the vaccine vesicles. On the fifteenth day all again in an active state. The variolous vesicle was truly splendid, and had acquired a magnitude greater than what the natural vaccine vesicle is apt often to attain, and an ample crust filled the centre. This was the period of greatest development of all the vesicles; the fifteenth day of variolation, and seventh of vaccination. It will appear, therefore, from this and the next experiment, that the variolous vesicle was retarded in its development several days; instead of reaching its acme on the tenth, as the vaccine vesicle does, it was the fifteenth. It was this tardy rising which induced me to give up all expectation on the ninth day, and vaccinate on the other side of the vulva—a happy mistake! On the sixteenth day decline in all was manifest, which was too palpable on the seventeenth to be doubted. The crust of the variolous vesicle was rubbed off prematurely, but the scar was deeper than is usually seen on the udder of the cow, and the surface rather more uneven;

the scars of the vaccine vesicles were less of course, nothing remarkable, but, like the scars attending Bryce's test-vesicles in man, exhibited induration and elevation of their margins much longer than the principal vesicle. Re-inoculation and re-vaccination were performed for obvious reasons. The effect of the lymph from the variolous vesicle, which will be detailed presently, was the production of the true vaccine. The lymph from the vaccine vesicles, taken on the fifth and seventh days of vaccination, the thirteenth and fifteenth of variolation, produced remarkably active vaccine vesicles on children. The differences require to be specially described.

In the second experiment (the first attempt) there was much promise, but no result. This I have several times met with; but re-inoculation has not been attended with the successful effects which ensued in this case. It was performed in *part* in a situation where the skin seemed thin and bled freely on puncture. On the fifth day the purplish or livid pimples, so much like the natural or casual vaccine on the thin skin of the teats, at this stage, announced the success of the operation *on* the lip of the vulva, and I certainly thought all the other punctures had succeeded on the thicker skin *near* the vulva; the want of colour in these elevations was attributed to the texture of the skin there. On the sixth day everything advancing, but the larger and colourless elevations seemed without lymph; the four glistening vesicles had a slight central crust, clearly announcing their character. Lymph was procured from one, with great difficulty, perfectly pellucid and adhesive. The seventh day the tubercular character of the four upper elevations quite manifest; they were *subsiding without a central crust;* the four vesicles had increased in breadth, and were less elevated. On the eighth day lymph was again taken from a vesicle which yielded it more readily than others; and, anxious not to interrupt their development, they were not again touched. All the vesicles were of a glassy resplendency; the tubercles were evidently passive. On the ninth day more lymph, perfectly pellucid, very scanty, was taken, the vesicles clearly advancing. On the tenth day, the day of maximum development of the vesicles, a slight areola round one of them; all had a very active appearance, and the lymph taken was perfectly limpid and quite as adhesive as before. The decline of the vesicles on the eleventh day was perfectly obvious, and precisely as in the natural, casual, and inoculated vaccine. This was confirmed by the appearances on the twelfth day. On the twenty-sixth day, the crusts having fallen a day or two, the smooth pale rose-coloured scars were observed. Re-inoculation and re-vaccination here also proved unavailing. The lymph taken on the different days was used with different degrees of effect; but, when successful, produced perfect vaccine vesicles, as will shortly be seen.

In the third experiment in neither attempt was there any satisfactory result; the skin was thick, and the animal seemed inaccessible both to variolation and vaccination, and affords a type of a great number of its tribe. The same chances in all respects as to time, season, circumstances, and manner of operating, were allotted to this animal, but entire failure was the result.

GENERAL OBSERVATIONS.

There was no apparent indisposition in either of the animals during the progress of the disease; the pulse, felt at the caudal artery, slightly accelerated at the acme, and increased heat and redness of the mucous membrane of the vulva, were the only symptoms noticed; eating and drinking went on as before. As these experiments were conducted in the same manner and on a similar description of animal as those for the purpose of ascertaining the susceptibility of the cow to primary and secondary lymph, by inoculation, they are capable of showing only comparative results. As in those, so in these experiments, no pains were taken to exclude the animals or defend the punctures from the external air or the weather beyond the precaution of confinement to the cow-house on the first night of the operation; at all other times the animals were allowed to roam about the field. It is true that during the progress of the disease I was engaged in an attempt, on the same premises, to infect the cow with blankets of a Small Pox patient, who, though weak and feeble, was prevailed upon to manipulate and frequently approach the nostrils of that animal, and, at the same time, walk amongst the sturks. The Small Pox, too, was prevalent, though not extensively so, around the premises, and the Cow Pox was in existence in some distant dairies. The atmosphere was moist but not very cold. The mean temperature of the month, indicated by the external thermometer, was 39·6; the mean pressure, by the barometer, 29·62. There was rain thirteen days in the month, seven days were overcast without rain, and eight fine with clouds. The prevailing winds were west, south-west, and north-west. I am thus precise in relating these facts, conceiving that where so little is known of the circumstances which favour the reception of variola by the cow, scarcely any particulars can be safely omitted in the description of a successful attempt.

Without attaching undue importance to any of the above circumstances, we may feel inclined to presume that the constitution of the atmosphere under which Cow Pox and Small Pox co-existed at the time of the operation, might possibly not be without its influence; but the utter failure of the experiment on the third animal clearly shows that far more importance must be attached to the temperament and constitution of the animal, and the condition and texture of its tissues, as influencing its susceptibility. At the same time it is right to state that many failures, more or less decisive, have occurred to me at different seasons and under different circumstances, in precisely or pretty nearly the same modes of operating, when the skin and general appearance of the animals have induced more favourable expectations. In about half the number of such cases, retro-vaccination, subsequently performed, at irregular intervals, has succeeded in a more or less perfect degree. In the remainder it has been as unsuccessful as the previous inoculation with variola.

These facts, and the promptness and precision (though of course under peculiar circumstances) with which the vaccine punctures in the first experiment answered, while only one of the variolous punctures tardily succeeded, afford striking proofs of the preference of these animals for the morbid virus natural to their kind. But the repeated though abortive attempts of the other variolous punctures on this animal to attain to the character of vesicles, and the final success of four out of eight variolous punctures, in concurrence with an equal number of lymphless tubercles in the second experiment, after the production of similar abortive tubercles in an immediately previous trial, plainly indicate also defect in the mode, the means, and the spot, and seem to declare that improvements in those particulars may be productive of better success.

Here we are forcibly reminded of the circumstances attending the communication of primary and secondary vaccine to cows and men, both casually and by the artificial method.* The rapidity and certainty with which the disease natural to the cow is propagated by the hands of the milker, and the difficulty and occasional futility of artificial attempts at such communication, especially with secondary lymph, the inferiority of our method on man with

* Vide *Progress of the Variolæ Vaccinæ*, p. 375; *Casual Cow Pox in Man*, p. 392; *Vaccination of the Cow*, p. 405; *Retro-vaccination*, p. 406; *Vaccination of Man with Primary Lymph*, p. 399.

a foreign virus, compared with the promptness and effect of the casual process, and the readiness with which such a virus, perfectly humanized, may be propagated from man to man by the artificial method, teach us that, to subdue or even to diminish the repugnance of the cow to a strictly human virus, we must have recourse to other means and measures than those by which, at times, we succeed in communicating its own. My experience has been too limited, my experiments insufficiently varied, to enable me to speak with precision on the best mode of retro-vaccinating, much less on that of variolating the cow. To acquire such knowledge, more time and ampler means than I have hitherto had at my disposal I am persuaded are absolutely necessary; but I will venture to throw out the following suggestions, which have reference to the selection of the subject, the season of the year, and the mode of operating.

There can be no doubt that the nearer we approach the practice of the "best vaccinators of the cow"—the milkers—the more likely we are to succeed; and although, if it were possible to employ a number of Small Pox patients to milk cows when their teats are chapped and cracked, we should not meet with the success that attends the manipulations of the former with a native lymph, yet it would not be unreasonable to expect a larger measure of success by this than by any other mode.* But the teats and udder of the milch cow, particularly with a thin skin, certainly should be selected in preference to any other part of the animal. It would be well not to have the animal too old, and the best possible assurance of its not having been the subject of the vaccine should be obtained. The back part of the udder, as being more out of the way of the milker, and more easy of access, would be preferable; but some part of the teat might be chosen which is least in danger of the casualties of milking—about the base, for instance. If, however, the sturk, the young heifer, or young bull must be the subject, either the prolabia of the vulva or the scrotum would afford the best prospect of success, especially if the animal be well bred and have a fine thin skin, and be of a light colour. I have found punctures on the skin, between the lip of the vulva and the tuberosity of the ischium, succeed better than those on other parts in that vicinity. It seems not improbable that some preparation of the parts might usefully be practised. The skin might be rendered more sensible

* According to Dr. Waterhouse (in a letter to Dr. Jenner), the casual communication of variola to the cow has thus happened in America. Vide *Report* of the Vaccination Section, p. 462.

and more disposed to absorb by covering it with some adhesive substance for a week or two before the operation. For instance, a mass of moistened clay might be affixed and carefully retained in a moist state.* I don't know that there is any advantage in a deep puncture, but the skin should be fairly incised. Superficial wounds, *if of long standing*, seem likely to answer very well; they might, therefore, be easily made in anticipation, and in imitation of the casual fissures on the teats of the cow.† Liquid Small Pox *lymph*, the earlier taken the better, not later than the seventh or eighth day, the fifth or sixth, seems preferable, and it should be used abundantly. We see points will answer, but the liquid lymph is obviously more advantageous and infinitely more convenient.‡ But as it is very probable that the success of the operation may be greatly affected by the state of the atmosphere, as influencing the system and particularly the condition of the skin of the subject, this must receive especial care. Extreme heat and extreme cold seem alike unfavourable to the success of inoculation, both of Small Pox and of Cow Pox, as they are to the spread of infection, especially if attended with corresponding dryness.§ Mildness and moisture would appear to be necessary. That condition of atmosphere which is well known

---

* I have often succeeded in procuring vaccine vesicles *without punctures*, on the skins of children especially and young persons, by keeping lymph in contact with the skin, and excluding it from the air by a coating of blood. Active lymph, blended with blood, casually trickling down the arm and drying in the most dependent part will often give rise to a vesicle. Not many days since I had a case where such a vesicle, at a distance of four inches from the inoculated vesicles, attained, on the twelfth day, the size of a small horse bean, and having no *firm* connection with the skin at its centre, like the casual vesicle on the cow, it acuminated on the eleventh day, as perfectly as on that animal. Vide p. 389, note. In our operations on animals we might take this hint.

† We are told by Dr. Jenner that Mr. Tanner succeeded best in retro-vaccinating the cow in an old superficial wound from which he had removed the crust. Such wounds, deluged with variolous lymph, and *excluded from the air*, might be highly serviceable.

‡ Variolous virus may be taken in bulbous tubes, or on small dossels of lint, and preserved between two plates of glass, one of which has a depression for its reception, such as Dr. Jenner used in sending liquid vaccine lymph to Bagdad, etc. They are very convenient. Vide *Baron's Life of Jenner*, vol. i., p. 420.

§ I have often observed the retarding effect of cold on vaccination, and particularly of a dry easterly wind, more especially on those who are much in the air. Dr. Adams gives a very interesting account of the effects of the *Leste*, or hot and dry south-east wind of Madeira, on vaccination, inoculation, and infection in general.—Vide *Medical and Physical Journal*, vol. ix., p. 314. Griva mentions the difficulty experienced in many parts of Italy of vaccinating in a dry and furfuraceous state of the skin. He successfully used emollient lotions preparatory to the operation.—*Epidemia Vajuolosa e Lavori Vaccinici*, p. 97.

to be favourable to the propagation and malignancy of Small Pox of course would be advantageous—warm, close, and moist—and such as an experienced inoculator of Small Pox would have *avoided* for his operations. His business was to mitigate; ours is to aggravate; we must, therefore, adopt the very means that he would studiously reject. Many punctures, much lymph, every natural advantage, and all the resources of art, seem necessary to ensure success to a moderate extent. Those who, like myself, attempt to sow a foreign seed in a soil with whose qualities and capabilities we are but indifferently acquainted, must not expect the same amount of product that doubtless will accrue to more expert, more favourably situated, and more experienced cultivators.

EFFECTS OF THE LYMPH.

Experiment first.—I need scarcely say that the effects of the lymph obtained from the above experiment were watched with intense interest, not unmingled with anxiety. Although some acquaintance with the physical characters of the natural and casual vaccine afforded sufficient assurance that I was neither rashly nor recklessly performing hazardous experiments on man, yet I could not be unmindful of the insidious but serious results of the very interesting and valuable experiments in India, performed by Mr. Brown, before alluded to, by which it appears that a vaccine disease, propagated from the cows at Silhet, had *ultimately and unexpectedly* been accompanied by a varioloid eruption, and had assumed a fatal character.*

My concern was not a little increased, *for a time*, by the following incident:—My assistant, Mr. Taylor, to whom I had entrusted the lancet used in opening the variolous vesicle in the first experiment, on the tenth day, while I was engaged in the tedious process of charging points therefrom, punctured the skin of his own hand, between the thumb and forefinger, with the instrument while moist with lymph, a circumstance with which at the time I was unacquainted. On the fourth day afterwards he directed my attention to a hard, deep red, papular elevation on the spot, stating the cause, and at the same time assuring me that he had been vaccinated in infancy, and had subsequently had modified Small Pox. On the fifth day there was a papulo-vesicular elevation, surrounded with a dark red areola, and much uneasi-

* *Quarterly Journal of the Calcutta Medical and Physical Society*, No. ii., April 1837. Also *Dr. Baron's Life of Jenner*, vol. ii.; Appendix.

[illegible]
[illegible]
[illegible]
[illegible] was
[illegible]
[illegible]
[illegible]
[illegible] was
[illegible] as
[illegible] parent.
[illegible] and
[illegible]
[illegible]
[illegible] he
[illegible] and
[illegible]
[illegible]
[illegible]

[illegible]
[illegible]
[illegible] airs.
[illegible] he
[illegible] the
[illegible]
[illegible]
[illegible]
[illegible] and the
[illegible]
[illegible] result
[illegible] the
[illegible] were

[illegible]
[illegible] in the
[illegible]
[illegible]
[illegible] peari-
Joseph
the [illegible]
did not
entirely
[illegible]

these cases the primary constitutional symptoms were very slight; the secondary proportioned to the extent and character of the areolæ: hence Joseph Woodbridge suffered severely, had vomiting and delirium. No eruption was observed in any of the cases except his; he had extensive roseola.

On three subjects, aged respectively eleven years, ten months, and two years and a half, some of the remaining points were employed; into these, also, were inserted, at the same time, points charged with ordinary vaccine lymph. In all three subjects the latter took effect in every puncture; while only five out of eight punctures with the new lymph answered, papulation being tardy as before; while the old lymph advanced as usual. As the areolæ of the vesicles from this lymph began to form, the sluggish vesicles from the new began rapidly to advance, and ultimately ran the same course, but did not eventually attain the same size, though perfectly well developed.

Six points, charged with lymph taken from the vaccine vesicle of the fifth day, on the variolated sturk, were inserted into two subjects at the same time as points charged with lymph from the variolous vesicle of the tenth day. One, Emma Churchill, aged five years, produced, from three punctures with the latter, two *papulæ* only; but from three punctures on the right arm, with the former lymph, two very fine active *vesicles*, in which the areola began on the ninth day, and was fully developed on the eleventh. In the other case, Richard Tompkins, aged four years, both sets of punctures took effect, but those with the retro-vaccine lymph were more early developed; the areolæ of both commenced on the ninth day, and declined after the eleventh. The symptoms in both subjects appeared on the approach of the areolæ, and were rather severe during its activity. In the subsequent removes of the lymph from the variolous vesicle and the retro-vaccine vesicles, and when propagated from arm to arm, it appeared rather more energetic than the ordinary lymph. Trials were made of both on the same and on separate subjects. In the subsequent removes of the new lymph, in the liquid state, by trials on the same and on different subjects at the same time, it was impossible to discover the slightest difference in its course and effects, whether derived from the variolous vesicle of the tenth day, or the retro-vaccine vesicles of the fifth or seventh day.

Experiment second.—The lymph from this experiment, on the sixth day, was employed on four subjects, viz., Mary Ann Hughes, aged two years and a half, fat, florid, but flabby and

base. On the thirteenth day the areola declined. Here sixteen punctures produced only seven vesicles, and one abortive lymphless tubercle. In these cases, also, the constitutional symptoms were scarcely noticed till the appearance of the areola, and with its increase they augmented, with its decline they disappeared; they were certainly severe. Some of the points, charged on the sixth day from the variolated sturk, were inserted into the same subjects at the same time as *liquid* lymph from Emma Churchill.* The vesicles resulting from these points, though for a time tardily developed, as above, were ultimately hurried on in their course by the promptness and activity of the *liquid* retro-vaccine lymph, so that on the eleventh day it was not possible to distinguish them, as in the case of Rebecca Walker, for example, aged one year and three-quarters. Points, charged with the primary variola vaccine lymph, of the sixth, eighth, ninth, and tenth days, were used on seven more subjects† with similar results—failure of some punctures, or more or less tardy or normal development of the vesicles, and all these phenomena occurred irrespective of the age of the lymph, whether of the sixth, eighth, ninth, or tenth days. I shall give two examples—one being the most successful, the other not without interest. Emma Jaycock, aged fourteen, dark swarthy complexion, thin skin, rather florid: two points of sixth-day lymph, and four of eighth-day lymph, were inserted into six punctures. Henry Jaycock, aged fourteen (twin brother), dark complexion, thin dusky skin: two points of sixth, two of eighth, and two of tenth day lymph, were used in six punctures. In Emma Jaycock, on the fifth day, four of the papulæ had ash-coloured summits, and seemed vesicular; two were doubtful. On the seventh day there were five small distinct reddish grey or ash-coloured vesicles, one very small; but I managed to take lymph, and inserted it by five punctures into a younger brother. On the eighth day the vesicles were advancing, of unequal size and of irregular form. Here I was forcibly struck with the strong resemblance some of these vesicles bore to those of the eighth day, depicted in Jenner's work,‡ on the arm of Hannah Excell, which he thought so remarkably like the results of Small Pox inoculation. My patient stated that she felt slightly indisposed on the fifth and sixth days, that the axilla was painful cn the seventh day, and that she was then giddy and sick, but felt

* Retro-vaccine from the variolated sturk.

† Three of them under the care of my colleague, Mr. H. Hayward, who kindly allowed me to observe the results.

‡ *Inquiry*, 1798. [Plate VI., vol. i.—E.M.C.]

worse on this, the eighth day. I charged points and glasses, and vaccinated an infant sister. On the ninth day the areola commenced, and she complained only of headache; on the eleventh day it was fully developed, when all her symptoms returned in an aggravated form. On the twelfth day it declined, but the turgid vesicles having burst the flimsy cuticle, renewed inflammation and induration with circumscribed sloughing and ulceration of the skin ensued, and rather deep scars are now visible. Henry Jaycock, on the fifth day, promised five vesicles for his six punctures; but being an irritable, intractable lad, he completely destroyed them with his nails, so that they were never properly developed. Subsequent vaccination, however, has been unsuccessful.* By this time I had succeeded in propagating, with the second remove of the first variola vaccine lymph, the retro-vaccine lymph from the same sturk, and the variola vaccine, sixth-day lymph, from the animal in the second experiment; and, desirous of comparing their character and effects, I selected a tractable though not a good subject, as regarded skin, for this purpose. Hannah Rogers, aged twenty-six, robust, florid, dark but thin skin, and inserted into six punctures, on her broad fleshy arm, lymph of the sixth day, from Rebecca Walker, and lymph from James Brown,† of the sixth and eighth day, second remove, of second variola vaccine. In each puncture two points,

---

* The *permanency* of the vaccine influence in this and in those cases mentioned by M. Bousquet (*Traité de la Vaccine*), where the incipient vesicles were destroyed by caustic, doubtless will be questioned by many. That the integrity of the vesicles is not essential to the production of the constitutional and preservative influence has been assumed from the experiments of that gentleman, and analogous cases to this now related. I have certainly met with not less than ten such cases, in which, at various periods, from fourteen to eighteen years afterwards, I have been unsuccessful in re-vaccinating. But this does not appear to be always the case. Out of thirty-five cases of ruptured vesicles, at the Nottingham Vaccine Institution (*Medical and Physical Journal*, vol. xvi., p. 137), three passed through the regular vaccine three or four months subsequently. If, as Jenner contended, the *primary* are the *essential* symptoms, then the integrity of the vesicle and the development of the areola are desirable only as probable indications of a fact which Bryce's test alone declares. I have met with seven or eight cases where the vesicles have been imperfectly developed, and where subsequent re-vaccination, after the same length of time, has been still less imperfect; but in one of these, who did not appear, as desired, for re-vaccination, a severe attack of Small Pox occurred ten years afterwards. One of the above cases has been exposed to Small Pox by inoculation once, and repeatedly to infection, without effect. Four patients, in one family, were vaccinated sixteen years ago by me; they had small vesicles prematurely formed, areola on the sixth day, which was extensive, and terminated on the eighth. All were indisposed, and have resisted re-vaccination to this very day. I have met with similar cases in other individuals, attended with similar results.

† Vide p. 438.

well charged with each lymph, respectively, were inserted and carefully retained.* On the ninth day nothing could be more uniform than the appearance of all the vesicles when the areola commenced; that uniformity they maintained throughout. On the eleventh day the areola declined, when the vesicles exhibited a remarkably blue tint, which increased till the thirteenth day, and was equal in this respect to any I ever saw in the casual Cow Pox on the hands of the milkers. The primary symptoms were slight on the fifth and sixth days, but acknowledged; her chief indisposition arose on the ninth day; severe headache, nausea, and general pain. The same identity of external character and general effects appearing in other trials, and believing it useless, and finding it inconvenient to keep up three stocks of lymph, I ceased to propagate from the two first after the fourth remove, when the vesicles were everything that could be desired, even on a puny, sickly, rickety child, aged two years and a half.† I then confined myself to the stock derived from Emma Jaycock. Her brother, Lewis Jaycock, aged twelve, was vaccinated from her vesicles on the seventh day; he had a dark, dusky complexion, and very thin skin, and was not so florid. He exhibited papulæ in every puncture on the fourth day, all of which were vesiculated on the fifth, on the evening of which day his axilla was sore; he felt headache, was giddy and sick. On the sixth day all these symptoms had rather increased, the vesicles were advancing; thirty-eight points were charged, and two children vaccinated from him, and he was re-vaccinated with his own lymph. On the seventh day he was in all respects better; vesicles advancing; took thirty-eight points and vaccinated a child. On the eighth day the areola commenced, and the *test* vesicles were forming. On the ninth areola pretty extensive, though pale, from the character of his skin, when headache, etc., returned. On the tenth areola increased, but only two vesicles were entire; the rest spontaneously burst or were rubbed; still complains. On the eleventh day they were nearly

* In all our experiments, doubtless, much must be allowed for the use of dry lymph, particularly in the use of that which is imperfectly assimilated. Here I thought two well-charged points to each wound would be more prompt than one.

† How often do we observe that those subjects from whom we expect the least, yield the most! Some of the finest vesicles I ever saw have been on rickety children not actually indisposed at the time. It is not the health and temperament alone of the subject, but the condition and quality of the dermic tissue that determines the development of the vesicle, and hence we never can predict beforehand the character of the vesicle without attention to this particular.

all destroyed. Here the vesicles were remarkably small, but not so on the subjects vaccinated from him; on the three children (two infants), all healthy and robust, with thick skins, nothing could be more satisfactory than the character of the vesicles, and the evidence of constitutional affection. As an example, I select the case of — Adcock, an infant four months old, vaccinated by Mr. J. H. Ceely, and consequently the third remove from the variolated sturk. Fretfulness and indisposition were manifest on the sixth and seventh day; but the active symptoms arose with the areola, which, at its height, had a bright damask hue. The vesicles were equal to any I ever saw, on similar subjects, from the early removes of primary lymph, and were not completely desiccated till the eighteenth day. The fourth remove to an infant four months old, with a plump, tense, thick skin, the vesicles were equally fine in all respects. From this was vaccinated — Slaughter, aged eleven months, where, on the fifth, sixth, and seventh days, slight indisposition was manifest; but on the eighth, when the areola commenced, smart symptoms of fever were present, which continued to the tenth, when it declined. Nothing could be more satisfactory or gratifying than the progress now made, which it would be needless further to detail; I shall therefore abstain from the description of individual cases, after adducing one example from the fourteenth remove, as a type of what might be produced in similar subjects, viz., an infant fourteen months old, florid, plump, and healthy, with a fine, clear, thick, smooth skin.

In the majority of instances, in propagating from arm to arm, distinct papulation was apparent on the second day; on the third it was not only visible, but elevated and well-defined; on the fifth and sixth, vesiculation was abundantly obvious, and lymph was often taken on those days; on the seventh day vaccination was frequently performed, and points were often charged; on the eighth the vesicle commonly exhibited a bold, firm, and glistening aspect;* between this period and the ninth day the areola generally commenced (but in young infants, with tense and sanguine skins, it appeared *early* on the eighth); by the tenth day the vesicle was commonly in its greatest beauty and highest brilliancy, glistening with the lustre of silver or pearl, having the translucency and appearance of crystal, or shining with a pale blue tint, occasionally of a dull white

* Although on this day most vesicles were abundantly yielding, many well-formed vesicles afforded an inconvenient and scanty supply till the ninth day.

or cream colour, bold and elevated, with a narrow centre and broad margin, or flat and broad in the centre with an acute margin, occasionally not raised above the level of the skin; on this and the eleventh day an extended and generally vivid areola existed, with more or less tension and induration on the integuments; at this time the lymph was frequently pellucid, and often perfectly efficient. From the eleventh to the thirteenth day, gradually increasing; in many individuals, both children and adults, sometimes the entire vesicle, at others only the central parts, reflected a blue or slate-coloured tint from the congested or ecchymosed subjacent adventitious structures, proportioned to the texture and degree of translucency yielded by its desiccating epidermis. On the thirteenth and fourteenth days, particularly on clear skins, moderately thick, the vesicles attained a considerable size, measuring often in their longest diameters six and a half or seven lines, and acquired a light-brown centre, from commencing desiccation, which was surrounded with an outer margin of dull white or pale dirty yellow, soft and flaccid, and still possessing fluid contents. During this period the areola, of a dull red or damask hue, would revive and decline again and again, and even to the sixteenth or eighteenth day, the period to which complete desiccation was frequently protracted. The crust commonly partook of the form of the vesicle; it was often prominent and bold, varying in colour from that of chestnut to that of a tamarind stone. It fell generally about the twenty-third or twenty-fifth day, often later.

The cicatrices were of variable depth and extent. When the vesicles remained unbroken on a thick sanguine skin, they were deep; but on a thin skin, shallow; they were not always proportioned in width to that of the vesicle, the smallest cicatrix often succeeding the largest vesicle; but the later the crust fell, of course the deeper the cicatrix, which on these occasions was often beautifully striated.* I need scarcely say that where the vesicles were accidentally broken, or spontaneously burst, much mischief ensued, deep sloughing of the skin, etc., etc. Spontaneous bursting did not often occur, except in those subjects possessing the before-mentioned and well-known obnoxious constitutional and dermic characteristics, upon whom we must always use active lymph with some risk.

When the lymph in the first remove produced normal vesicles,

* Inspection of many scars, caused by this lymph, shows that in a few months little is to be learned in many subjects, with thin skins, of the degree to which the vaccine influence has been exerted on them.

all destroyed. Here the vesi
so on the subjects vaccinated
(two infants), all healthy an
could be more satisfactory th
the evidence of constitutiona
the case of Adcock, an in
Mr. J. H. Ceely, and cons
variolated sturk. Fretfulne
on the sixth and seventh
with the areola, which, at
The vesicles were equal t
from the early removes
pletely desiccated till th
to an infant four month
the vesicles were equal
vaccinated - - Slaughte
fifth, sixth, and seven
but on the eighth, wh
of fever were present
declined. Nothing co
the progress now m
detail; I shall theref
cases, after adducin
as a type of what
an infant fourteen
a fine, clear, thick,

In the majority
distinct papulation
third it was not
the fifth and si
lymph was oft
vaccination was
changed; on th

the slightest approach to anything of a varioloid character. Roseola, strophulus, lichen, were the principal eruptions.

The papular eruptions, as observed by Jenner, frequently became vesicular. In a robust infant, aged six months, vaccinated at the sixth remove from the second experiment, at the incursion of the primary symptoms, an eruption of strophulus volaticus appeared of unusual severity, attended with much constitutional disturbance. The summits, both of the solitary and clustered papulæ, were vesiculated to an extraordinary degree; and the eruption being so thickly strewed on the face and body, I found it difficult to convince the parents, their friends, and neighbours, that it was not Small Pox. It disappeared and reappeared for three weeks. The other species of strophulus, particularly albidus, often assumed the same character as did those of lichen. In a few instances a vesicular eruption of a pemphigoid character, either in large bullæ, or closely resembling lenticular varicellæ, was observed, both in a solitary and in a grouped form. This seems to me to be strictly a vaccine eruption. It is seen on the cow, and often on young dogs, during or after the secondary vaccine symptoms. It will subside in a few days, or continue for some weeks in children.* In one case actual varicella appeared on an infant, aged fifteen months, six days after vaccination at the sixth remove. The vaccine vesicles became suddenly flattened, and the disease was impeded for two days.†

---

second experiment. A male child, aged two years, very fair, born eight weeks after his mother's recovery from a dangerous attack of Small Pox sixteen years after vaccination, and at birth covered with a multitude of shrivelled variolous pustules, the marks of which were long in disappearing, was vaccinated in December last, and yielded perfect vaccine vesicles, and one supernumerary vesicle, with the usual symptoms. From him I vaccinated a female child, aged five years, whose mother had been affected with mild casual variola four months before her birth, at which time she exhibited no marks. Here the vaccination was modified, the areola appearing on the seventh day, and subsiding on the ninth. An infant vaccinated at the same time showed perfect vaccination from the first subject. But I have known such cases as the above male child resist variolous inoculation; and others are stated to have been equally insusceptible of the vaccine.—Vide Bousquet, *Traité de la Vaccine*, p. 51.

* Vide p. 389; also *Willan on Vaccine Inoculation*, Appendix, No. 7.

† I failed in my attempts on several eligible subjects to inoculate with the pellucid lymph of these varicellous vesicles. The disease was prevailing in the village at the time; and two children of the same family, from one of which this infant was vaccinated, became infected with varicella soon after the infant recovered. This disease—called in Buckinghamshire "the blisters"—is continually met with, both sporadically and epidemically, without any connection with variola. I have often seen it, not only after Small Pox, but soon after vaccination, and in one instance a month after direct vaccination from the cow. Dr. Thomson has shown that variola assumes a *varicelloid* character; but it does not appear to me that he has succeeded in disproving the distinct and independent nature of varicella.

Supernumerary vaccine vesicles were often met with in, near, or distant proximity to the seat of vaccination, from the practice of free incisions and a liberal allowance of lymph;* but small *eruptive* supernumerary vesicles were observed in several cases at the period of full development of the areolæ, and within its sphere, when *points only* were used. In one case a vesicle appeared on the shoulder, and one on the neck. In two other cases two vesicles appeared on the abdomen, all during the early removes of both stocks of lymph.

The effects of the lymph have been well observed at Cheltenham, where it has been extensively used† by Mr. Coles and many other surgeons. It was in use many months at the Small Pox and Vaccination Hospital in London; and has been attentively observed at Bristol by Mr. Estlin;‡ also at the Cow Pock Institution of Dublin;§ and by many private practitioners.

GENERAL OBSERVATIONS.

In the transfer of the above lymph from the animals to man, my attention was forcibly arrested by the difficulties attending the process; and in the entire failure of so many punctures, the production of so many lymphless papulæ, and the formation of so few perfect vesicles, I recognized phenomena so common in similar trials with primary lymph.‖ In some instances the difficulties were not completely overcome even in the second removes. The marked improvement, in subsequent removes, in the development of the vesicles, and the active manifestation of the primary and secondary symptoms, were not less apparent than in the use of natural lymph under corresponding circumstances, except that in very few instances, and those principally in later removes and in peculiar subjects, there was not observed that disagreeable, inconvenient, and mischievous acrimony so peculiar to the former lymph. The lymph from the vaccine vesicles on the first experiment seemed to have acquired activity without causing the same amount of difficulty in its transmission.

These experiments with the variola vaccine lymph on man, show the necessity of having a number of subjects of different temperaments on which to employ it, on its first removes to ensure success. It seems highly probable, too, that the direct transmission

* Vide p. 389, note.

† Vide *Report of the Vaccination Section of the Provincial Medical and Surgical Association*, p. 464.

‡ *Medical Gazette*, December 27th, 1839.

§ Vide *Report*.

‖ Vide p. 399.

of the liquid lymph from the animal to children will save much trouble and conduce to greater success.

It has been justly observed by Dr. Adams,* "that diseases in one class of animals, when communicated to another, seem to alter many of their properties;" and no more appropriate illustration can be adduced than the *vaccine modification of variola.* The wonderful sagacity of Jenner taught him first to believe and announce the important fact of the affinity between vaccine and human variola; and through the brilliancy of his genius, his unwearied industry, and boundless philanthropy, it has been made subservient to the welfare of mankind. Hence the fact in question proves deeply interesting to all. But the physiologist cannot fail to desire some knowledge of the probable causes of such remarkable modification. In the prosecution of enquiries of so interesting and comprehensive a nature, of course he will not confine himself to the physiology and pathology of the cow; but, in considering the structure of this animal, and its functions in health and in disease, his attention is arrested by many remarkable peculiarities. The abundance of its cellular and adipose tissue, its low vital energies, its sluggish habits, the tendency of its diseases to pass into the chronic state, the difficulty of exciting suppuration in an abscess and in setons, clearly evince the antiphlogistic and lymphatic temperament.† Hence the insidious nature of many of its maladies, and their tendency to pass under favourable circumstances into the adynamic state. The well-known proneness of this class of animals to carbuncular, gangrenous, epizootic, and enzootic typhoid diseases, will greatly diminish therefore our surprise at the fact of their liability, in certain situations and under certain circumstances, to malignant vaccine, and even to variola. It would ill become me to do more than allude to this highly interesting subject, and point attention to the valuable records of such facts which are accessible to all.‡ I shall therefore conclude

---

* *Observations on Morbid Poisons*, p. 51.

† *Je puis errer, mais il me semble que, comme je viens de le dire, l'abondance des tissus cellulaire et graisseux, l'energie vitale toujours moindre, toutes choses égales d'ailleurs, dans le bœuf que dans le cheval, les habitudes lentes de cet animal, la tendance qu'ont ses maladies à passer à l'état chronique, la difficulté qu'éprouve la suppuration à s'établir dans les abcès, les sétons, démontrent évidemment l'association de la prédominance plus ou moins marquée du système lymphatique sur l'appareil vasculaire sanguin, et prouve l'existence du tempérament mixte que je viens de signaler.—Pathologie Bovine.* Par P. R. Gellé.

‡ *Dr. Baron's Life of Jenner*, vols. i. and ii.; *Quarterly Journal of the Medical and Physical Society of Calcutta*, No. 2, April 19th, 1837; *Report of the Vaccination Section of the Provincial Medical and Surgical Association;* and *Asiatic Journal*, December 1839.

REPORT OF THE VACCINATION SECTION

OF THE

PROVINCIAL MEDICAL AND SURGICAL ASSOCIATION.

JOHN BARON, *Chairman.*

[*Reprinted from the "Transactions of the Provincial Medical and Surgical Association." Vol. VIII.*]

1840.

REPORT OF THE SECTION

APPOINTED TO ENQUIRE INTO

THE PRESENT STATE OF VACCINATION,

AS READ AT

THE ANNIVERSARY MEETING

OF THE

PROVINCIAL MEDICAL AND SURGICAL ASSOCIATION

HELD AT LIVERPOOL, JULY 25, 1839,

AND ORDERED TO BE PRINTED FOR GENERAL CIRCULATION.

CHAIRMAN:

JOHN BARON, M.D., F.R.S., CHELTENHAM.

SECRETARIES:

WILLIAM CONOLLY, M.D., CHELTENHAM.
A. T. S. DODD, ESQ., CHICHESTER.

COMMITTEE:

Joseph Brown, M.D., Sunderland.
Joseph Bullar, M.D., Southampton.
Henry Coles, Esq., Cheltenham.
John Conolly, M.D., Hanwell.
S. Cox, M.D., Edinburgh.
John Green Crosse, M.D., F.R.S., Norwich.
King Ellison, Esq., Liverpool.
J. Engledue, M.D., Portsmouth.
Thomas Evans, M.D., Gloucester.
George Goldie, M.D., York.
R. T. Gore, Esq., Bath.
— Greenhow, Esq., Newcastle.
G. Gregory, M.D., London.
— Heathcote, M.D., Rotherham.
Christopher H. Hebb, Esq., Worcester.
James Kendrick, M.D., Warrington.
— Loe, Esq., Leeds.
David M'Crorie, M.D. Liverpool.
Jonas Malden, M.D., Worcester.
Daniel Noble, Esq., Manchester.
Roger Nunn, M.D., Colchester.
Frederick Ryland, Esq., Birmingham.
Thomas Shapter, M.D., Exeter.
R. I. N. Streeten, M.D., Worcester.
T. P. Teale, Esq., Leeds.
T. O. Ward, M.D., Shrewsbury.

PRELIMINARY REMARKS.

THE subject committed to our care is one of deep importance to the safety and well-being of the community. We have entered upon it with an earnest and anxious desire to discover truth, and to lay it before our brethren in the most simple and perspicuous manner. The number and variety of the questions involved in the investigation increased the difficulties of our task; these we have endeavoured to surmount by fixing our attention upon the great and leading features, and thus to find a place where all the subordinate parts might take their station without disorder. The diversified character of our materials, and their intimate relations with each other, rendered this partition and separation both perplexing and laborious. We dare not hope that we have completely realised our own wishes, but our brethren, we trust, will believe that our endeavours have been both diligent and sincere. It will be seen, as we advance, that some of the information about to be communicated is highly interesting and valuable. It has happily enabled us to carry out the arrangement with greater precision than could otherwise have been attained. This benefit, considerable though it be, is small when compared with the practical results that flow from it.

The first division of the Report embraces those points that have received what we take to be a satisfactory demonstration. The other divisions, all more or less dependent upon it, have been drawn up from authentic documents, and set forth the past and present experience of many of the most respectable professional gentlemen in this country, in a faithful and condensed form; this at least has been our aim. It must, at the same time, be admitted that the testimony has not always accorded. In arriving at conclusions we have been compelled to weigh and balance evidence; but as the facts which have guided us are fairly stated, our opinions can at once be brought to the test, and of course will avail no more than as they appear to be conformable to the truth. With this admission we desire it to be understood that nothing has been introduced of an hypothetical or speculative nature; nothing has been kept back unfavourable to the cause of vaccination; neither has anything been withheld that was calculated to produce an impression of a different kind. While arguing either for one side of the question or the other, we have studied to confine ourselves within the limits of a strict impartiality. At the outset we would claim credit for this intention, the nature of the evidence being occasionally of a jarring and contradictory description; to sift and examine that evidence made up no trifling part of our duty. It would have been gratifying had this necessity not existed; but to have shrunk from the difficulties arising out of it would have rendered the present undertaking equally inconclusive and unsatisfactory. We have endeavoured on the one hand to moderate and regulate public expectation where needful; and on the other to prevent undue apprehensions from damping confidence in a practice that has already been fraught with such wondrous benefit to mankind; and when perfectly understood and carefully followed, we humbly hope may still be permitted greatly to bless our race.

Valuable information, from whatever source derived, has not been overlooked; but we have ever borne in mind that after having accomplished the most important part of our labour, the next was to confine our enquiries, as much as with propriety could be done, to the present state of vaccination in these kingdoms. To have detailed, even in the briefest manner, the opinions that have been published in other countries, would have swelled this Report to a very needless magnitude. These opinions are also often of a contradictory nature, the experiments by which they are supported are not less so, and we have had no inclination to enter on this disputed ground, because we flatter ourselves that the sources of these contrarieties are likely to be removed.

The gentlemen who have favoured us with their returns, may rest assured that they have been most carefully scanned; and though every individual name has not been mentioned, all will perceive how much the value of our Report depends upon their respective communications. We will only add, that from the method of conducting vaccination in Great Britain, accurate registers are not in general kept, and it has therefore not been possible to construct such tables as could have been desired.

Having premised these observations, we shall now state the order in which we mean to arrange the different heads or sections. The first will treat of the affinities between human Small Pox and Cow Small Pox. The second will contain what we deem essential to render Vaccination correct, with some observations on the impediments to that practice. We will then proceed to consider the protecting power of Vaccination. Our fourth section will comprise remarks on Small Pox after Small Pox; which will be followed by a brief examination of the question of re-vaccination. Lastly, we shall enquire into the state of the population generally, both with regard to Small Pox and Vaccination; the means at present employed for the dissemination of the former, with suggestions for restraining it, and promoting genuine effectual Vaccination.

AFFINITIES BETWEEN HUMAN SMALL POX AND COW SMALL POX.

In pursuing this investigation, we have especially directed our attention to the nature of the *variolæ vaccinæ*, their origin, their history, their affinities with the *variolæ* of the human species, and the foundation on which confidence may rest as to their lactic virtue. This portion of the subject may well oc attention of the Association, as upon a due understand everything that is valuable in the practice of vaccination de Formerly it was supposed to be obscured by difficulties an certainties; now we have the satisfaction of being able to sa such difficulties are removed, and that the great problem resp the nature of the security afforded to man by the communi of the vaccine disease, is solved. We cannot refer to this mo tous event without paying a passing tribute to the genius discrimination of the magnanimous and most distinguished a of vaccination. He called the disease the *Variolæ Vaccinæ*, good reason he had for this most correct and pregnant designa Many of his contemporaries derided it, but he wisely adhere his own views, remarking, with admirable sagacity, that this appellation contained in it the germs of a theory which fu observations would illustrate and verify. That verification ha been obtained; and we deem it of so much importance, that w place it in the most conspicuous part of our Report, well assur that it influences every question that can arise respecting th object of our researches.

Let us, therefore, recur to the idea involved in this designati It implies that one genus of the inferior animals is liable to a disease of a kindred nature with that which attacks man, the latter, for the most part, being pestilential and fatal; the former often mild, and scarcely pestilential at all. The practice of in-oculation had long been in use to diminish the mortality of human *variolæ*, and it had been ascertained, by casual observation, that an affection derived from the cow protected from subsequent attacks of that disease. This, and other facts, led Dr. Jenner to conclude that the protecting power arose from the impregnation of the constitution with a mild species of Small Pox instead of the malignant and virulent sort, which is for the most part propagated from man to man, whether naturally or by inoculation. This idea, which he very early took up, guided him through all his investigations, and led him at last to the great result of his labours, namely, the successful transmission, by inoculation, of the mild and safe affection from the inferior animals, instead of the contagious and malignant disease which for so long a period had devastated mankind. His confidence in this practice arose from his unalterable conviction that these two disorders, how different soever they might be in some particulars, were in reality identical.

These conclusions, resting upon a very wide induction, drawn both from the history of human Small Pox, as well as from accurate observation of Small Pox among cattle, were published by him in every possible form, as his reasons for recommending the inoculation with *Cow Small Pox* instead of *human Small Pox;* but his doctrines were disregarded and contemned, and the majority, we believe, of the public, as well as of the profession, to this hour imagine that the benefit derivable is not because these diseases are alike in essential properties, but because they are in all respects dissimilar and opposed the one to the other—the disease arising from the cow being imagined to be an antidote, not a safe and effectual substitute for a more malignant form.

Things continued in this state nearly up to the time of his death; and the controversy which sprang from his discovery had very little reference to this fundamental part of his doctrine, but consisted rather in assertions and counter-assertions respecting the alleged virtue of the disease derived from the cow. Some of those who have followed Dr. Jenner have laboured to bring back the question to its proper basis, and to prove that the opinions which he promulgated were capable of demonstration, both from the medical and literary history of *human Small Pox* and *Cow Small Pox.* The light thrown upon the whole subject by these enquiries respecting the diseases of the inferior animals is very striking and peculiar, and they must be specially brought forward in this place, in order to enable us to complete that chain of evidence which leads us to our great conclusion. We will begin, therefore, by stating that it has been shown, by unquestionable evidence, that cattle and other animals have for centuries been known to be affected with Small Pox or *variola.* This latter appellation has unhesitatingly been given to the disease by every different writer who has seen it; by Dr. Layard, in England; and, long before him, by Fracastorius, Lancisi, Lanzoni, Ramazzini, and others, in Italy. We believe that these facts were unknown to Dr. Jenner; but, be this as it may, they give an authority to the language employed by him, corroborated as it will be by still more explicit evidence.

The disease described by the authors above named was of a malignant character, and destroyed the cattle almost as extensively as Small Pox did the human race. It is not known how often it may have raged in England, but it is certain that it was introduced into this country in 1745, and again in 1770, and appeared among the horned cattle, with more or less violence, so late as 1780. At this time Dr. Jenner was carrying on his investigations; and it was in this very year that Dr. Layard

nothing but the misery of a ruined grazier, and the whining piety of a methodist." He adds in a note, "There was something wonderfully pathetic in the mention of the horned cattle." Could this bold and unfeeling writer have caught the slightest glimpse of the wonderful consequences arising from this disease "of the horned cattle"—could he have seen, in the most remote degree, its affinity with a like distemper in man (and history and experience were not silent on this point, even in his day)—he might have perceived that the sufferings as well as the safety of his fellow-creatures were deeply involved in the question. The party politics of the hour might then for a moment have lost their influence, and a nobler sentiment have taken possession of his soul. But notwithstanding the sarcasms of Junius, his Majesty recurred to the subject on the opening of the ensuing session, Tuesday, November 13th, in the same year. Both Houses of Parliament in their addresses alluded to it, and talked of "the fatal contagion which has of late appeared in some of the distant parts of Europe." It was not to be expected that our senators should be accurate medical historians; but we know, from the clearest evidence, that the appearance of this disease had not been of recent date, as we have descriptions of it hundreds of years before.

Whether the great increase of mortality from Small Pox which occurred during the latter part of the last century had anything to do with this epizootic, we cannot tell; the coincidence, nevertheless, deserves notice. From the year 1731 to 1772, the proportion of deaths from Small Pox compared with those that arose from all other causes was as eighty-nine in a thousand; whereas, from 1770 to 1800, they were as ninety-six in a thousand. This increase has been attributed to the general practice of Small Pox inoculation during the latter period. Such may have been the case; but still it is true that when the cattle were scourged by the variolous disease, mankind were in like manner great sufferers. One of our correspondents, Mr. Bree, of Stowmarket, makes an incidental remark applicable to this point. "During the prevalence of Small Pox in this neighbourhood," he observes, "several dairies became affected with Cow Pox; which supports the opinion of the identity of the two diseases, the latter being probably modified by being developed in the cow."

The history of these epizootics shows also that horses as well as cows are liable to this affection. This interesting fact illustrates and explains one of the most difficult and perplexing events in the practice of vaccination. It was known that a disease from the horse was sometimes communicated to the cow by men employed in dressing the heels of the one, and afterwards milking the other. This disease was supposed to be what is vulgarly called *the grease*, and was imagined by Dr. Jenner, in the outset of his enquiry, to be the origin of Small Pox. This idea he lived to correct; but the prejudices it excited, and the erroneous views to which it gave birth, have unhappily been perpetuated. It is ascertained that the horse is liable to a vesicular disease of a variolous nature as well as the cow; and that lymph taken from the horse and inserted into man will produce an affection in all respects like that derived from the cow, and equally protective. The error consisted in believing that this affection was *the grease*, and that it required to be transmitted through the cow to give it efficacy. A misapprehension of this kind may well be excused in the infancy of so complicated an investigation—the disease appearing for the most part on the thin skin of the heels of the horse, and the traditions among the farriers in the country, leading to the mistake. We now know that the vesicle may appear on other parts of the animal's body; and that the horse as well as the cow has in different ages and in different countries suffered both from the mild and malignant *variolæ*.

These variolous epizootics may be traced in the most authentic medical records for several hundred years, and the connexion between them and pestilences, which have ravaged both man and the inferior animals throughout the ages of the most remote antiquity, may be discerned with much greater accuracy than at first might be imagined. It is likewise worthy of remark, that the countries where the disease has of late years been found, either on cows or horses, are those where it has formerly been known to have existed among them in its most virulent form. But its ravages are not confined to one region of the earth; it has been discovered in the valleys of England, on the mountains of the Andes, on the elevated ranges of the Himalayan chain, in the plains of Lombardy, and the green pastures of Holland and Holstein. What it was formerly in the days of Lancisi and Lanzoni in Europe, it is at this moment in Asia.

The cows in Bengal have long been affected with this complaint; and it is a point not to be overlooked on this occasion, that the natives describe it by the very same terms by which they designate the *variolæ* in the human subject, namely, *bussunt*, *mhata*, or *gotee*. In August, 1832, Mr. Macpherson found this disease among some cows at Moidapore. The description which he has given so entirely agrees with what is recorded by Fracastorius and the other Italian writers already mentioned, that it is impossible to doubt that they were all delineating one and the same disease. We have farther to observe, that an affection of a precisely similar character has been witnessed in a dairy in Gloucestershire so late as 1825. The veterinary surgeon who saw it described it as an aggravated case of Cow Pox, the whole skin from the base of the horn to the end of the tail, and to the hoofs, being covered with the disease. It destroyed the animal, and spread through all the other cows in the dairy, between forty and fifty in number. Now, all this exactly agrees with the variolous epizootic described by Dr. Layard, in 1780, which, he said, "bore all the characteristic symptoms, crisis, and event, of the Small Pox." We will connect this subject with the experiments conducted by Mr. Macpherson in Bengal, who observed the disease among the cows in its topical, as well as in its more malignant and pestilential form. Thus, he found two small pustules on the teats of one cow. From the crusts obtained from these pustules, he inoculated eleven children. It failed in the majority of instances, but in one it produced the true vaccine disease. Not the least impressive event in this history is yet to be mentioned. In 1837, another series of inoculations was performed with virus from diseased cows; on which occasion an eruptive complaint of the true variolous nature was produced. The same phenomena have been observed in the course of the last year at Gowalpara by Mr. Wood. In several of his cases the symptoms were so severe as to excite apprehension that the disease would terminate fatally. He was so strongly impressed with this fact, that he thought it would be better to take human Small Pox rather than Cow Small Pox for inoculation, when the latter assumes its dangerous and fatal form.

It is thus incontestably proved, that a severe variolous disease may be communicated from the inferior animals to man, as well as a more mild and benignant affection. The event in either case seems to depend upon the state of the disease in the animal from which the virus is taken; and had inoculations been performed on man with lymph taken from the cattle as they were afflicted in the middle and latter part of the last century in England, we should probably have witnessed the very same results that have recently taken place in Bengal.

We have already alluded to the simultaneous existence of Small Pox among men and the inferior animals in this country, and as this is a peculiarly interesting and important branch of our inquiry, we must endeavour to establish it by a few additional facts. That the pestilence was very fatal, both to the horned cattle and to the human species during a great part of the last century, admits of no dispute. The remark likewise of Mr. Bree, of Stowmarket, that the prevalence of Small Pox in his neighbourhood, at the same time that the disease appeared in the dairies of Suffolk, ought to be had in remembrance while we mention that many other parts of England have lately borne witness to the same truth.

During the late epidemic the affection among the cows has certainly been more observed than at any period for many years. In Gloucestershire it has been seen by many persons, and it is from this county, we believe, that Mr. Estlin derived the lymph which he has so assiduously diffused. In Dorsetshire it has been found by Mr. Fox, of Cerne Abbas, and within these few weeks by Mr. Sweeting, of Abbotsbury, both of whom have successfully propagated the affection on man. In Buckinghamshire, likewise, it prevailed extensively, and enabled Mr. Ceely to institute some of the valuable experiments which we shall shortly notice. We have no doubt at all that had attention been generally directed to this point, much more information might have been obtained. We are happy in being able to supply deficiencies of this kind, by a short reference to facts recently derived from other regions of the earth.

In a General Sketch of the Province of Guzerat, by A. Gibson, Esq., published in the first volume of the *Transactions of the Medical and Physical Society of Bombay*, which has just reached us, is the following passage:—"Variola, or Small Pox, carries off annually many persons, particularly in the more remote and unfrequented districts, out of the line of the great roads, or at a distance from large towns. I believe that in the midland country, beginning at Surat and ending at Ahmedabad, in the whole of which range vaccination is thankfully received, and often eagerly sought after, the frequency of variola has been greatly lessened, and the results appear evident in the increase of population. *The same disease is at times very fatal among the cattle;* they become so weak and feverish as to be unable to eat in consequence of the effect of the pustular eruption on the lips, tongue, and throat."

Let us now take another quotation from a letter written by Mr. Macpherson (to whom we have already alluded), dated at Murshidabad, May 1st, 1836:—"The disease is said to make its appearance among the cows here generally about the breaking up of the rains; but no cases, so far as I have been able to ascertain, have occurred for the last two years; and I am happy to add, that very few cases of variola have been known within the same period. From these circumstances we may infer (as I have remarked in former letters on this subject) that the unknown causes which favour the disease in the human subject, have the same tendency in the cattle; in fact, that *variola and mhata, or gotee, owe their origin to the same cause.*"

This observation is eminently deserving of consideration; and that constitution of the atmosphere which promotes the dissemination of the disease, either among men or the inferior animals, ought to be particularly watched, when it is attempted to inoculate the latter with human Small Pox. We believe that many unsuccessful experiments may be ascribed to the neglect of this precaution.

Mr. Lamb, who wrote from Dacca on May 9th, 1836, and described the disease among the cattle with great accuracy, although he did not frequently observe the co-existence of human Small Pox and Cow Small Pox, nevertheless mentions, that when the former was prevalent at Dacca, the latter appeared in one *Muhalla* and carried off fifteen or twenty cows. He attempted to inoculate the cows with human Small Pox, after the manner practised by Dr. Sonderland, but without success. The virus was then inserted on the udder, and about a dozen irregular pustules made their appearance, but he was unable to produce any effect from them by repeated trials on the human subject.

We will now advert to a letter from Mr. Brown, addressed to S. Ludlow, Esq., Superintending Surgeon, of Barrackpore. Mr. Brown, who was stationed at Silhet, where the variolous disease was prevalent among the cows, selected from one of them some of the dark brown scabs scattered over the back and abdomen. These he reduced to a pulp with water, part of which he inserted into the arms of four children. In all, correct vaccine vesicles were said to have been produced, the constitutional disturbance, however, being on the *eighth day* more severe than usual. From this stock, the disease was propagated during two months without any suspicion as to the genuineness of the affection. After this time, children in whom the virus was inserted were on the *eighth day* attacked with fever, followed by an eruption which spread over the whole body, and in one case proved fatal. Mr. Furnell, whose own child perished by the disease, describes it as a true Small Pox in its worst form. Connected with this detail we find the following interesting case:—Mr. T., about eighteen years of age, was first vaccinated in India in his infancy; he was re-vaccinated in Scotland, whence he had returned about eight months. Two days after his arrival in Silhet he was attacked with severe rigors, nausea, vomiting, and slight delirium. These symptoms were followed by a copious eruption, which spread over the whole body, and was evidently of a variolous character. The origin of this disease attracted the attention of Mr. Brown, and he observes, "we can only ascribe it to one or other of the two following sources of infection :—the eruptive disease which attacked the European children above referred to, or that which prevailed epizootically among the cattle.*

In the present argument it is of little moment to which of these scources we ascribe the disease. The case is brought forward merely to show the feeling in the mind of the writer, that it might have arisen from the pestilence which was then raging among the cattle.

These facts have all but proved that the vaccine disease is not a preventive of Small Pox, but the Small Pox itself. In order to complete the demonstration, it is necessary to show that the ***human Small Pox*** can be communicated to the cow in like manner as the disease of the latter has been communicated to man. There are good grounds for believing that many of the variolous pestilences that have at different times laid waste the various regions of the earth have been common both to man and the brutes. It would be improper in a report of this kind to enter into historical details illustrative of this point; but they are to be found in abundance in the writings both of the physicians and the chroniclers of the earlier and middle ages. We shall, therefore, at once proceed to mention other events that tend to confirm the opinion respecting the identity of the ***human Small Pox*** and the ***Cow Small Pox***. The first we shall notice occurred many years ago in America, and is recorded by Dr. Waterhouse, of Cambridge, Massachusetts, in a letter to Dr. Jenner. His words are, "At one of our periodical inoculations, which occur in New England once in eight or nine years, several people drove their cows to an hospital near a populous village, in order that their families might have the daily benefit of their milk. These cows were milked by persons in all stages of Small Pox; the consequence was, the cows had an eruptive disorder on their teats and udders, so like the Small Pox pustule, that every one in the hospital, as well as the physician who told me, declared the cows had the Small Pox."

No inoculations were performed with the virus from these cows, but it is impossible, we conceive, to doubt the fact that

* See the *Calcutta Quarterly Medical Journal*.

on this occasion the Small Pox had been conveyed from man to the cow, just as it has been communicated, in the dairies of Gloucestershire, from the cow to man.

Many unsuccessful efforts were made by different individuals in England to put the question beyond all dispute, by directly inoculating the cow with human Small Pox. This experiment is said to have succeeded at the Veterinary College, in Berlin, so early as 1801; and M. Viborg declares that he communicated the disease likewise to dogs, apes, and swine. It is mentioned in the *Saltzburgh Medico-Chirurgical Journal*, for 1807, that Gassner was equally successful in imparting the Small Pox to the cow by inoculation. Similar information is detailed in a paper read before the College of Physicians, by Dr. McMichael, in 1828. "Vaccine matter having failed in Egypt, medical gentlemen were led to institute certain experiments, by which it has been discovered that by inoculating a cow with Small Pox from the human body, fine active vaccine virus is produced." It is added that several children had been vaccinated with this virus with complete success. Professor Sonderland, of Bremen, took another method to inoculate the cows. He covered them with sheets on which persons labouring under Small Pox had lain, and in this manner, it is said, conveyed the infection.

It has been customary to treat all these examples as unworthy of consideration. This scepticism might have been justifiable at one period, but to persist in it after the direct corroboration about to be offered, would be to act in the spirit of Pyrrhonism, rather than in that of philosophic caution and candour.

What many gentlemen in this country failed to accomplish, we are happy to say has been at length achieved by one of the members of our Association, Mr. Ceely, of Aylesbury. Influenced by some of the facts and reasonings mentioned above, he resolved to attempt to ascertain whether he could, by inoculation, impregnate the cow with human Small Pox. Twice he has succeeded in accomplishing this important object after many previous fruitless trials. His experiments were conducted in the presence of five medical men and one veterinary surgeon. He produced five vesicles on the cows, from which source several hundred patients have been vaccinated, who have exhibited all the phenomena of vaccination in the most perfect form and complete degree; there was no attendant eruption, nor any thing that could lead him to suspect that he had not in this manner propagated the genuine *Variolæ Vaccinæ*. He kindly transmitted

FURTHER OBSERVATIONS ON THE VARIOLÆ VACCINÆ.

CEELY.

[*Reprinted from the "Transactions of the Provincial Medical and Surgical Association." Vol. X.*]

1842.

FURTHER OBSERVATIONS ON THE VARIOLÆ VACCINÆ.

BY ROBERT CEELY, ESQ.,

Surgeon to the Buckinghamshire Infirmary.

THE imperfect knowledge which we at present possess on many points connected with the natural history of the *variolæ vaccinæ*, and the numerous and formidable impediments to the improvement and extension of that knowledge, demand the continuance of vigilant, patient, and diligent inquiry. The inherent and contingent difficulties which attend many of our investigations into the remote, predisposing, and exciting causes of this interesting disease, though in many respects not under control, in some measure admit of very material mitigation. The infrequency of the disease must always prove one of the greatest obstacles to the rapid accumulation of facts of a really valuable character; but there is good reason to believe that an increase of the number of competent observers, will abate much of this difficulty, by leading to more frequent detection. An increase of the number of competent observers, however, without the diffusion of a greater amount of discriminating knowledge among the proprietors and attendants of the subjects of the disease, will be but an imperfect approximation to the amount of means indispensable to the success of our inquiries. The careful record of every fact bearing immediately or remotely on the points above mentioned, irrespective of any theory—the improvement and perfection of the means of diagnosis, by the study of the exanthemata of the lower animals, particularly those of the cow—and the diffusion of such knowledge, in the proper quarters, by those whose time, situation, and circumstances will admit, seem to me to be essential to the successful promotion of our object.

With a conviction of the value of these investigations to medical science—not I trust overrated, and under the influence of the encouragement offered by this Association, manifested by the distinguished, but I fear unmerited, reception which it has given to my former observations, I am induced to offer a few additional facts which I have lately had occasion to witness, and which, from their importance, have been investigated with all the care and impartiality of which I am capable. I am desirous also of adding some additional observations, illustrative of some particulars contained in my former communication, which required time to furnish.

For the opportunity of making the following observations, and investigating and recording the facts, I am indebted to the very great kindness and intelligence of my friend, Mr. Thomas Knight, surgeon, of Brill, who has on former occasions rendered me invaluable assistance in the prosecution of similar inquiries.

Cases of Variolæ Vaccinæ occurring in Cows and Milkers.—On Friday, October 22nd, 1840, my friend Mr. Knight informed me, by letter, that he had on that day seen on the hand of a patient (Mr. Pollard), aged fifty-six, who had never had Small Pox or vaccine, two broken vaccine vesicles, which the patient stated he had caught while milking his own cows, some of which he knew were affected by the same disease, and were then very difficult to milk. Mr. Pollard at the same time expressed his conviction "*that his cows had been infected from human Small Pox effluvia*, to which he considered they had been exposed."

On the following day I proceeded, in company with Mr. Knight, to the farm of Mr. Pollard, in the village of Oakley, about two miles from Brill, at the extreme and north-west end of the Vale of Aylesbury, and about sixteen miles from the town of Aylesbury. We saw the ruptured vaccine vesicles, with their central sloughs, on the hand and fingers, which were apparently between the second and third week of the disease, and carefully examined the cows. The cows were ten in number: eight milch cows and two sturks. On two of the milch cows there were the vestiges, on each, of not fewer than twenty-five to thirty vaccine vesicles on the teats, and the remains of one vesicle on each udder. On two others we noticed the remains of not more than half that number of vesicles on each; and on the fifth milch cow there was evidence of only one vesicle on the hinder part of the teat, which, being out of the way of the milker, was completely desiccated and entire, forming a characteristic blackish-brown oval crust. This crust on the teat, and two crusts on the udders of the other cows just mentioned, were the only perfect crusts observed. On the teats all the imperfect crusts had been casually and prematurely removed by the manipulations of the milkers, and, hence, were visible florid ulcerations, many of which were manifestly depressed in the centre, and *all* surrounded with the more or less circumscribed, indurated, and elevated integumental boundary which marks the vaccine disease. Upon the udder of one of the affected milch cows was observed an abundance of the sub-epidermic vesicles or bullæ, which not unfrequently arise during the acme and after the decline of the vaccine disease. Three of the milch cows, although carefully and repeatedly inspected at that time and at subsequent periods, indicated no external trace of the disease. One of the sturks, not then supposed to be in calf (but subsequently proved to have been so two months), appeared to have several dark brown partially adherent crusts on the teats; but was very wild and intractable, and could not be caught and carefully inspected at the time. The other sturk appeared, like the three milch cows just mentioned, to have entirely escaped the disease.

After the inspection of the cows we were fortunate enough to find another milker, Joseph Brooks, aged seventeen (who had had neither Small Pox nor the vaccine), with a very fine vaccine vesicle on the right temporo-frontal region, another over the last articulation of the thumb, and a third on the radial aspect of the ring finger, all just past their acme, as the diffused areolæ had evidently disappeared.* From the first vesicle we obtained lymph, and immediately used it.

In reference to the presumed origin of the disease on the cows, from Small Pox effluvia, as intimated by the proprietor, we obtained some remarkable facts; but previously to detailing the particulars of his statement, and that of the milkers, it is necessary to remark that both Mr. Knight and I were aware that the Small Pox had been casually introduced into the village in which this farm was situated, about the commencement of the preceding June; but this being met, on the part of Mr. Knight, by prompt vaccination, only twelve cases of Small Pox had occurred up to the time when the above cows exhibited their disease. Of this number of Small Pox cases the last three were, a woman, aged forty, who had been satisfactorily *inoculated* in infancy by the celebrated *Sutton*, a young child, and a woman rather beyond the middle period of life. The two cottages in which these three patients resided during their illness were situated on each side of, and closely connected with, a long narrow meadow or close, comprising scarcely two acres. The first-named patient, though thickly covered with pustules, was not confined to her bed after the full development of the eruption; but

* [Vol. I., Plates XI. and XII.—E.M.C.]

frequently crossed the meadow to visit the other patients—the woman and child, the former being in great danger with the confluent and malignant form of the disease. She died on Monday, the 7th of September, and, according to custom, was buried the same evening. The intercourse between the cottages, across the close, was of course continued after this event. On the following day the wearing apparel of the deceased, bed-clothes, bedding, etc., of both patients, were exposed for purification on the hedges bounding the close; the chaff of the child's bed was thrown into the ditch; and the flock of the deceased woman's bed was strewed about on the grass within the close, where it was exposed and turned every night, and for several hours during the day, till the 13th of September—eleven days. On that day the above-mentioned eight milch cows and two sturks were turned into this meadow to graze. They entered it every morning for this purpose, and were driven from it every afternoon to be transferred to a distant meadow to be watered and milked, where they remained through the night. Whenever the cows quitted the meadow in question, in the afternoon, the infected articles above-mentioned were again exposed on the hedges, and the flock of the bed spread out on the grass and repeatedly turned, where it remained till the morning, when the cows were readmitted. It appears however that the removal of the infected articles was not always accomplished so punctually as had been enjoined; for both the proprietor and the milkers affirm that on one occasion, at least, they observed the bed flock on the grass, and the cows amidst it and licking it up. The proprietor positively declares, and the milkers corroborate his statement, "that the animals were in perfect health on their first entering this close; but within twelve or fourteen days of that event five of the milch cows appeared to have heat and tenderness of the teats, upon which, embedded in the skin, were distinctly felt small hard pimples, which daily increased in magnitude and tenderness, and in a week or ten days rose into *blisters*, and quickly ran into brown and blackish scabs. At this period, when the teats were thus *blistered* and swollen and very tender, the constitutional symptoms were first observed, viz., sudden 'sinking,' or loss of milk, drivelling of saliva from the mouth, and frequent inflation and retraction of the cheeks, staring of the coat, 'tucking up of the limbs,' and 'sticking up' of the back, and rapid loss of flesh. The process of milking was now very difficult, disagreeable, and even dangerous; and on the 14th of October, the middle of the third week, the detachment of the crusts and loose cuticle, and the abundant discharge of pus on attempting to milk, compelled the milkers to desist for the purpose of washing their hands. Soon after this period the cows became by degrees more and more tranquil as the tenderness and tumefaction of the teats subsided, and, finally, milking was performed with comparative facility;" and at the period of our visit scarcely any trouble arose in the performance of the operation, though here and there a teat seemed still tender.

Cases of Casual Vaccine in the Milkers.—Case 1.—Mr. Pollard, æt. fifty-six, had never had vaccine. He had been, some years previously, exposed to Small Pox infection with impunity; while his companion, a young man, took the disease and died. Mr. Pollard had since that held himself exempt from risk of Small Pox.

The vaccine vesicles, when first seen by Mr. Knight, on the hand and finger, had burst, the secondary constitutional symptoms were declining, and the centres of the vesicles, as usual, were in a sloughing state. The patient says, that about ten days after the discovery of the disease on the cows, he observed two itching small pimples on the site of the present ulcers, which, according to his account, ran the normal course of the vaccine vesicle; that as soon as the areolæ commenced, having felt scarcely any indisposition before, pain and tenderness of the axillary glands, with the usual constitutional symptoms, arose, and gradually increased for four or five days, but were never severe enough to confine him to the house. They had entirely ceased on the day Mr. Knight and I saw him, and the topical inflammation was rapidly departing; the vesicles were quite broken up, and a blackish brown slough adhered to their centres, their base being surrounded with an elevated induration of a livid red colour.

Case 2.—Joseph Brooks, æt. seventeen, a fine, healthy, intelligent young man. Had not been the subject previously of variola or the vaccine. Stated that he commenced milking on Friday, the 9th of October, and that his milking was confined to four cows, only *one* of which had the disease—from four to six vesicles on each teat. He milked those four cows occasionally, and continued to do so till the 18th of the same month—ten days, having milked them in that period six times.* On this day (the 18th) he felt the cervical absorbent glands and lymphatics stiff and tender; and on the 20th found a pimple on the temporo-frontal region, which he could not resist scratching. On the day before that, he observed on his finger a red pimple, of the size of a pin's head; the next day one on the thumb, very small. In neither situation was he aware of

* The milker who attended in his absence having been vaccinated by Mr. Knight with variola vaccine lymph, (with which I had supplied him,) did not receive the disease from the cows.

the pre-existence of any visible wound or abrasion of the cuticle. On the 21st he had headache, general uneasiness and pains of the back and limbs, with tenderness and pain in the course of the corresponding lymphatic vessels and absorbent glands, particularly of the axilla, which increased till the 23rd, when nausea and vomiting took place. His right eyelids became swollen, and were closed on that day; but after this period he became better in all respects, never having been confined to the house, although disabled from work. The engravings* represent the vesicles as they appeared on the 23rd, when the constitutional and local symptoms were subsiding. The vesicle on the temporal region had a well marked central depression, with a slight crust, a general glistening appearance, and was of a bright rose or flesh colour, with a receding areola; and there was an inflamed, tumid, and completely closed state of the corresponding eyelids.

On the finger † the vesicle was small and flat, with a slightly depressed centre, containing a minute crust. It had a beautiful pearly hue, and was seated on a bright rose-coloured slightly elevated base. On the thumb the vesicle was also flat and broad, but visibly depressed towards the centre, where there appeared a transverse linear-shaped crust, corresponding, doubtless, with a fissure in the fold of the cuticle. The vesicle was of a dirty yellowish hue, and visibly raised on an inflamed circumscribed base. Lymph was obtained from the vesicle on the temple, in small quantity, by carefully removing the central crust, and patiently waiting its slow exudation. In this, as in most other respects, it strikingly resembled the vesicle on the cow, and appeared as solid and compact. The lymph was perfectly limpid, and *very* adhesive. No lymph was taken from the vesicles on the finger and thumb, with a view to avoid any interruption of their natural course.

On the 26th and 27th, when the redness and elevation of the base of the vesicles had materially diminished, the vesicles themselves had become greatly enlarged. On the thumb and finger they were loosely spread out at the circumference, each having a dark and deep central slough. On the temple the margin of the vesicle (as on the cow) was firm and fleshy, its diameter being nearly ten lines, and its centre filled with a dark brown firmly adherent slough. In about seven or eight days, with the aid of poultices, the sloughs separated and the deep ulcers healed, leaving cicatrices like variola, deep, puckered, and uneven, which were seen on the 25th of

* See Plates XI. and XII. † See Plate XII.

November. The scar on the temple was nearly as large on the 5th of December as the vesicle represented in the engraving.

Vaccination with the Lymph taken from Joseph Brooks.—It was directly transferred to three of his younger brothers, a lad older than himself, and two infants. The primary symptoms in his brothers and the young man, aged nineteen, were manifest on the seventh day, but were mild. After the appearance of the areolæ, the secondary symptoms were promptly excited, and gradually increased till their decline. There was nothing remarkable in the character of the vesicles till the full development of the areolæ, when they became remarkably broad and flat, spreading outwards, turgid with lymph, bursting their walls, and, like those from which they were derived, followed by sloughs and deep slowly healing ulcerations. In the infants, fine and healthy, with thick compact skins, the usual fretfulness and feverishness appeared on the evening of the sixth or seventh day, remitting in the morning and increasing in the evening, in proportion as the areolæ advanced, and declining with them. As usual, nothing remarkable before the eighth day in the appearance of the vesicles; in one the vesicles burst and sloughed; in the other they remained entire, were fine and satisfactory, leaving characteristic crusts, and moderately deep finely reticulated cicatrices.

In the subsequent transfers of the lymph the effects varied according to circumstances. In infants with tense thick skins, the vesicles, though active, were perfectly free from inconvenience, yielding fine "tamarind stone" crusts and regular scars. On children and adults, where the skin was thin, vascular, or irritable, upon the full expansion of the areolæ, the vesicles spread out broad and flat, and, yielding to the distending influence of their *diluted* contents, burst and terminated in sloughs, more or less deep, followed by a corresponding extent of ulceration; but where the skin was pale and thick, and especially if the patients were also pale and dark in complexion—the conditions in every respect most suitable for the use of *new* lymph—then the vesicles were more compact, restricted, bold, and better defined, with proportionately less areola, and often not distinguishable at any period of their course from those induced by ordinary lymph. Here the crusts were of the ordinary size and form, and the cicatrices of the common depth and extent.

The constitutional symptoms varied not less. In many *infants* the *primary* were scarcely noticed; the *secondary*, proportioned to the texture and vascularity of the parts, the local inflammation, and the temperament of the individual. In *children*, as usual, both were more [illegible] noticed: the *primary*, on the sixth or seventh day [illegible] at an early period, were marked with [illegible] fever, and occasional delirium. In [illegible] the same early [illegible] of constitutional symptoms, though not always, were [illegible]; and during the *secondary*, as usual, [illegible] was made, some few keeping their beds a day or [illegible] and secondary constitutional symptoms were [illegible] in many individuals of the three classes [illegible].

At the expiration of [illegible] patients were tested with variola, by [illegible] than a trifling fugitive inflammation at the [illegible] vesicle resembling the modified vaccine [illegible] containing a *limpid* [illegible] lymph, [illegible] and terminating on the eighth or ninth day [illegible] brown crust, and unattended throughout [illegible] any constitutional symptoms.

Remarks.—The cases of [illegible] above detailed are interesting in many respects, and we were particularly happy in having to collect the [illegible] with them from persons possessing more than the usual share of intelligence and acuteness of observation. The [illegible] animals, though occasionally practising as the [illegible] had not the remotest idea of the medical [illegible] the nature of the disease, and consequently had no [illegible] in favour of the opinion he spontaneously suggested on first exhibiting his hand to Mr. Knight. He assigns as reasons for this opinion, first, the fact of the state of [illegible] the cows entered the close; secondly, the existence of variolous effluvia within its precincts; thirdly, the [illegible] from the exposure of the cows to such influence and the appearance of the vaccine disease on them; and, fourthly, the simultaneous or nearly simultaneous attack of all the [illegible].* I need scarcely say that we spared no pains [illegible] as to the validity of the statements in support of this [illegible] and the accuracy of the facts upon which they were based. Hence the information [illegible] detailed was not deemed [illegible] till after thorough investigation and minute inquiry, [illegible] visits to [illegible] and the sources of it.

[illegible] could be no doubt of the existence of variolous effluvia [illegible] and precincts of the close [illegible] to the

---

* [illegible]

propagation of the disease among human beings, had they been exposed; but whether sufficient to excite the vaccine in cows I really cannot pretend to say, having failed myself in attempts to infect *two* or *three* such animals *at a time*, with means not less potent, and under a closer atmosphere. The period at which the disease was stated to have been developed on the six animals was certainly remarkable, and called for careful scrutiny. The result of close and repeated inspections of *all* the cows, both at our first visit and several subsequent visits, was a conviction of the correctness of the alleged simultaneous occurrence of the disease on all the subjects at the time specified, a circumstance which increases the probability of the operation of *one* common cause. And here it is necessary to observe that, although the vaccine disease is sometimes epizoötic, and attacks one or two cows, *at different farms*, about the same time, I never remembered to have seen so many cows simultaneously attacked in one farm as in this instance. Most frequently we find the disease break out on a single cow, and spread slowly, by direct contact of the hands of the milkers, through a dairy. It is also important to add that the vaccine was not then epizoötic in the Vale or neighbourhood, and of this fact I had the best possible assurance. The *aphtha epizoötica*, as the disease is called, was then prevailing, and my knowledge of the state of the dairies in general, both from daily inquiries and frequent personal inspection, for the purpose of observing the phenomena of that disease, was more perfect than it had been for at least twenty years; in fact, I had altogether despaired of seeing the vaccine disease for some length of time, in consequence of the existence of the epizoötic.

Another circumstance too requires to be particularly noticed in estimating the value of the opinions put forward by Mr. Pollard, and which might be adduced in support of his reasons of belief. It is the fact of the occurrence of the vaccine disease on a young sturk, which of course could not have been induced by those casualties which commonly propagate it amongst milch cows, but simply by the cause which originated the disease in the other five animals, whatever that may have been. The sturk is not considered liable to the vaccine, at least so it is inferred in this neighbourhood, because no one has ever seen the animal affected by it. I have shown, however, that by inoculation the disease may be communicated to the sturk, and I have also adduced several reasons for its not having been otherwise detected on that animal.* In Germany, however, I believe it has been, on two

* Page 372.

or three occasions, seen on the sturk without probable contact. From personal observation I know also that both the sturk and heifer are liable to a vesicular disease of the teats and udder, which is very common on milch cows in this neighbourhood. I have called it the *verrucous* or *wart* vesicle, and shall describe it at a future period. I will merely mention now that, although occasionally these vesicles are as large as vaccine vesicles, most commonly they are far below the average size of them. They commence on the teats or udder as small red vesicles, sometimes scarcely perceptible on a coloured skin, raising the cuticle, with an amber or saffron coloured lymph, which concretes into a solid mass, into the base of which vessels shoot, by which it becomes organized, and continues to augment and grow, as a prolongation of the cutis, in the form of a wart; these warts vary in shape, according to the shape and size of the vesicle from which they spring. Now and then both small and larger verrucous vesicles are covered with a thin flimsy crust, of a light yellowish or saffron colour, never like the solid blackish brown crust furnished by the vaccine vesicle. Hence, although I could not obtain at the time so close an inspection of the teats of the sturk in question as I wished, I could not hesitate to pronounce the crusts vaccine, from the size, shape, and colour. About a month after the occurrences above described, this sturk having been accidentally found in the cow-house, and seeming quiet, was carefully examined by the proprietor's intelligent nephew, who found the teats covered with numerous scars as large as horse-beans, and bearing, as he said, an exact resemblance to those on the other cows. I had an opportunity myself, nine months afterwards, of inspecting these scars, and comparing them with those on the other animals; I could see no difference.

Whatever may have been the source of the vaccine in these animals, the phenomena attending it, so correctly described by the proprietor and the milkers, and the facts observed by us, are very instructive, and need a few remarks. The ages of the cows affected were *two* four-years, and *three* seven-years. Of the three milch cows which remained free from the disease, *two* were three-years, and *one* probably four-years old. That they really did escape was obvious enough, as far as careful inspections, from time to time, of the teats and udders could enable us to declare; and the total absence of any symptoms of indisposition removed all doubt of the fact. Now these three milch cows were shown to have been equally exposed to the same primary cause as the others, and, as we ascertained, were exposed also to the chance of casual inoculation in the process of milking; yet they escaped. These and similar facts, which have often fallen under my notice, induce me to believe that there exist among cows, as well as among men, different degrees of susceptibility to the vaccine. I never recollect to have seen a dairy visited by the disease in which two or three cows, equally exposed to casual infection, have not escaped. Moreover we know, by direct experiment, that some cows may be *vaccinated* or *retro-vaccinated* with facility; others with the greatest difficulty; some not at all. The phenomena of the disease were well described by the milkers. The primary or incursive symptoms were so slight as scarcely to attract notice, as is most commonly the case; though in two instances—one some years since, the other more recently—there was considerable precursory indisposition. The heat and tenderness of the teats, with the presence of *small hard pimples, deep in the skin,* which gradually increased daily, with their inevitable and obvious concomitants, *for more than a week* before "blistering" or *acumination,* were not less indicative of the vaccine than the correctness of the observers. At this period—the acme—they notice the constitutional symptoms, developed in all their intensity, and describe them with more than ordinary accuracy and precision; they certainly were more clearly marked than usual. Many contingencies, however, affect the development of the incursive and secondary symptoms; the chief are the season of the year and the actual condition of the animal, and the quantity and quality of food. The retraction and expansion of the cheeks is not always noticed by the careless unobserving milker; nor is the drivelling from the mouth. This last sign was so well marked that the proprietor feared the animals were about to be attacked by the aphtha epizoötica (which was then prevailing in the adjoining farms), where it is one of the first signs noticed, though not actually the first in existence, and depends on positive inflammation and vesication of different parts of the mucous membrane of the mouth. In the vaccine disease, however, this is not the case, at least here, where the disease is generally mild; for no vesicles are observed in the mouth, nor difficulty of mastication. The drivelling appears to be the effect of topical irritation in the seat of the disease—the teats and udder; for it is very well known that such a symptom does attend similar degrees of irritation from other causes and in other parts. The secondary constitutional symptoms were noticed in all the patients, including the sturk, and were proportioned in each to the amount of topical irritation. It was remarked, however, that the appetite seemed very little impaired, notwithstanding the wretched appearance of the animals, during the presence of the constitutional symptoms, and the sudden and notable loss of milk. To form some idea of the quantity of milk lost, we ascertained, from the dairy records, that in the first week of indisposition, six pounds of butter were deficient; in the second week, two pounds; in the third week, none. These may be deemed trivial and unimportant particulars, but their utility will be presently shown.

It is hardly necessary to observe that a correct knowledge of the vaccine disease on the cow in its *early* stages is of much importance in many points of view, and that too much pains cannot be bestowed on the minutiæ of the local phenomena by those who are desirous of acquiring the means of a safe and accurate *diagnosis*, if it be important to avoid the inconveniences of propagating from spurious vesicles, or to prevent disappointment when non-contagious lymph is erroneously employed. But to those who think themselves better engaged in investigating the nature and causes of the disease than in hunting after new lymph, a careful study of the latter or ulcerative stage will not be less interesting and productive, and more so than many would probably suspect, though at times it must be admitted the difficulties attending this part of the diagnosis are scarcely to be surmounted with safety and satisfaction. In this place I can only point out the general characteristics of the ulcerative stage, in so far as it is necessary and practicable for comparison at a future period with the ulcerative stage of some other vesicular diseases. It must be obvious that in proportion to our ability to form a judgment for ourselves, *by these means*, concerning the nature and stage of the disease whose history we may be desirous to investigate, and of which we may be able to acquire very interesting facts, in that proportion is our history perfect, and our information valuable. From the nature of things we are indeed compelled to depend too much and too often on the imperfect observations of ill-informed persons, and therefore we should cultivate every opportunity of rendering ourselves less dependent on such sources. The general points of recognition of the vaccine disease in its other stages, as already indicated, being borne in mind, we shall often be able to remark some of their vestiges in the stage of ulceration; but the extent to which we shall be able to do so, in individual cases, depends upon many contingencies. As there is nothing discriminative in the site, figure, or size of the vaccine vesicle, it will follow that when all vestiges of cuticle and crust are removed, in the stage of ulceration, we can then derive no aid in our diagnosis from the mere consideration of these circumstances. It is true that the distinct or solitary vaccine vesicle never attains the extreme magnitude, nor assumes the irregular shape, not unfrequently acquired and exhibited by some other vesicles in the same parts, but, on the average, falls far below in size, and is most commonly more perfect in form than such vesicles; yet, in many instances, the former are equal in size to some of the latter, and whenever vaccine vesicles are coalescent and ultimately interfluent, or have been closely and thickly grouped with intervening erysipelatous vesications, the resulting ulcerations are of considerable magnitude, and most commonly irregular, and consequently cannot by such characters be distinguished. Our main reliance in forming a diagnosis in the ulcerative stage of the vaccine disease must then be on the phenomena and effects connected with the seat and elementary character of the eruption.

Vaccine ulcers are generally distinguishable by a rounded elevation, more or less manifest, of their outer margins, and a circumscribed induration, of greater or less extent, of their base, with a proportionate depression in their centres of deeper ulceration, sometimes caused by a slough. But these characters are obviously influenced by several circumstances which must be taken into account when attempting our diagnosis; the principal are—stage of the disease, texture of the tissues, site of the ulcers. It is necessary to know that in the early ulcerative stage of the severer forms of some other vesicles nearly as much induration, &c., is occasionally found, especially if the texture of the tissues is lax, and much mechanical irritation has been inflicted. If we can be positively assured that the above-mentioned diagnostic conditions have existed in any given ulcer for three or four weeks, or even longer, especially if it be removed from *severe* casualties, we may fairly presume that it is vaccine; and this presumption will be strengthened, if, under the circumstances, the ulcer be small, for such sized and circumstanced ulcers of most other vesicles, being for the most part superficial and sub-epidemic, speedily heal. But as the texture of the parts in which vaccine vesicles appear varies so much, and as their seat is not uniform in depth, and as elevation of the margin and induration of the base and depression of the centres of the consecutive ulcers are sometimes merely questions of degree, (since time or stage is not always determinable,) it is clear that uncertainty in judging of an individual ulcer must now and then happen. Out of this difficulty we often escape by finding a group of characteristic ulcers on the same animal, or a series of animals, clearly infected one from another. And when we have an opportunity of inspecting ten or twelve, to say nothing of thirty or forty, subjects we seldom fail to detect on some of them the elements of a safe and correct diagnosis, as late as the fifth or sixth week. Such condition of parts very rarely occurs in connection with ulcers resulting from other contagious vesicles, except on peculiar subjects, where the subcutaneous cellular tissue has suppurated and sloughed, and the cicatrizing ulcer has a puckered surface and indurated margin. Most commonly this result is confined to the first subject attacked, which continues also to furnish a succession of milder vesicles for four or five weeks. It must be borne in mind however that the vaccine ulcer also is found co-existent with small superficial vesicles or bullæ, both on the teats and the upper, back, and hairy parts of the udder, as in one of the above subjects at Oakley; of the same nature and possessed of the same harmless contents as the vesicles and bullæ which appear (at the acme, or on and after the decline of the vaccine,) on the face, trunk, and limbs of children in high health, and in a few adults with irritable skins.*

These remarks, arising out of the above circumstances, which to my mind are not altogether destitute of interest and importance, will not, I trust, be considered ill-timed or misplaced; and I will merely add that on our visiting and inspecting these cows on the 25th of November following, more than two months after the outbreak of the disease, we found on some of them a few superficial irregular sores, but all character was gone. The scars were pale and smooth.

I must not however, in spite of the length of the above remarks, omit to give a brief statement of what had befallen the above animals between this and our last visit, because the particulars involve pathological facts of considerable value, and, as far as I know, are of some novelty. We were informed that on the 14th

* A few months ago I had vaccinated a remarkably fine, florid, plump, vivacious infant, aged eight months, with an active lymph, about eighty removes from the cow. At the acme of the areolæ of the two vesicles nearly the whole surface of the skin of the face, trunk, and limbs, was suddenly covered with large and elevated erythematous patches and spots, which speedily became surmounted with vesicles and *pemphigoid* bullæ of various forms and sizes, exciting considerable and intolerable irritation; but this was not all, for nearly the whole of the mucous membrane of the lips, cheeks, mouth, and fauces, as far as the eye could reach, was affected in like manner; the whole exhibited a most deplorable sight, and was certainly not without danger. Five or six weeks elapsed before these vesicles and bullæ ceased to appear, and the child was restored to comparative health and comfort.

of November all the animals, including the sturks, were attacked with the *epizoötic aphtha*, which had long prevailed in the Vale, and for some weeks also in the village. The difference in the nature and phenomena of the two diseases was well marked, and the comparative severity of their constitutional effects not less striking. It would be out of place here to enter into a detailed description of the epizoötic aphtha; but as there are circumstances attending the development of this disease which contribute to the elucidation of some of the obscurities of the incursive phenomena of the vaccine, I shall in a very few words state the chief symptoms of the former for the purpose of comparison and explanation. This epizoötic seems to be a specific febrile eruptive disease, with catarrhal and rheumatic characters, comprising a cold, a hot, and a critical or eruptive stage. Its invasion is generally sudden. The cold stage is very short—a few hours—*often unobserved;* the stage of febrile reaction is quickly followed by patches of inflammation on the mucous membrane of the lips, gums, cheeks, tongue, and fauces, and about the nostrils and mouth, with congestion of the conjunctiva. These red patches, which are often overlooked or rarely observed, quickly run into irregular vesications or bullæ, containing a limpid pale amber-coloured fluid, and are attended with profuse salivation, difficult and even temporary inability to masticate, with proportionate constitutional disturbance. Similar vesications are often seen on the teats, especially on the involutions of the skin at their apices, also on their bodies.* Still more frequently they are seen on the skin where it joins the claws, as well as on the interdigital membrane, whence they often extend under the horn, creating much mischief and causing excruciating pain by its detachment, etc.; but all these parts are seldom equally affected in the same subject. The constitutional symptoms continue for four or five days, when the topical irritation abates, and mastication is restored. It attacks all ages, and is often suddenly fatal to the very young.† In the milch cow there is a notable diminution of milk, arising, in

* Inflammation and suppuration of the mucous lining of the milk ducts and reservoirs is not unfrequent, and too often subsequent *mammitis* and all its consequences.

† In these cases of sudden fatality, and in some others of longer duration, the *post mortem* appearances were chiefly excessive pulmonary and cardiac congestion. In an *ox* which survived the acute stage, but wasted with *hæmaturia*, and was ultimately killed, the whole of the subcutaneous cellular tissue was occupied by patches of *purpura hæmorrhagica*. The sub-serous tissues of the lungs and costal pleuræ, and the sub-serous and sub-mucous tissues of the fourth stomach, small intestines, and bladder, were in the same state; liver softened.

the first instance, from fever; secondly, inability to masticate—for the appetite soon returns or is not long absent; and, third, topical irritation. Now in the milch cows at Oakley there was this manifest difference in the severity of the constitutional impression produced by this disease—the aphtha epizoötica—indicated by the greatly diminished secretion of milk; the quantity of butter lost in the first week was thirteen pounds; in the second week seven pounds. The suddenness of the invasion of the disease, as well as its severity, were demonstrated by the fact that on the morning of the 14th, the day of attack, the usual quantity of milk, "*two bucket-fulls*," was obtained; but, in the evening of the same day, "*scarcely a quart.*" At this time the salivation, erection of the hair, "tucking up of the limbs," &c., were obvious enough, though in the morning—an interval of eight or nine hours—no symptoms of illness were observable. The loss of flesh also was greater, and the animals were longer out of condition; but the season of the year was not without its influence in this respect, as well as in the restoration of the secretion of milk, which was then hopeless.

In Respect to the Casual Vaccine in the Milkers.—It is difficult at all times, for obvious reasons, to determine the precise period of incubation of the disease; and we know also, by direct experiment,* that the stage of papulation is often later in *primary* than in subsequent vaccinations. Judging however by the period of cessation of the *secondary* symptoms, and the decline of the areola on the 23rd, it seems not improbable that, in the case of Brooks, the *primary* symptoms, which were first felt on the 18th, were manifested on the sixth or seventh day of infection. The same may probably be said in the case of Mr. Pollard. Be that as it may, however, it is quite clear that in both cases we have again additional evidence of the correctness of Jenner† concerning the mildness of the symptoms, under such circumstances, compared with the secondary or topical symptoms. The vesicle on the temporo-frontal region in Brooks was produced, in all probability, by the casual application of the infected hand during or immediately after milking, or the resting of that part on the side of the cow which he might occasionally have touched in his endeavours to save his milk pail from the restive movements of the animal. He thought he had scratched a pimple on this part; but it appears the pimple in question was really the vaccine pimple. It

* Page 400.
† *Further Inquiry*, p. 171.

seems to have run a parallel course with the vesicles on the thumb and finger. It certainly is not necessary that there should have been a visible breach of surface, from what we know in these two cases, and not unfrequently observe among milkers, who not only become infected themselves from the cows, without any known wound, but convey the infection to their wives and families, on whom the results appear on parts where there is no probability of such breach of skin.* The bursting and sloughing of the vesicles on the hand and fingers of the milkers is partly the result of the acrimony of the lymph, partly a consequence of the organization of the tissues affected. I have never yet seen a crust on the hands or fingers of such persons, but always the condition of parts here described. The slough from the vesicle on the temple was the largest I ever saw; but even here the *secondary* symptoms, it will be observed, were by no means severe.

In the subsequent removes of the lymph we again observe the same mildness of the primary symptoms, and the same average uniformity in the period of their approach, the variable intensity of the secondary symptoms, and the extent to which the special organization of the individual tissues influenced the development of the vesicles, and how much age and temperament, in conjunction with these accidents, determine the amount of the attendant constitutional disturbance. We see also that in some cases it was very difficult to distinguish the local and general effects of the lymph from those of the *variola vaccine* lymph, which was obtained by experiment in February, 1839, and which had been in constant use from that period.

Cases of Variolæ Vaccinæ occurring in Cows and Milkers at the Village of Dorton.—On Wednesday, the 2nd of June, 1841, my kind friend, Mr. Knight, brought with him to Aylesbury, for my inspection, a young man with two fine casual vaccine vesicles on the left hand, which he had caught from milking some cows at his master's dairy, in the village of Dorton. When Mr. Knight first saw the boy's hand, the day before, he remarked the areola was commencing; and then ascertained that other milkers had been affected, and that the disease had been prevailing in the dairy for some weeks. At the time the hand was presented for my observation, it exhibited a fine specimen of casual vaccine just

* Not long since I saw a wife and five children labouring under a *pustular* disease of six weeks' standing, and infected by the father, who had caught the disease from the cow, which was in a terrible condition. It was of the character of ecthyma, but communicable, affecting the face, trunk, and limbs, and could be propagated by inoculation.

before the acme, the areola not having arrived at its full expansion. The boy was then under the influence of the secondary symptoms, and being unable to work, I prevailed on him to remain at Aylesbury that drawings might be taken of the vesicles in all their subsequent phases, and the phenomena, both local and constitutional, more carefully noticed, as I had done in the former case of Joseph Brooks; but I must defer the description of the present case of Joseph White till I have detailed the particulars of our visits on the same day and at subsequent periods to the dairy alluded to.

On our arrival at Dorton, about twelve miles to the westward of Aylesbury, at the dairy of Mr. Tompkins, we found cows in all stages of the vaccine disease, and abundant evidence of its existence there for at least three months. It was a large dairy farm, though at the time there were not more than forty-eight cows in milk; and there were three sheds for milking at different parts of the farm. The disease had visited, in succession, all the sheds, and we found that only three milch cows had escaped the contagion, to which all had been equally exposed. It had evidently existed in very different degrees of severity, in different subjects, from first to last; for we found many of the cows which had been attacked at an early period, with much severity, perfectly well, with depressed and puckered scars; and many others, affected at a much later period, with smooth uniform scars; and there were some still troublesome to milk, for the most obvious reasons, that had been ill four and five weeks. A careful inspection of all the animals enabled us to furnish the following particulars as to the state of the dairy, and enabled us, at the same time, to form an opinion concerning the probable duration of the disease therein. We noticed :—

1. *Cicatrices, perfect:* a few irregular, puckered, and uneven, but in general regular and well-defined; oval or circular, of various sizes, some scarcely perceptible, others as large as a chestnut; their outer margins slightly elevated, and gently rounded off, and their bases a little indurated. On a coloured skin the *whole* of these parts were obviously without pigment.

2. *Cicatrices, imperfect:* some irregular and puckered, but most with small, florid, granulating, depressed centres; *imperfect,* with small, bloody, black, thin, flat crusts in their centres; *imperfect,* with small, brown or blackish brown, thin, secondary or tertiary crusts in their centres. In most of these cases the elevation of the rounded margin and induration of the base were generally more marked, especially when large and irregular.

3. *Ulcers, granulating,* of all sizes; others *partially covered* with thin irregular incrustations of a bloody black colour; all having pale, more or less rounded, margins, and hard bases.

4. *Crusts:* large, flat, dark brown, *secondary,* many covering coalescent ulcers; large, flat, dark brown, *primary,* covering interfluent vesicles, with corresponding appearances of the margins and bases; long, oval, thin crusts, not distinguishable from crusts of spurious vesicles, but by the often repeated condition of the margin and base to which they adhered.

5. *Vesicles, passive,* but not desiccated; *passive,* and in progress of desiccation; *passive,* and recently desiccated. Some in all these states on the same animals. *Sizes,* smaller than half a vetch, or larger than an orange pea.

The parts chiefly affected were the *bases* and *bodies* of the teats; around the former, on many cows, the vesicles had been very numerous; on the latter, in many instances, they had been thickly grouped, often confluent. In two cows vesicles were found on the *apex* of the teat; in one of them the inflammation and swelling of the vesicle had obstructed the termination of the milk tube, and caused much pain and difficulty in milking. In several cases there had been large vesicles on the *udder,* near the bases of the teats, many of which, at the time of inspection, were covered with light or dark brown crusts, eight or nine lines in length; some others with thin and secondary and blacker crusts, with characteristic margins. In one of the cows, which had been severely affected for not less than six weeks, as was manifest by the swollen and tender teats, full of imperfect and puckered cicatrices, with very hard and elevated margins, surrounding deep irregular, and waving fissures, we observed a sub-epidermic, half desiccated, half broken vesicle, as large as an almond, containing some light amber-coloured fluid, which was without any elevation or induration of the base, or the slightest degree of tenderness. It had arrived at that stage, in three or four days, from a reddish slightly raised spot or pimple, as had several similar vesicles before it, and as did another about a week afterwards, while the heat and tenderness of the teats continued. After these had subsided no more of these vesicles or bullæ appeared, as far as I could learn. On the farm we observed sturks and dry cows free from the disease, although they had continued to graze and herd with the milk stock during the whole period of its duration. The drivelling from the mouth, the inflation and retraction of the cheeks, "dry rumination," staring of the coat, sticking up of the back, &c., had been noticed in several of the subjects, particularly those which had been severely affected. But no loss of appetite amongst any of them had been observed by the milkers; nor had the proprietor detected any material diminution of the quantity of milk. In this respect, and in the comparatively trifling and temporary influence on the general health and condition of the cows, they afforded an agreeable contrast, in the recollection of the proprietor, with the injury he and most of these cows had sustained by the *epizoötic aphtha*, with which they had been affected many months before—about the autumn of the previous year. Here, as in many other dairies, examples of two at least of the evil *sequelæ* of this disease had occurred—protracted lameness and loss of condition from sinuses of the hoofs; and secondly, inflammation and consequent partial or complete loss of the functions of the udder.*

In prosecuting our inquiries relative to the period when the disease was first observed, and as to the subjects on which it probably first arose, we were not so happy as at Oakley. There had been changes and interchanges of milkers; there were three places of milking; there had been changes and interchanges of the animals to and from the three sheds, all creating difficulties which the accustomed carelessness of observation of ordinary milkers did not enable us satisfactorily to surmount. Although the milkers and proprietor all agreed that the disease first appeared in the "home shed," and was by degrees propagated and conveyed to the cows in the other two sheds, yet some of them frankly admitted that the disease had been in this shed some time before they suspected it, a circumstance which we have before stated as of frequent occurrence. Others thought that they first observed the disease in February on three cows which grazed together in a separate close, but were milked in the "home" shed.

Now it was curious enough that Mr. Knight had been in attendance on a young man who, arrived from London, had fallen ill with modified Small Pox. The patient was sent on the 26th of December previous from his home, situated on this farm, to the parish pest-house, where he remained a month. We could not ascertain, however, whether during that period he had left the

* In several instances of this disease, though the *milk* was greatly diminished in quantity, the *cream* was considered to be relatively more abundant, and the *quality superior*. In other instances, however, both pus and blood were blended with the milk, probably from inflammation and suppuration of the mucous membrane of the ducts and reservoirs. The former were often obstructed (needing constant attention and relief) by incrustation of their extremities, and pus and blood were often the precursors and accompaniments of the milk.

house for air or exercise; it was believed that he had not. After this period, and when convalescent, he certainly did go among the cows, and was seen in February at the "home" milking shed. Beyond this, we could obtain no other information that could be relied upon; and the time that had elapsed, added to the circumstances and difficulties above enumerated, made further satisfactory investigation utterly hopeless.

Cases of Casual Vaccine in the Milkers at Dorton.—We found two milkers had received the infection in a mild and modified form, both having been formerly vaccinated.

A man, aged forty, who had been vaccinated twenty years previously, on the present occasion was infected through a puncture which he had accidentally inflicted some time before with a pointed steel instrument. Some swelling and glandular enlargement, with early constitutional symptoms, attended the development of the modified vesicle; but there was no remaining vestige of the latter on our visit. Another man, aged thirty-two, who had been vaccinated thirteen or fourteen years before, had on this occasion some modified vesicles, which gave him very little local or general inconvenience; they also had disappeared before our arrival.

Case of Joseph White, æt. eighteen; fair complexion, thin skin. Had never before had variola or vaccine. He had not been long engaged in milking at Dorton before he received the infection; he first noticed the pimples on the thumb and dorsum of the left hand on the 25th of May. On the 30th, the sixth day of papulation,* he first felt the mild constitutional symptoms and the axillary swelling and tenderness. The next day these symptoms increased; but on the following day, the eighth of papulation, they abated; yet, as his hand was more painful, and he found himself incapable of work, he called on Mr. Knight for advice. Lymph was then abstracted and used by that gentleman; the areolæ were just commencing. On the 2nd of June, the ninth day of papulation, he came to Aylesbury, when the following appearances were observed. On the side of the thumb, between the root of the nail and above the last articulation, was a flat vesicle, raised on a hard, red, tumid base. The vesicle was of a dirty white hue, with a slight central *discolouration* rather than *depression*, and a pale red areola extended around the vesicle and beyond the last joint of the thumb. On the back of the hand there was a smaller vesicle, of a different colour and

* From our inability to determine the precise period of infection, we are obliged to reckon from the earliest period of recognized papulation.

character; it was visibly raised, overlapping at the outer margin, and depressed in the centre, on a less circumscribed but obvious base. The vesicle was of a light flesh colour; its central crust dark brown; and a moderate light rose-coloured areola and some tumefaction surrounded and raised the whole. A small red imperfectly vesiculated pimple was seen on the left cheek—noticed by the patient now for the first time. The axillary glands and absorbent vessels were very tender; and though early in the morning the patient felt generally better, in the evening there was increase of all the symptoms.

June 3rd, tenth day of papulation.—To-day worse in all respects; both vesicles considerably enlarged, and the areolæ much increased.* There was considerable tumefaction of the thumb and the back of the hand; and the absorbent vessels, highly inflamed, could be traced by the eye into the axilla.

June 4th, eleventh day of papulation.—The vesicles enlarging; areolæ rapidly subsiding; constitutional symptoms less in the morning, but in the evening augmented; the areolæ then quite gone, but much puffiness of integuments remaining; and some red absorbents still visible on the arm. The vesicle on the face now contains a light amber crust.

June 5th, twelfth day of papulation.—Better in all respects; less tumefaction of the hand, &c.; vesicles expanding. That on the thumb was of a dull dirty white horn colour, and it had still a dull red areola around the raised and tumid base; the centre of the vesicle, scarcely depressed, was of a dirty yellowish brown colour. On the hand the vesicle was of a dull pearly hue, though rather more glistening than before; it was much puckered at the centre and the margin: the centre was deeply depressed, and contained a small dirty yellowish brown crust. The areola was dull, but brighter than that on the thumb.

June 8th, fifteenth day of papulation.—The vesicle on the thumb† was still characteristic, though it had acquired a vesicated margin. The vesicle on the hand ‡ was also characteristic, though puffed exceedingly at its circumference. The vesicle on the face was now capped with a hard light brown crust.

June 12th, nineteenth day of papulation.—The stage of ulceration was fully developed,§ and the extent of topical disorganisation was now sufficiently manifest.

In about a fortnight the ulcers were perfectly healed, leaving

* *Vide* Plate XIII.
† *Vide* Plate XIV., figure 2.
‡ *Vide* figure 1.
§ *Vide* Plate XIV., figures 3 and 4.

scars like those succeeding variolæ or any other disease attended with entire destruction of the corium.

Vaccination with the Lymph taken from Joseph White.—Lymph was taken from the vesicle on the thumb on the afternoon of June 3rd, the tenth day of papulation, and at the time the areolæ were declining. The *centre* of the vesicle was opened by displacing a dirty fragment of concrete lymph, when there issued forth a turbid serous fluid. After wiping this away, by repeated dossils of lint, the lancet was directed to the deep centre of the vesicle, where some *tenacious limpid* lymph was found; but it was impossible to extract this unmingled with some of the turbid opaque fluid. Lymph was taken the next day, when the areolæ were nearly gone; it was then chiefly turbid, though the centre of the same vesicle still contained a more adhesive lymph than the circumference, which was avoided as much as possible. After this period no further attempts were made to procure lymph, with a view to avoid damaging the vesicle; though efficient lymph might have been subsequently obtained with the exercise of proper care directed to the central seat and source of it.

The lymph taken on the 3rd was employed on three children, aged respectively three, four, and five years, florid, plump, and in good health; and on a young girl, Sarah Horwood, aged twelve, selected for the purpose, with dark hair and eyes, and pale thick skin, but perfectly healthy; she was vaccinated in four punctures.

On the eighth day her vesicles were without areolæ, were of a pale rose-colour, and yielded a *very* adhesive lymph, but in *exceedingly* small quantity. She denied having felt any indisposition.

On the ninth day very moderate pale rose-coloured areolæ; vesicles still but scantily supplied with lymph, yet that is very adhesive. Charged a few points and vaccinated her brother, æt. two years, and her elder sister, aged fourteen. She complains of tenderness, &c., in the axilla, and has some headache, but is up and engaged in straw plaiting.

Tenth Day.—States that yesterday afternoon she was obliged to go to bed, and was very bad with headache and general pain all night; but better in all respects to-day. There is nothing remarkable in the size or character of the vesicles; the areolæ have coalesced, very moderate in extent, and of a pale rose-colour. The vesicles are flat, pale rose-colour, and rather brown in the centres.

Twelfth Day.—The areola quite gone; very little induration at the base of the vesicles, which are now completely desiccated.

The crusts were very fine, *not large*, but very perfect, and separated on the twenty-first day, leaving a moderate reticulated pit.

The three children vaccinated on the same day as the above patient did not reappear till the fourteenth day, but their vesicles seem to have been moderately active; some were broken, but none were very inconvenient, and little complaint was indicated or made by either of them till the development of the areolæ.

In the cases of *William Horwood*, aged two years, florid, plump, and sanguine, with tense skin; and *Ann Horwood*, aged fourteen, very dark complexion, pale, white thick skin: in the first, on the *ninth day*, no visible indisposition; the four vesicles had a bluish hue: in the second no indisposition, five vesicles small, no areolæ. Took very adhesive lymph, which was scantily secreted, and vaccinated her mother.

Tenth Day.—W. H.: ash-coloured vesicles on a damask base, areolæ commencing, lymph very scantily furnished; no appearance of constitutional symptoms till the evening, then fever with diarrhœa. A. H.: vesicles pale flesh-colour, small; areolæ commencing; lymph very adhesive, perfectly limpid; topical but not general uneasiness.

Eleventh Day.—W. H.: very feverish; diarrhœa; refuses food; deep rose-coloured areolæ; vesicles silvery. A. H.: vesicles pale rose-colour; areolæ coalescent, bright rose-colour; headache and nausea.

Twelfth Day.—W. H.: vesicles bright and glistening, one blue, one partly abraded, not remarkable in size; fever, anorexia, and diarrhœa. A. H.: four vesicles burst, one has a bluish tint; areolæ declining; better to-day; engaged in straw plaiting.

Desiccation of the vesicles in the child was late—*sixteenth* and *seventeenth days*; but on the elder patient it commenced on the *thirteenth day*, and rapidly advanced. In the latter case the crusts fell on the *twenty-first* and *twenty-fourth days*, leaving shallow striated pits; in the former the irregular crusts fell later, and the scars were larger and deeper.

Horwood, Mrs., æt. thirty-five, fair, florid, thin skin. *Fifth day.* —Scarcely any signs of papulation; yet on the *seventh day*, the headache, pain of the back and limbs, commenced, with fever, and increased till the *ninth day*.

On the tenth day felt better; has five very fine rose-coloured vesicles, considerable areolæ, and much œdema of the arm, which increased till the *eleventh* and *twelfth days*, on both of which days the constitutional symptoms were much aggravated, and bitterly complained of; after this period merely local uneasiness.

Seventeenth Day.—Flat dark brown crusts, deeply imbedded in the hard and inflamed integuments; when the crusts separated they exposed the subcutaneous cellular tissue, the corium having sloughed.

Vaccination with the lymph taken from the milker on the 4th of June was performed on two boys, brothers, aged respectively eleven and six, both very fair, with light hair, blue eyes, *red tarsi*, and consequently thin irritable skins. *On each subject* two vesicles were raised with this "*Dorton*" *lymph*, two with the "*Oakley*" *lymph*, and two with the "*variola vaccine*" *lymph*. They all advanced in both subjects, *pari passu*, and could not be distinguished either before or after the *eighth day*. On the younger boy slight headache arose on the *seventh day*. Both complained of local and general symptoms when the areolæ were extending on the *ninth day*. There was nothing remarkable in the size of the vesicles on the *tenth day*, when the disease was at the acme, and the areolæ were extensively diffused. *Eleventh day*: areolæ below the elbows. *Twelfth day:* the elder boy had a very bad night, arm much swollen and inflamed; the younger had a good night, though his arm was as bad as his brother's. After this period the general symptoms abated; but all the turgid vesicles burst the thin cuticle, corium sloughed, ulcerated, and threw up loose spongy granulations not easily repressed.

From these was vaccinated a younger brother, of precisely similar temperament, complexion, and dermic organisation. In him the vesicles were equally indistinguishable at all periods; and as more care was taken to preserve their integrity, though not completely successful in the endeavour, less topical mischief was the result. Scarcely any constitutional symptoms appeared till the *tenth day;* from this period till the *thirteenth* they were severe, attended with anorexia, fever, and delirium.

Vaccinations were continued from these sources on a series of fine, healthy, plump infants, and fine active vesicles resulted, with corresponding manifestations of the constitutional symptoms, chiefly at the approach of the areolæ, though not unfrequently a day or two before, always increased at their full development. Then the subjects were favourable and the season was warm; but it was perfectly satisfactory to all who observed them that no visible difference could be detected between the vesicles or the effects produced by the "Dorton," the "Oakley," or the "variola vaccine" lymph, on the same or on similar subjects.

Remarks.—The occurrences at Dorton, above recited, will afford a fair specimen of the general difficulty which besets investigations connected with the origin of the vaccine disease in a large dairy. The disease, in existence some time before it is suspected by the proprietor or the milkers, has generally extended in all directions before the medical observer casually becomes acquainted with the fact, when he finds the incidents attending its outbreak so imperfectly remembered, carelessly noted, or altogether disregarded, that after all the pains he may bestow on a thorough investigation, he will too frequently conclude with dissatisfaction and regret as far as regards the chief points of his inquiry. Unsatisfactory however as many of these investigations often prove, they can seldom be altogether unprofitable. Many valuable facts are often obtained, to say nothing of the acquisition of greater precision in the diagnosis of the exanthemata of these animals, which is the only safe basis for future successful investigations. Those who cannot conform to the required "toil," may as well abandon the pursuit altogether; they will either be disappointed themselves, or mislead others. Disappointment of some kind, on most occasions of this nature, *all* must expect; errors to a certain extent, in many instance, *few* will escape. Hence the absolute necessity of vigilance, care, and caution, directed by judgment, derived from *personal* experience; and when it is recollected how few are the opportunities which occur to furnish the latter qualification, it must be obvious that we never can safely neglect to make ourselves intimately acquainted with every particular, however trivial and commonplace it may at first sight appear. The repetition of our visits is often indispensable, if only for the reinvestigation of our facts; and experience teaches us that it will seldom be unattended with advantage. We shall often discover new facts, and find it necessary to qualify and correct the old ones; and at least we shall, by this proceeding, always have the satisfaction of having done everything that was practicable.

Although our visits and investigations at Dorton were on some points unsatisfactory and inconclusive, yet on others they were highly valuable and very instructive. Here we had an opportunity of observing, on a large scale, the vaccine disease in its later stages, under almost every variety of condition and circumstance; and were thus enabled to correct, qualify, or confirm former observations, and to make juster comparisons with the corresponding phases, phenomena, and effects of the more common but not less contagious eruptions on the same parts; to collect, in fact, additional materials of diagnosis, or acquire increased confidence and precision in their application. The manner in which I have detailed the facts thus obtained, as well as the lengthened observations already made on the Oakley cases, will, I am sure, supersede the necessity of any further remarks in this place; and I shall now only observe that the *regular* vaccine cicatrix on the cow (though destitute of some of the characters by which it may *frequently* be recognized in man) does often furnish us, when *recent*, with some points by which it may be distinguished from the *regular* and *recent* cicatrices of other vesicles on the same parts. It will be manifest that most of the diagnostic points are involved in those appertaining to the ulcerative stage of the regular and perfect vaccine vesicle, and may, with their exceptions, be safely deduced from that source, due allowance being made for the obvious effects of the progressive changes which time produces and reveals. Hence many of the characteristic phenomena of regular vaccine ulcers may be found in the last stage—that of cicatrization—though of course in a very subdued degree. The *recent irregular* cicatrix presents the same comparative difficulties as the irregular ulcer, and, *mutatis mutandis*, must be judged by the same means.

The cow in which the *bullæ* appeared in succession, after the decline of the vaccine, had been very difficult to milk, the teats being studded with large deep ulcers, much swollen, and excessively tender, and but imperfectly healed at the expiration of the sixth week. It was therefore not surprising that when these organs, throughout their whole cutaneous surface, were so irritable and congested, such an eruption should appear, and attend the irritating but necessary tractions of the milker. He of course considers these vesicles or bullæ as a continuance of the original disease, though nothing is more manifest than their difference in nature, seat, and course; and that they partake of the character of those vesications which often arise on the same parts when in an inflamed and congested condition from various common causes.

The difference in intensity of the constitutional symptoms and effects of the vaccine disease observed in the dairy at Dorton, as compared with those noted at Oakley, was indicated chiefly in the absence of any signal *general* deterioration of condition of the animals, and in the inability of the proprietor to discover any material loss of milk. Both these apparent discrepancies may, in a great measure, be accounted for from the following considerations:—In the Oakley dairy there was a *simultaneous* attack of nearly the whole *small* milch stock, and the attack was at the period of decline of the milk season, when the cows were daily losing succulent food; hence the secretion of milk would be not only more easily influenced, but its loss more readily detected. In the

Dorton dairy, on the contrary, the mode of attack was quite the reverse—probably solitary, or nearly so; and the disease was propagated slowly by contact through a series of forty-eight cows, by the hands of the milkers, at a season too when the condition of the animals was gradually improving by a progressive increase of more succulent food. Here the probable diminution of milk in the early individual cases, often varying from other and obvious causes, could hardly attract much attention in estimating the average aggregate of so large a supply; and the less significant loss in the later cases, as the grass season advanced, would be compensated by an increase of secretion of those which had recovered. But allowance too must also be made for the difference in effect between the *primary* disease at Oakley and the *casual* at Dorton.

The outbreak of the *epizoötic aphtha* in both dairies was nearly contemporaneous: at Oakley only a few weeks after, at Dorton some months *before*, the vaccine. These are interesting pathological facts, and at once show the difference in *nature* of the two diseases. Other points of difference may probably be indicated at a future period. But we must not neglect this opportunity of deriving very useful instruction which may serve to guide us in our pathological investigations, particularly in regard to the exanthemata. In the great majority of instances of this epizoötic, though prevailing for many months, we find that proprietors, milkers, and attendants in general of cattle, failed to observe the preliminary stages of the disease—those preceding the critical or eruptive stage. Till the topical symptoms, the salivation, inability to feed, or lameness, were visible, no suspicion of disease existed in their minds. It was only by the intelligent veterinarian that the incursive febrile symptoms and the topical precursors of vesication were ever detected. It is true that the former are of short duration, and the latter are, for the same reason, difficult to detect; yet that both might be recognized by the intelligent and observant was abundantly evident, and is beyond dispute. Here we have another proof of the difficulty of confiding in the uninstructed and unobservant ordinary attendants of these animals, and a striking illustration also of the insidious approach and sudden aggravation of important disease in this class of animals, and of the truth and pathological value of the observations so frequently made, especially in reference to epizoötic and enzoötic maladies, by the most experienced British and continental writers on the subject. "*Enfin*," says M. Gellé in the conclusion of the able "*Considérations préliminaires*," prefixed to his valuable but unfinished work,* "*les maladies de ces animaux out presque toutes un caractère trompeur qui en impose facilement aux jeunes vétérinaires. Un calme trompeur, une espèce d'insensibilité, de stupeur même masquent les affections les plus graves, etc. etc. Les maladies charbonneuses et typhoides épizootiques et enzootiques, présentent souvent aussi des symptômes insidieux qui peuvent faire méconnaître leur véritable caractère, surtout* dans leur principe ; *aussi le vétérinaire a-t-il besoin de beaucoup d'expérience et d'habitude d'observer ces maladies, pour éviter des erreurs de diagnostic et de prognostic qui pourraient nuire à sa réputation.*"

The facts above mentioned, and the remarks here quoted, must teach us caution in denominating disorders of the bovine species "*topical*," in which the preliminary indications are seldom or never detected by incompetent observers, especially when we know that both in Europe and Asia the vaccine in a more acute form is attended by palpably incursive symptoms. Our inability to discover the subjects on which the disease first appeared in this dairy, as is the case in too many instances, compels us to be content with the simple statements already made, with these additional remarks : that, before the disease broke out, there was no evidence of ill-health in any of the animals ; that, from the absence of grass at that season, they were chiefly fed on dry food ; and that, as in the Oakley cases, no fresh purchases had been added to the stock, and consequently no infection could have been derived from that source. Subsequent inquiry has not enabled us to trace any direct communication between the Small Pox patient and the cows at a time when infection might have been presumed from such a source, upon some individuals at least, out of a large herd of forty-eight cows. The duration of the disease on the farm for more than three months is not difficult to account for, considering the number of cows affected and the circumstances in which they were placed. Of its occurrence, at the latest, in the month of February, not only the testimony of the milkers, but careful and repeated inspection of the cows, leave on the mind of Mr. Knight and myself not the shadow of a doubt.

I omitted to stated that at *Oakley*, Mr. Pollard believed the vaccine had occurred in the village twelve years before. At *Dorton*, Mr. Tompkins had not previously seen it on his farm ; but he had resided there only a few years. Mr. Knight informs me

* *Pathologie Bovine ou Traité complet des Maladies du Bœuf, par P. B. Gellé, &c. &c., tome* 1, *p.* 43;—*Dictionnaire de Médecine de Chirurgie et d'Hygiène Vétérinaires, par M. Hurtrel d'Arboval; Art. Enzootie et Epizootie;* —also *British Cattle*, &c., &c.

that during fourteen years' residence at Brill he has several times seen the disease on the hands of the milkers from the surrounding villages, which are all situated in the midst of a large tract of pasture land, devoted almost exclusively to the dairy. He assures me also that he has a perfect recollection that on some occasions the Small Pox and the vaccine have been co-existent, in others the latter has immediately succeeded the former. In this village of Dorton, for example, the Small Pox and Cow Pox were *co-existent*, and *endemic*, and *epizoötic*, in the latter part of the year 1831, at which period the Cow Pox was not known to prevail in the other villages. The Small Pox had been in the village for some time, and was supposed to have been introduced, by infected clothing, from a distance. About the latter end of December of that year, the weather being mild and moist, both diseases were in existence on this *identical farm* before Mr. Tompkins was the occupant.*

Both Dorton and Oakley partake of the general topographical characteristics of the Vale of Aylesbury,† at the western extremity of which they are situated, forming part of an extensive dairy district. The former is rather more than a mile to the southward of Brill, the latter about two miles to the south-west; both are placed at the base of the immense triple hill on which Brill is erected, and from which there is a grand, enchanting, and extensive prospect. The soil of both villages is heavy and tenacious, yet there are some particulars in which they differ. *At Oakley*, under a thin stratum of vegetable matter, lies a stiff clayey loam, about two or three feet deep. In some places gravel and loose rubble are also found. Immediately underneath lies the *impenetrable* dark blue clay. There are several chalybeate springs in the village; a very powerful spring mingles its waters with the drainage of the village at the south-west; but these springs are far inferior to those at Dorton. Besides other fossils, at a depth of one hundred feet, multitudes of pyritic ammonites have been brought up. *At Dorton*, although there is the same general character of the soil, based upon the unfathomable blue clay, there are several very interesting points of difference in certain localities. This village has within the last four years risen into considerable repute from the existence of a powerful chalybeate spring, which has been wasting

* On this occasion the Small Pox occurred in a cottage on the farm. In the family affected, one of the members, a milker, had just recovered from the casual vaccine; he slept with those members of the family who had the Small Pox, and was also inoculated with it, but with no other result than slight topical irritation and some fever for about a day's duration.

† Page 367.

its waters in the precincts of the village from time immemorial. It would seem to be unrivalled in England, and inferior only to that of Toplitz, in Germany. The following analysis by Professor Brande will not be uninteresting. In an imperial pint are contained—

Carbonic acid	a trace.
Nitrogen gas	
Sulphuric acid	
Silicia	
Sulphat of lime	11·5
Muriate of soda	1·4
Sulphat of alumine	2·1
Sulphat of iron	10·0
	25 grains.

It reddens vegetable blues from a slight excess of sulphuric acid, which amounts to about 0·8 per cent. The imperial pint yields an evaporation of twenty-five grains of dry saline matter. The specific gravity of the water at the temperature of 60° is 1004. The well is situated in the corner of a meadow adjoining the grounds of Dorton House, near the bottom of the hill, where a handsome and spacious pump-room is erected. To the distance of twelve acres around the well the following is the character of the superficial and deeper seated soil. Within a foot it is loam, thickly interspersed with shattered shells, inclined to moulder; still deeper by another foot, clay—short, unctuous, and friable—in layers, each layer having an intermediate body very like precipitated sulphur, or more properly "*lac sulphuris*," to which it answers in smell and colour; numberless crystals of gypsum; and thick patches of moist brown accumulations of iron pyrites. This extends to the depth of sixteen feet. The water given up by the spring is upwards of ninety gallons per day. Dorton lies about five miles and a half north-west of Thame; twelve miles north-east of Oxford; and fifty miles from London.

In Respect to the Effects of the Lymph obtained at Dorton.—The lymph taken from the milker on the 1st of June, just as the areolæ were commencing, Mr. Knight informed me, failed to produce any effect on some younger members of Joseph White's family and another eligible subject. With me the lymph taken on the 2nd and 3rd of June succeeded in every subject, not more than two *punctures* failing, which may be in a great measure attributed to the precautions taken in abstracting it,—precautions which are often necessary and successful in the employment of natural and casual vaccine in cows and milkers. By this method we may often succeed, in very distant removes, with *active* lymph, especially on subjects with substantial *moderately* vascular skins and *compact* cellular tissue, even as late as the twelfth day, or after the decline of the areola; and *always* when the lymph, in the deep centre of the vesicle, is *quite limpid* and *thoroughly adhesive*. But such proceedings under ordinary circumstances are not to be recommended, for disappointment is not always the only penalty. There can be no question that the lymph of some subjects is more active and efficient at the tenth, eleventh, and even the twelfth days, than that of some others at the eighth day, and that *perfect limpidity* and *viscidity* or *adhesiveness* are infallible indications of the fact; yet I should be the last to impugn the general truth of the remark that the earlier is the more active lymph, or that there is anything but prudence, propriety, and advantage, in the general rule of taking lymph on the eighth day, or before any material amount of areola is present.

From the lymph of the Dorton milker (as well as many others I might mention at the same stage) the resulting vesicles were perfectly normal, varying only as above described, according to the quality of the tissues in which they were generated, affording another proof—if indeed such were needed—that the activity or acrimony of such lymph is not manifest on all subjects, but that in *many* instances neither the local nor constitutional effects appear to differ from those induced by good lymph which has been some time in use; and, lastly, that we have no better standard of comparison of the local and constitutional symptoms of efficient vaccine than that originally furnished and so beautifully illustrated by Jenner—a standard to which we may at all times confidently appeal.

Within the last three years I have had occasion to observe and note the local and constitutional effects, on a variety of subjects, of more than *fifteen* different stocks of vaccine lymph, of which *six* have been direct from the cow or the milkers, and *seven* artificially produced on the cow. They have all varied in their effects, both locally and constitutionally, according to the circumstances so often alluded to; but none have lacked the essential qualities and properties, nor have any possessed them in a superior degree, to those indicated in that description and those illustrations which I have just mentioned. I have seen also as much local inconvenience, in some subjects, from the *oldest* as from the *newest* lymph.

Here I will beg to remark that the comparisons which I have thus been enabled to make with the *variola vaccine* lymph—some of which have been detailed and illustrated in my former communication, others in this—may be deemed by many, as they are by myself, to afford sufficient proofs of the identity of this lymph with genuine vaccine, particularly when so many practical observers, both in England and on the continent, have had opportunities of comparison, by employing it on many thousand subjects. But I think it right, for the satisfaction of others, to state that the variola vaccine lymph has been submitted to the test of variolous inoculation on twenty-two subjects, at various periods, after vaccination. In order that a fair parallel may be presented of the effects of this test, it will be convenient and necessary to adduce authentic descriptions of the results of variolous inoculation after vaccination at a corresponding period —within three years, as furnished by the records of the time when such test was deemed necessary, and was employed for the Jennerian lymph. Dr. Willan* has not only furnished us with many details of such cases, but has drawn up a concise summary of the results of variolous inoculation at different periods after vaccination. This I shall perhaps be allowed to quote, although his coloured illustrations will be found very interesting and necessary to be referred to. "The most frequent result," he observes, "of variolous inoculation after vaccination is a small pustule,† not attended with disorder of the constitution; but some of the following circumstances and appearances take place after it in particular constitutions:—1. A pustule resembling those exhibited,‡ but having in some cases a more diffuse inflammation or efflorescence around it. 2. Slight febrile symptoms, such as a pulse somewhat accelerated, a whitish fur on the tongue, languor and heaviness, but without any eruption. 3. A red efflorescence on the skin, which continues for a day or two. 4. Febrile symptoms for two days, attended with an eruption of some hard minute pustules, which usually disappear in three days. 5. Purpura or petechiæ sine febre on the seventh day after inoculation."

Dr. Willan adds "that similar symptoms take place after Small Pox in persons who have been inoculated with variolous matter, *especially in children* of an irritable constitution who have

* *On Vaccine Inoculation:* London, 1806, p. 69.
† Plate 1, No. 2, *ibid.*
‡ Plate 4, No. 5, *ibid.*

a *delicate skin.*"* Of such he quotes and details several instances, adding, "These, with other similar cases on record, should warn us against the indiscriminate use of variolous inoculation as a test of the correctness of vaccination, or for any other purpose."†

Dr. Jenner mentions similar facts ;‡ and in his very interesting paper,§ detailing two cases of Small Pox conveyed to the fœtus in utero, the parents at the time being free from variola (by which he endeavours to show that the *continued* susceptibility to variola remains in all through life, though in all it is not equally manifested) remarks, "My principal object in the foregoing observations is to guard those who may think fit to inoculate with variolous matter, after vaccination, from unnecessary alarms: a pustule may sometimes be thus excited, as on those who have previously undergone Small Pox; febrile action in the constitution may follow, and, as has been exemplified, a slight eruption." ‖

At a very early period after the production of the variola vaccine lymph, I had an opportunity of testing *both stocks* by variolous effluvia, having to vaccinate several children who were living and sleeping in the same rooms with patients labouring under variola, and in every instance the vaccinated escaped. Very soon after the introduction of the second stock of lymph into use at the Small Pox and Vaccination Hospital in London, Mr. Marson very kindly tested one patient, soon after vaccination, by variolous inoculation, without any local or constitutional result. Subsequently to that time I have tested twenty-one patients at different periods, the chief particulars of which will be found in the following table.

* Do we not over estimate the results of revaccination in many subjects, *particularly children*, who often appear *especially* susceptible of its influence?

† To this I may add that I have seen variola propagated by the short and trivial fever induced in a child by variolous testing. The child had no eruption; a small vesicle, like a modified vaccine vesicle, on the arm, with some areolæ on the eighth day, with a few hours' fever, and no subsequent inconvenience. The mother, who had been vaccinated twenty-three years before, was evidently thus infected, and had a mild varioloid attack. We see therefore that not only the *limpid* and *adhesive lymph* of these "*test*" *varioloid* vesicles will produce variola by inoculation; but that the *fever*, though slight and fugitive, which sometimes attends such "testing" is occasionally specific and infectious. But these warnings *now* are needless; the 3rd and 4th of Victoria, c. 29, will doubtless altogether supersede them.

‡ *Further Observations on the Variolæ Vaccinæ*, 1799;—also *Continuations of Facts and Observations on the Variolæ Vaccinæ*, 1800.

§ *Medico-Chirurgical Transactions*, vol. i., 1809, p. 269.

‖ See also *Medical and Physical Journal*, in 1803-4-5, &c.;—Dr. Labatt's *Address to the Medical Practitioners of Ireland on Vaccination*, &c. &c., p. 103.

Table showing the sex, age, period after vaccination with variola vaccine *lymph, number and kind of scars, and results of the test of variolous inoculation of twenty-one subjects.*

No.	Sex.	Age.	Period after vaccin.	Number and kind of scars.	Results.
		Years.	Months		
1	Girl	11½	5	8 very fine scars	Two papulæ from the 3rd to 5th day, then declining; 6th, gone.
2	Girl	8½	5	5 very fine scars	Three papulo-vesicular elevations on the 4th day; declining on the 5th day; desiccating on the 6th day; dark brown crusts on the 7th day.
3	Boy	8½	5	2 large, 2 small	Two papulo-vesicular elevations on the 5th day; declining on the 6th; desiccating with brown crusts on the 7th.
4	Girl	8	5	4 fine scars	Two papulo-vesicular elevations on the 5th day; enlarged, with slight areolæ, on the 6th; small silvery white vesicles, with bright red areolæ, containing a few drops of limpid adhesive lymph, on the 7th; bluish vesicles, with pulsating areolæ, on the 8th; declining on the 9th; desiccated on the 10th.
5	Boy	7½	5	4 fine scars	Two papulo-vesicular elevations, enlarging with tawny jagged areolæ, on the 6th; declining, with yellowish brown crusts, on the 7th; incrusting on the 8th; small brown crusts, like modified vaccine, *forcibly* removed on the 12th; numerous hard warty papulæ on the face, trunk, and limbs, on the 14th; several suppurated on the 16th day; all decadent on the 18th. Very slight fever for a few hours at commencement of eruption.
6	Boy	7½	5	3 small scars	Three papulo-vesicular elevations on the 7th day, with small areolæ; took a few drops of adhesive limpid lymph; declined on the 9th; yellowish crusts on the 10th.
7	Boy	1½	5	4 very fine scars	Two papulo-vesicular elevations on the 5th day; large glistening vesicles like vaccine on the 7th day, with small areolæ; pale flesh-coloured vesicles, with patches of brown crust on hard bases, on the 8th; very fine vesicles (like vaccine of the 14th day) this 9th day; "tamarind-stone" crusts on the 10th day.
8	Girl	4	12	4 small scars	Three papulo-vesicular elevations on the 5th day; increasing with areolæ on the 6th; declining on the 8th, with minute brown crusts.
9	Girl	7	13	4 good scars	Three papulo-vesicular elevations on the 5th day; with areolæ on the 6th; and limpid adhesive lymph on the 8th; declining on the 9th, with yellowish brown crusts.

No.	Sex.	Age.	Period after vaccin.	Number and kind of scars.	Results.
		Years.	Months		
10	Girl	6	13	4 good scars	Precisely the same.
11	Girl	4	13	4 very good scars	Nearly the same; but vesicles larger with more areolæ on the 8th day; with a few hours' fever and pain in the arm; all declining on the 9th day.
12	Boy	11	14	4 fine scars	Trivial fugitive inflammation for two days.
13	Girl	7	26	2 good scars	Two papulæ on the 4th; on the 6th gone.
14	Girl	2½	29	4 fine scars	Two papulo-vesicular elevations on the 6th day, with slight areolæ; declining on the 8th; desiccating with brown crusts on the 10th day.
15	Girl	5	29	2 small scars	Two papulo-vesicular elevations on the 6th day; with slight areolæ on the 7th; declining and desiccating on the 8th and 9th days.
16	Boy	4	29	1 small scar	Two papulo-vesicular elevations on the 5th day; slight areolæ on the 6th; declining on the 8th; encrusted on the 10th.
17	Girl	5	30	2 small scars 1 large scar	Two papulæ on the 6th day; vesicular on the 7th; ash-coloured vesicles on the 8th, on dark red base; decadent and encrusted on the 10th day.
18	Boy	5	30	1 fine scar	Two vesicular tubercles on the 5th day, with areolæ; encrusted on the 7th day.
19	Boy	2½	30	1 fine scar	Two fugitive inflamed spots; 6th day, gone.
20	Girl	17	30	5 good scars	Four small tubercular vesicles on the 5th day; decadent on the 6th day, no lymph; 9th day, brown crusts.
21	Boy	14	31	5 fine scars	Two vesicular tubercles on the 6th day, with areolæ; advancing, with pain in axilla and head, and slight fever, on the 8th day; rapidly decadent on the 9th day; with brown crusts on the 10th.

Observations.—The boy, 5, was the only patient on whom any eruption appeared. It was of the form described by Willan in the above summary (4),* for it partook of the double character: hard elevated papulæ; hard elevated papulo-vesicular eminences, some desiccating, some rapidly suppurating, all disappearing on the fourth day. The vesicles from inoculation having encrusted, like modified vaccine, the crusts were removed before the skin was sound; and two days afterwards he was shown to me in the state described. He had had no indisposition at any period of

* *On Vaccine Inoculation,* Plate 2, No. 6, and Plate 2, No. 2.

the testing process, but seemed rather hot just before the eruption; but was cheerful, and with reluctance kept within doors, taking his accustomed diet. The greater part of the eruption resembled the vesicular lichen occasionally seen after vaccination. This boy had four remarkably fine vaccine vesicles; but never showed during their rise, progress, or decline, the slightest constitutional disturbance, not even acceleration of the pulse. The child, 7, was brother to the above. The test vesicles were very fine, and could not be distinguished from large modified vaccine vesicles; he had no fever; his vaccine vesicles were remarkably fine, and the constitutional symptoms were well marked. Both patients had very clear florid skins. The children, 9, 10, 11, were of one family; all had clear florid skins, on which their vaccine vesicles had been beautifully developed. No. 11 had the finest vesicles, and suffered most from fever; she indicated also most influence from the variolation, but had no eruption; the others had no fever. The girl, 15, had but *one* good variola vaccine vesicle; she was vaccinated direct from the *first* variolated sturk,* and had scarcely any indisposition; but was tested with Bryce's test with a satisfactory result. The boy, 16, was vaccinated from the same *direct* source; he was attacked with gastro-intestinal fever soon after vaccination; his only vaccine vesicle rose very tardily and languidly, but ultimately acquired a large size.† The subjects, 18 and 19, soon after vaccination from the early removes of the second variolated sturk,‡ were attacked with fever of dentition, and one retarded small vesicle only rose on each. The boy, 21, had shown early and well marked symptoms from his vaccination—the second remove from the second variolated sturk. He complained of pain in the arm and axilla from the test vesicles, had distinct fever and slight loss of appetite from the seventh to the ninth day, but stated that his symptoms were *trifling* compared with those which he felt from the vaccination.

In none of the other cases was there the slightest constitutional disturbance, the patients running about and playing with their companions, eating and drinking, and enjoying themselves in all their accustomed ways, unconscious, like their friends, of the nature of the process to which they were subjected, and insensible of anything but topical trivial inconvenience. No suspicion could arise in the mind of any one; for it was impossible to distinguish the vesicles when they did appear from modified

* Page 423. † Page 436. ‡ Page 424.

vaccine of different degrees of perfection; the limpidity and adhesiveness of the few drops of contained lymph, and the small dark brown "tamarind-stone" crusts, when the vesicles were unbroken and unirritated, deceived several medical men to whom I exhibited the patients. Under the microscope the concrete lymph exhibited the beautiful reticulated appearance said to be characteristic of efficient vaccine.* But I have seen this and the *linear* appearance, mentioned by the same author, in the *concrete* lymph of the *verrucous vesicle* of the cow before alluded to.† The variolous matter employed was recent, taken on the sixth and seventh day, perfectly limpid, and some from the confluent and malignant variety; it was taken in tubes, or dried on *large* "store" points, repeatedly charged. In applying the test, clusters of superficial scratches were made on the skin, over an area as large as an orange-pea or a horse-bean, from two to four such patches on each patient; the variolous lymph was then discharged from the tubes, or rubbed off the points on the abraded surface.‡ In *every* instance *some effect* resulted, as above described.

I need scarcely say that I did not venture to use any of the limpid adhesive lymph from the *variolous test vesicles* on subjects which had not undergone vaccination; but I did, in three or four instances, employ it on the same arm with the other variolous matter. It was clearly possessed of inferior power; for while the latter was capable of exciting a papulo-vesicular result, the former or modified lymph scarcely excited on the same arm more than a slight fugitive inflammation, or a hard, red, lymphless tubercle. These experiments, though necessarily

* *Recherches microscopiques sur la composition du fluide vaccin, par M. Dubois (d'Amiens).—Bulletin de l'Académie Royale de Médecine, Avril* 30, 1838.

† See p. 480.

‡ This method is adopted by many in vaccinating. It is, as pointed out by Mr. Estlin, of Bristol, the only sure mode of successfully vaccinating with dry lymph which has been kept some time. He recommends broad and long points—(*Medical Gazette*, December 27th, 1839,)—to be *repeatedly* charged from good vaccine vesicles, *from time to time*, and carefully excluded from the air. When required for use, the lymph may be carefully rubbed off on such clusters of scratches by the aid of the serous or slight sanguineous exudation therefrom. By this means I have repeatedly revived the variola vaccine lymph after three, four, six, and nine months, in all its potency. "Store points," thus properly charged from *good and early lymph*, (not the draining of vesicles,) may form an efficient substitute for crusts, and are more convenient. Some of Mr. Badcock's *variola vaccine* lymph—(*Brighton Herald*, March 20th, 1841,)—with which he kindly favoured me, I thus revived, in admirable perfection, after four months. It was wrapped up in gold-beater's skin, and enclosed in tinfoil. I usually roll mine up in cotton wool, and enclose it in a small corked phial full of the same material.

limited by time and circumstances, it is presumed will suffice to prove the main point for which they were instituted, and thus furnish the only remaining evidence required to establish the identity of the *variola vaccine* artificially obtained and the vaccine naturally or casually yielded by the cow.

General and Concluding Observations.—In the foregoing cases, as well as in many others embodied in my former "Observations," it will be seen that endeavours have been made, not only to acquire information relative to the phenomena of the casual vaccine, but to accumulate facts illustrative of the pathology and ætiology of the disease in its primary form. That for this purpose, especially, the course of inquiry has necessarily been directed to the investigation of facts bearing on the age, state of health, condition, and circumstances of the animal or animals affected; the character of the incursive, eruptive, and secondary symptoms of the disease; the season of the year, and the state of the weather when it has been observed; the nature and character of the soil, and the condition of the pasturage where it has been found. Whether sporadic, epizoötic, or enzoötic; whether prevalent during epidemic or endemic variolous conditions of atmosphere; whether clearly or presumably traceable to the direct contagion or infection of human variola. But no one can be more sensible than myself of the small amount of positive information at present obtained from this locality on many important points of this enquiry, and of the utter inadequacy of these *contributions* to furnish more than a mere fragment in the history of the subject. But if they were far more extensive and complete than time and circumstances and the various' difficulties so often indicated and deplored have allowed, they would still be insufficient for such purpose; for it must be manifest that the history of this disease cannot be complete unless it embody the results of the most comprehensive investigations, made under far better auspices, in various localities, in other countries, and in different climates. Hence it is greatly to be desired that members of our profession, favourably situated, should earnestly direct their attention to the subject, and emulate the practice of many distinguished human and comparative pathologists on the continent, and some of our brethren in the East. Comparative pathology has engaged the attention of the most eminent human pathologists of ancient and modern times, with acknowledged benefit to humanity and unquestionable advantage to science; and it is truly gratifying to know that talents and attainments of the highest order are at this time directed to these pursuits, at once furnishing incontestable evidence of their interest and importance, and conveying the best assurance of eventual success. "*De même que l'anatomie et la physiologie comparées*," say the distinguished pathologists alluded to,* "*jettent une vive lumière sur l'anatomie et la physiologie humaines, de même l'étude des maladies chez les animaux servira à dissiper bien des doutes et des incertitudes qui regne encore dans la pathologie de l'homme.*"

If comparative anatomy be necessarily allied to that of man, if the relations of organisation that exist between all the mammalia establish between the larger animals and the human species evident analogies in all the physiological and pathological changes which take place, comparative pathology must offer results highly useful to the study of general medicine. The knowledge of the diseases of animals, when it becomes more advanced, will contribute to diffuse new light on the diseases of man, and perhaps bring to perfection methods of cure or prevention, owing to the facility of multiplying on the inferior animals experiments which we cannot attempt on man. These sentiments, expressed by one of the ablest and most accomplished of modern veterinary practitioners and writers,† are well worthy of our attention, and it is hoped that their correctness may be abundantly established by the zeal and ability of enlightened pathologists of the present era; and although the genius and patient research of a Jenner may be required for the complete realisation of all these hopes, yet in so ample a field there are few who may not be usefully and advantageously occupied. In the department of comparative pathology, comprehending the exanthemata, much remains to be accomplished, notwithstanding its diligent and successful cultivation in some parts of the continent since the time of Jenner. What has hitherto been effected there cannot suffice however to supersede, much less to paralyse, the efforts of his countrymen. But they must arouse themselves, and no longer exhibit a practical indifference to the researches to which he so successfully devoted the energies of his great mind. A comprehensive study of the exanthemata of the mammalia, especially of the bovine species, is not less essential to a correct diagnosis of the vaccine disease, than to the formation of a just estimate

* *De la Morve chez l'homme, chez les solipèdes et quelques autres mammifères, par MM. Breschet et Rayer.—Bulletin de l'Académie Royale de Médecine, le* 10 *Fevrier*, 1840.

† *Dictionnaire de Médecine, de Chirurgie, et d'Hygiène Vétérinaires, par M. Hurtrel d'Arboval. Tome deuxième; Art. Epizootie.*

of its nature and causes. It is greatly to be lamented that, in England at least, veterinary instruction is generally confined to so limited a range, and that, of course, so little is conveyed relative to *general* pathology, and particularly in those branches which relate to the history of epidemics and human exanthemata. On the other hand, it is not less to be regretted that a comprehensive knowledge of comparative pathology is not made an integral part of a sound medical education.

It has been well observed by the author above quoted, in an able and enlightened article on this subject:* "*Nous croyons qu'on ne s'est pas encore assez occupé de la vétérinaire sous le rapport de la médecine générale et comparée, et que lorsqu'on se sera livré à ce genre de recherches et d'études avec tout le soin, toute l'attention, et la persévérance nécessaires, on pourra découvrir des analogies qu'ont échappé jusqu'ici à toutes les investigations.*" Such interchange of knowledge would be reciprocally advantageous, and productive of incalculable advantages to the sister science. Many of the difficulties which at present attend the formation of a generally satisfactory theory of the vaccine influence appear to me to admit, and likely eventually to receive, a more complete solution from comparative pathology than some persons are disposed to expect or believe. It behoves us at all events to prosecute these and analogous enquiries to a successful issue, aided by an attentive consideration and careful study of the valuable information which modern veterinary medicine is now capable of affording. The rapid advances which this science has made of late years, the zeal, the learning, and the ability now devoted to its cultivation, are not only highly creditable, but must prove equally beneficial to science and humanity. Hence we are encouraged to believe that the hopes so fervently and so eloquently expressed by the late M. Hurtrel d'Arboval may at no distant period be amply realised:—"*Espérons que des hommes instruits, profitant de l'analogie qui existe entre les propriétés organiques et vitales de l'homme et des animaux, parviendront un jour à transporter dans la vétérinaire les faits et les documens qui servent de base à la médecine humaine, et que leurs efforts parviendront à reverser sur celle-la les trésors de celle-ci, en comblant quelques unes des lacunes qui restent encore dans notre art.*"

* *Dictionnaire de Médecine, de Chirurgie, et d'Hygiène Vétérinaires. Tome sixième; Art. Vétérinaire.*

A Detail of Experiments

CONFIRMING

THE POWER OF COW POX

TO

PROTECT THE CONSTITUTION

FROM

A SUBSEQUENT ATTACK

OF

SMALL POX,

By proving the identity of the two Diseases.

BY

JOHN BADCOCK,

CHEMIST,

BRIGHTON.

1845.

PROPER VACCINE VIRUS;

How to produce it upon the Cow, and the probable advantages of fresh supplies, &c.

FROM whatever cause it may arise, the fact has been of late years already ascertained, that the ordinary vaccine virus has lost a great deal of its protective power against Small Pox. A greater number of cases in which that disease has occurred after vaccination are met with than formerly, and in some instances these are very severe, and occasionally even terminate fatally.

Several reasons have been assigned for the failure of the vaccine virus, the principal of which are, the probability of its becoming modified by age, or influenced by passing through so many constitutions, during the lengthened period of half a century, or even deteriorated by want of the necessary care in the selection of the lymph for vaccination; this latter reason being supported by the fact that Dr. Jenner himself found that lymph taken from a genuine vesicle at too late a period, either failed entirely, or produced a spurious vesicle. It is not at all improbable that all these causes may have operated in lessening the value of vaccination, as a means of protection against Small Pox.

Dr. Gregory, Physician to the Small Pox Hospital in London, in a report which he made some time since, gives additional weight to one of these reasons, by the remark that vaccine lymph, passed through many persons, loses, in process of time, much of its activity. His statement has been confirmed by several eminent medical men on the Continent; and I believe there are but few practitioners who would, at the present day, venture to gainsay the statement.

Be the cause what it may, the fact is now beyond a doubt, that the vaccine lymph, *that most precious boon of Jenner to a suffering world*, has become greatly impaired in value, and is even still advancing in the process of deterioration. Medical men repeatedly find in practice that vaccination with the old stock of lymph requires to be repeated more than once, and occasionally as often as four times, ere a genuine vesicle is produced, and that even when they have used great care in the selection of the lymph they employ. In other cases again, besides the direct evidence of the failure or loss of protecting power in the lymph, afforded by a subsequent attack of Small Pox, it has been ascertained that the existence of a proper cicatrix, usually relied upon as the test of perfect vaccination, offers no proof of its permanent protection.

The fact that re-vaccinations, practised as they have been on a very extended scale in the Prussian army and elsewhere with success, and the formation of a genuine vesicle, despite the existence of a proper cicatrix, as shown, clearly demonstrate that, at all events in a large proportion of the population, the lapse of a certain number of years has been sufficient to exhaust the influence of the previous vaccination on the system, and to render it liable to the invasion of the disease, against which it was intended to guard.

To remedy, or rather prevent the increase and spread of, this formidable disease, re-vaccination has been practised very extensively on the Continent, and has been strongly recommended by many practitioners in this country, some of whom go so far as to state that the limit of protection afforded by the operation is seven years, and that at the end of that time it should be repeated. Without admitting this doctrine in its fullest extent, there cannot be a doubt that, unless some means be adopted to secure a more effective virus, re-vaccination at stated periods must be generally had recourse to.

A proposal has been made to meet the wants of the population occasioned by the failure of the old stock, that recourse be again made to the original source; but the formation of the genuine vesicle in the cow is of such rare occurrence, the animal is subject to so many spurious pustules, and, being generally in the hands of ignorant persons, the true disease, where it does occur, is so likely to be overlooked, or mistaken, or else the proper time for taking the lymph allowed to pass by, that the hope of thus procuring it is almost illusory. If it could be readily procured, so as to form a large and efficient supply, there is but little doubt that it would soon supersede the use of the old stock.

M. Bousquet has published the particulars of some comparative experiments which he instituted with vaccine virus obtained from a cow at Passy, near Paris, in 1836, and some of Dr. Jenner's which had then been in use about forty years. He showed, by beautifully engraved illustrations, the daily appearance of both vesicles, and clearly proved the greater activity of the new lymph. Dr. Trompeo, also, at a meeting of the Scientific Congress at Lucca, in 1844, remarked on this subject, "that it is of great importance to resort frequently to the primary source of the virus by re-taking it from the cow, in order to obtain durable results."

An important document, published by the Minister of Commerce, on vaccination, as performed in France in 1843, strongly confirms the views which have been just advanced. After furnishing us with calculations on the durability of the vaccine influence, it concludes by advising us how to obtain active virus. It appears that in that year, there were 547,646 vaccinated, and of those 11,773 were attacked with Small Pox. Of the latter 1,294 became disfigured or infirm, and 1,379 died in consequence of the disease. The report contains, as well, the following information: first, that vaccination loses its efficacy with time, but the Small Pox seldom attacks the vaccinated before ten, sometimes twenty or twenty-five years;—secondly, the cases of Small Pox are less severe in subjects who have been vaccinated than others;—thirdly, the only mode of renewing the vaccinating virus, is by application to the cow.

On the Continent it has been deemed expedient to try a fresh stock of vaccine, and I believe I am correct in stating that the Neapolitan Government has at this time agents seeking new supplies in Gloucestershire, where Dr. Jenner originally obtained it.

Why it is that in our own country similar propositions are unheeded, and fresh supplies of vaccine, however efficient, are refused, I am at a loss to conjecture.

The statements issued periodically by the officers of the National Vaccine Institution "of continued confidence in their vaccine," etc., may certainly lead many to suppose no change is necessary; but that supplied from this establishment has not for years past given perfect satisfaction; and, if we refer to the Government returns of death from Small Pox during the last year, we shall be led to the conclusion that our system of vaccination is at present very defective. The returns published from the registrars of the several districts for the year 1844 are not sufficiently clear for correct calculation, from omissions in some of them; but those of the Metropolitan District will answer my purpose.

In London, or the Metropolitan Districts, 1804 deaths from Small

Pox were registered in that year. Of this frightful mortality, I have not been able to ascertain how many of the victims had been previously vaccinated, but without doubt a considerable number of them, as I find of 151 fatal cases in the London Small Pox Hospital during the same year, 24 had been vaccinated; and of the 647 patients admitted with Small Pox, 312 had received the promised protection of vaccination, 7 of them at that Hospital. The returns from some of the country districts were not more satisfactory, for I observe at Blackburn in the last quarter of that year (viz., the thirteenth week ending in December), the number of deaths from Small Pox amounted to 118, of which 36 or nearly one-third, had been previously vaccinated. With these authenticated statements before our eyes, it is but natural we should lose confidence in the old vaccine; for if it has undergone no change with age, how can we account for the singular fact that, when Dr. Jenner petitioned Parliament for a reward, some years after his discovery had been tested, the subject underwent a most rigid and searching investigation before a Committee of the House of Commons, and no satisfactory evidence could be brought forward by his strongest opponents of one death from Small Pox after proper vaccination. It would be a serious reflection on the profession, if the numerous failures of the present day were to be attributed to their carelessness, for vaccination is now almost entirely performed by medical men, when formerly the operation was practised so successfully by many who had but very little pretensions to medical knowledge.

The facts thus brought forward are sufficient to show that the old stock of vaccine lymph has from some cause lost in a great measure its protecting power, and it becomes necessary to seek for some means to supply its place with a better virus. I have already observed that the disease shows itself naturally on the cow but rarely, and from various causes a considerable period of time might elapse ere a supply from that animal could be obtained. It becomes therefore necessary to endeavour to produce the disease in her, and in that I have succeeded by inoculating her with the matter of Small Pox. I should say that my attention was directed to this experiment from circumstances which I am about to mention.

Towards the end of the year 1836, I suffered severely from a dangerous attack of Small Pox, which happened but a few months after re-vaccination, and my mind having previously been impressed with an idea that the *old vaccine* had lost its protective influence by passing through so many constitutions, during the long period of forty years, I was exceedingly anxious to procure some fresh from the cow, for the purpose of having my own children re-vaccinated. On enquiry, I found that the true disease seldom prevails among cattle; and I also learned, from very excellent authority, that disastrous consequences have arisen from inexperienced persons communicating other pustular diseases of the animal in mistake. The only satisfactory mode of obtaining, with certainty, the *true* vaccine that presented itself to my mind was, therefore, to inoculate a healthy cow with Small Pox matter, as the result of that operation, if any, must be cow Small Pox. I must here mention that this method of obtaining vaccine is opposed to Dr. Jenner's theory; for he informs us that the origin of vaccine was a disease on the heel of the horse, called the *grease*, which was communicated to the cow by the milkers. But perhaps it will be best to quote his own words:—"The *grease*," says Dr. Jenner, in a work published in 1798, "is an inflammation and swelling in the heel, from which issues matter possessing properties of a very peculiar kind, which seems capable of generating a disease in the human body (after it had undergone the modification which I shall presently speak of), which bears so strong a resemblance to the Small Pox, that I think it highly probable it may be the source of that disease. In this dairy county (Gloucestershire, and the surrounding counties), a great number of cows are kept, and the office of milking is performed indiscriminately by men and maid servants. One of the former having been appointed to apply dressings to the heels of a horse affected with the *grease*, and not paying sufficient attention to cleanliness, incautiously bears his part in milking the cows with some particles of the infectious matter adhering to his fingers. When this is the case, it commonly happens that a disease is communicated to the cows, and from the cows to the dairy maids, which speads through the farm until most of the cattle and domestics feel its unpleasant consequences. This disease has obtained the name of Cow Pox. With respect to the opinion adduced, that the source of the infection is a peculiar morbid matter arising from the horse, although I have not been able to prove it from actual experiments conducted immediately under my own eye, yet the evidence I have adduced appears sufficient to establish it."

But this doctrine of Jenner's does not appear to be well supported. It is known that the lower animals have a variolous disease, resembling our Small Pox, and it is more than probable that the cows were labouring under that disorder or human Small

Pox. In searching for information on this subject, I found the following in an old work written by Dr. Fuller:—" Mr. Mather, in his letter from Boston, in New England, saith that Dr. Leigh, in his Natural History of Lancashire, reporteth that there were some cats known to catch the Small Pox, and pass regularly through the state of it; and at last he telleth us, we have had among us the very same occurrence. For, in like manner, there was, about the year 1710 or 1711, upon the South Downs in Sussex, a certain fever raging epidemically among the sheep, which the shepherds called the Small Pox; and truly in most things it nearly resembled it. It began with a burning heat, and unquenchable thirst; it broke out in fiery pustules all the body over. These maturated, and, if death happened not first, dried up into scabs about the *twelfth day*. It could not be cured, no, nor in the least mitigated, by phlebotomy, drinks, or any medicines or methods they could invent or hear of. It was exceedingly contagious and mortal, for, where it came, it swept away almost whole flocks; but yet it could be in no wise accounted the same as our human Small Pox, because it never infected mankind."

Having, as I have already stated, lost some of my confidence in the old vaccine, and being desirous of avoiding the risk of taking the casual disease from the animal, I solicited some of my medical friends to inoculate a cow of mine with Small Pox, but their want of leisure from professional duties disappointed me in that respect, and, after waiting nearly three years, I undertook the experiment myself.

In the month of December, 1840, I commenced operations on a fine young cow, with Small Pox matter taken from a strong healthy girl, and was singularly successful. My own little boy was the first vaccinated from the cow, and from this and subsequent operations I have carefully kept up the supply of vaccine. In these proceedings the utmost caution was observed for the public safety, as well as to make the experiment interesting to the profession. Three days after inoculation with Small Pox, the cow was inspected by medical men, the vesicle was watched in its progress, and the lymph taken in their presence. I also placed all my early cases of vaccination under the inspection of medical practitioners, and a great number of them visited my little boy during the progress of the disease. After my success in this experiment, the next was to inoculate a pony with Small Pox, but without any result. I was equally unsuccessful with three cows which I inoculated with grease (the reputed source of Dr.

Jenner's vaccine), for in all I failed to produce anything like a vaccine vesicle. It was not until some time after the commencement of my investigations, nor, in fact, before I had succeeded in my object, that I became acquainted with the experiments of Mr. Ceely, of Aylesbury, made a few months previous, and so beautifully illustrated in the eighth volume of the Transactions of the Provincial Medical and Surgical Association.

Dr. Jenner's writings clearly evince his belief in the identity of Cow Pox and Small Pox—that, in fact, they have one common origin; for he not only contends that the Cow Pox was derived from the grease of the horse, conveyed to the cows by the milkers, but he also thought it highly probable that that disease was the source of Small Pox in the human subject.

The following extract from a lecture by Mr. Erasmus Wilson confirms the opinion that Cow Pox and Small Pox are identical: "We may," says this clever surgeon, "regard *vaccine* in another and its true light—namely, as identical with variola, and consequently the operation as the same with inoculation with Small Pox; the only difference being the greater mildness of *vaccine*, resulting from its transmission through the cow. In this sense it is clear that variolation, after vaccination, is re-vaccination in all excepting in name."

In a work published by Mr. Pruen in 1807, entitled "A Comparative Sketch of the Effects of the Variolous and Vaccine Inoculation," the opinion of a Mr. Birch is quoted that "Cow Pox was nothing but Small Pox transmitted through the cow." All these authorities, therefore, favour my view of the question, and tend *a priori* to show that the lymph obtained from vesicles produced on the cow by inoculation with Small Pox matter, would cause on the human subject the usual effects of a perfect vaccination. This fact, as I have before stated, I have repeatedly demonstrated by direct experiment.

I have already remarked that my own little boy was the first human being whom I vaccinated with the lymph which I obtained from the cow. The operation was perfectly successful, and one of the medical gentlemen who had witnessed the development of the vesicle upon the cow, became desirous to vaccinate his child from mine.

Although I had the greatest confidence in the lymph thus produced, and infinitely preferred it to the old stock of doubtful origin, which appeared to be worn out; yet, as it was the first experiment of the kind I had ever heard of, I naturally watched its transmission with some anxiety.* My little boy's novel case excited considerable interest, for more than thirty medical gentlemen of Brighton and the neighbourhood, including six physicians, visited him during the first ten days.

Notwithstanding the unanimous opinions of all regarding my child's case, I thought it advisable to subject most of the patients of the first and second removes from the cow to the same scrutiny; the results were equally gratifying. Good vesicles were produced, and the children did not appear to suffer more constitutional disturbance than is usual from the ordinary vaccine. By the kind co-operation of the profession in furnishing me with frequent supplies of Small Pox lymph, I have been able, during the last four years, to repeat this experiment upon upwards of ninety cows; and from occasional successful cases, am obtaining fresh supplies of vaccine. The experience I have now had in several thousand cases of vaccination with this virus, and in numerous instances when exposed to Small Pox contagion (some of which, as they are remarkable cases, I shall refer to), would justify me in recommending it for general use. But as I have not the presumption to think the public mind would be satisfied upon such an important matter by my individual statements, I shall proceed to give such confirmation of them as appears necessary. Among those of the profession in this neighbourhood who have favoured me with their opinions, I must first mention the name of Sir Matthew Tierney, as many are aware he has taken great interest in vaccination ever since its first introduction.

Much of Sir Matthew Tierney's valuable time was devoted to the examination of patients in all stages of the disease at his own house; and in proof of his confidence in my vaccine, he not only recommended it to his own patients, but as Vice-President of the Brighton Dispensary, proposed its use to that Institution, as will be seen by a letter from the House-Surgeon, in an Appendix to these remarks. Others of the profession are no less entitled to my sincere thanks, as, by their valuable testimony, I have been able more satisfactorily to establish a fact in medical science which has hitherto been much disputed—namely, the identity of Small Pox and Cow Pox.

Mankind are indebted to the illustrious Jenner for a knowledge of the fact, that the human constitution is protected from an attack of Small Pox, by being impregnated with a vesicle of a given character, arising upon the udder of the cow, called Cow

* Mr. Ceely's similar experiment was at this time unknown to me.

Pox. The similarity in the protective powers of Small Pox and Cow Pox led to the conjecture that the two diseases are the same.

This identity, however, has hitherto been a mere matter of surmise; their points of difference being such as sufficiently to indicate their dissimilarity, and to stagger our belief in their essential unity. Thus, Small Pox is infectious, but Cow Pox is not so; Small Pox diffuses itself over the whole surface of the body, but Cow Pox does not do so. Cow Pox is characterised by a double areola surrounding the vesicle, which is not the case in Small Pox. Small Pox is attended with violent fever and severe pain in the head and back; Cow Pox is attended with a fever of a much milder character. The Cow Pox vesicle is depressed in the centre of a pearly appearance, and contains a transparent crystal fluid; the Small Pox pustule, on the other hand, soon suppurates, and becomes conical in its figure. The crust of the Cow Pox is of a dark brown colour, like a tamarind stone; but the crust of the Small Pox is of a lighter colour, like he honey-comb. It has been noticed, that when the variolous and vaccine fluids are mixed together, and thus inserted, sometimes the vaccine pustule, at others, the variolous, has been produced, each of them retaining its characteristic marks throughout.

Again, it has been found that when the two fluids are inserted separately and so near together that the two pustules which follow spread into one, by inoculating with the fluid taken from one side of it, the vaccine pustule alone will be produced, while the fluid taken from the other excites the genuine variolous pustule with the general eruption of the Small Pox on the body. Thus, while the similarity of the two diseases was indicated by their equally exerting a protective power over the constitution, their dissimilarity was sufficiently evident to require some further proof of their being the same. In proof of the protective power of vaccination over the constitution, we might refer to the instances of immunity which have occurred, and to the fact, that you cannot induce inoculated Small Pox in a vaccinated individual; but its mode of action is not explained, and, upon a partial failure of the process, individuals might be induced more readily to relinquish their confidence in the protection of vaccination, from its not being accounted for on rational principles.

Up to the period of the experiments performed by Mr. Ceely and myself, I believe, there is no authentic record of an individual, in this country, having succeeded in inoculating the cow with Small Pox matter; but I have already shown she may be so inoculated, and that a vesicle thus produced yields a fluid which, being transmitted to the human subject, produces all the appearances which Dr. Jenner has described as the true vaccine vesicle; thereby demonstrating the identity of the two diseases, and that, notwithstanding the several points of dissimilarity, they are, indeed, the same,—that Cow Pox is Small Pox which has passed through the constitution of the cow, having lost its *infectious qualities*, but retained its *protective power*. This demonstration of the identity of the two diseases establishes the protective power of vaccination upon a substantial basis, proving, that as one attack of Small Pox will prevent a subsequent attack, so will vaccination, for they are the same disease; and this identical nature of the two will afford a rational explanation of the protective virtues of the Cow Pox.

I shall now briefly notice some of the cases which have been under my care, and in the Appendix shall give a selection from numerous letters received from members of the medical profession, approving the lymph which I have thus ventured to bring under the notice of the profession and the public.

The first opportunity I had of testing the protective power of this vaccine was on the 11th of March, 1841. Four children, by the name of Callam, of the respective ages of two, six, nine, and eleven years, residing at 32, Kensington Gardens, Brighton, were brought to me to be vaccinated, in consequence of another child of the family, living in the same room, having the Small Pox. This was the *fourth day* of the eruption. One of my patients entirely escaped the infection; the vaccine vesicle progressed properly with the other three, but on the *tenth day* a slight eruption came out, without much fever, and began to desiccate on the *third day* satisfactorily, thus showing the effect of tne new vaccine in modifying the disease.

The next case was that of Charles Carter, seventeen months old, No. 6, Gloucester Terrace, vaccinated by me on the 18th of February. This child's brother, a few months after, died from Small Pox. The two children were constantly together, and slept in the same bed. My patient escaped the disease.

Mary Johnson, two and a-half years old, residing at 30, Gardiner Street, was vaccinated by me on the 21st of January, 1841. The child was exposed to the contagion of Small Pox, without being the least affected by it. It is worthy of remark—her sister, five years of age, who died from the Small Pox, had been vaccinated with the old stock of vaccine a few months previously.

Maria Busby, ten years of age, residing at No. 4, Cumberland Place, not having been vaccinated, applied to me for that purpose on the 20th of September, 1841, in consequence of two of her sisters being dangerously ill with Small Pox. She continued in the same house with them, and was entirely protected by vaccination.

John Dendy, aged twenty months, No. 1, Little Norfolk Street, was brought to me to be vaccinated, at the request of Mr. Dill, surgeon, on the 11th of January, 1844, another child of the family having a severe attack of Small Pox. This patient, as in the other instances, I observed sleeping in the same bed with the infected child, and yet did not show the least symptoms of the disease.

Four children, named Tugwell—Phillis, seven, Peter, four, Sarah, two years, and David, six weeks old,—residing at No. 4, Thomas Street, were vaccinated on the 18th of July, with the new virus.

I understood at the time, that their father was confined to his bed with Small Pox.

On the 26th (eight days after vaccination) the children were brought to me for examination. The father had died that morning. I found the first three going on very satisfactorily, but in the infant's case the vaccine had produced no visible effect. I then re-vaccinated him, from his brother's arm.

Three days afterwards I saw the children again. All, excepting the infant, were doing well. One small pustule was observable on Sarah's ankle, which had something of the appearance of a variolous pustule, but the child having no constitutional symptoms to confirm it. On the contrary, being in perfect health, I was not disposed to consider it as such. Circumstances compelling me to leave home, a week elapsed before I had an opportunity of seeing these children again, when my suspicion regarding the infant was confirmed. He had died from Small Pox. The others remained in perfect health.

The mother then informed me that another daughter (Rhoda), nine years of age, vaccinated in infancy with the old vaccine, took the Small Pox, but had it mildly.

Brighton Dispensary, 1844.

The cases of the above four children, named Tugwell, were under my observation, and I can answer for the accuracy of their relation.

(*Signed*) *S. R. SCOTT,*
House Surgeon.

Victoria Trott, aged twelve months (32, Upper Gardiner Street), was vaccinated by me on the 1st of August, with virus obtained from the cow in 1841.

The child's father informed me her twin sister was ill with Small Pox. I examined the child on the 4th, and eight days after vaccination she was rather feverish; but not more so than is usual. The vesicles were very perfect. On the tenth day the mother counted eight or nine pimples on different parts of the body, which remained for three or four days, then desiccated; but, to use her own expression, "the child was neither sick nor sorry." The sister died of Small Pox, three days after Victoria was vaccinated. It is singular this child should have escaped the contagion, for the mother, having lost one nipple, suckled both her infants from the same breast up to the hour of her sister's death.

Brighton Dispensary, Nov., 1844.

The above case of Victoria Trott, and also that of her twin sister, who died of Small Pox, came under my observation. The facts of those cases were exactly as related by Mr. Badcock.

(*Signed*) *S. R. SCOTT,*
House Surgeon.

Thos. Oliver, four years, and Henry Oliver, eight months old (24, Upper Gardiner Street), were vaccinated by me with the new virus. As in this instance another of the family had just been taken ill with Small Pox, I had an additional proof of the efficiency of my vaccine. The sick child died about a week after these children were vaccinated. They were constantly in the same room exposed to the infection, and one slept in the same bed with the Small Pox patient until the day of its death; but both escaped the disease.

Brighton Dispensary, Nov., 1844.

The above cases of Henry and Thomas Oliver were under my observation. I have much pleasure in attesting their accuracy.

(*Signed*) *S. R. SCOTT,*
House Surgeon.

Mary Ann Mitchell, at three years of age, was vaccinated by me on the 13th day of January, 1842, with vaccine of a former supply from the cow.

In September last, three of her sisters—Henrietta, twelve,

Susannah, ten, and Emily, eight years of age, were taken ill with Small Pox. Each had been vaccinated, in infancy, with vaccine from the old stock; but Mary Ann alone escaped the infection.

Brighton Dispensary, Nov., 1844.

It gives me much pleasure to be able to confirm Mr. Badcock's relation of the above cases of Mary Ann, Henrietta, Susannah, and Emily Mitchell.

(*Signed*) *S. R. SCOTT,*
House Surgeon.

——— Rusbridge, two years of age, No. 16, Francis Street, was vaccinated on the 13th of February, 1845.

The child's father, at this time, was dangerously ill with Small Pox; and about a week subsequently a younger child died of the disorder.

As the parents had no means of separating the children, my patient was constantly exposed to the infection; and when I visited the family, I observed her myself rocking the cradle of the dying infant in perfect security.

Dr. Kebbell attended the Small Pox patients.

Ruth Clout, four years of age, Mercy Clout, two years, and Sophia Clout, seven months, were vaccinated by me on the 7th of April, 1845, in consequence of a lodger's child having Small Pox. Vaccination was equally successful in all these cases, for neither of the children were in the least affected by Small Pox.

William Henry Gould, 33, Essex Street, aged ten months, was vaccinated the 30th of May, 1845. Four days subsequently to this his mother, who had been unwell several days, was found to have Small Pox. The child, up to this time, was nursed by the mother; but her situation rendered it necessary to take him from the breast. The vaccine went through its course satisfactorily, and the child was not the least affected by the mother's disease.

CORRESPONDENCE

FROM

MEMBERS OF THE MEDICAL PROFESSION,

RELATIVE TO

RECENT SUPPLIES

OF

VARIOLÆ VACCINÆ,

OR

MODIFIED SMALL POX.

London, George Street,
January 5th, 1841.

Dear Sir,—I beg to thank you for your communication respecting the experiment on vaccination. I think it would be well if you were to communicate the circumstance to the Vaccine Board here; and it might, I think, be well, if the medical men of Brighton are fully satisfied of the success of the experiment, to use the virus from the new source *alone* at Brighton: that is, adopt this new stock of virus *to the exclusion of all others at Brighton;* this would be a means in some degree of putting in view what you have obtained so satisfactorily to the test, as the *Brighton stock* might in future be referred to as evidence of the efficiency of a virus more recent and closer to the cow; of course you will take care to keep up your stock of virus by successive vaccinations. I shall be glad to hear your further observations on the experiment, and am,

Dear Sir, yours truly,
JAS. CLARK.

9, *Old Steine,*
January 7th, 1841.

Sir,—Having seen two children vaccinated by you with lymph recently obtained from the cow; having marked the results, and heard from you the particulars of the experiment, I have no hesitation in saying that I consider the experiment to be perfectly successful, and that as it is always desirable to fall back upon recent lymph, when it can be procured, I consider the obtaining of a large quantity of lymph, similar to that which you have just obtained, an object much to be desired both by the profession and the public; and shall therefore be happy to assist in any manner in my power towards the accomplishment of it.

I am, Sir, yours truly,
P. M. LYONS.

London, January 8th, 1841.

Dear Sir,—I enclose you a letter which I have just received from Mr. Estlin, of Bristol, who, as you no doubt know, has taken great interest in vaccination, and introduced a recent lymph. You no doubt also know Mr Ceely's experiments.

When the weather is milder I think you might send Mr. Estlin some of your stock of virus, in order that he might compare it with his own. You should pay great attention to the progress and appearance of the vesicle, and keep accurate notes on the subject. Do not trust to memory.

It is most desirable that the old and new virus should be closely watched in their *effects* locally, and their *influence* as a protection. The first may be soon observed, the latter will take time. You will very likely hear from Mr. Dodd, of Chichester, to whom I desired Mr. Estlin to send your letter. Be careful to keep up your stock.

Yours truly,
JAS. CLARK.

Brighton, 10, *Devonshire Place,*
January 9th, 1841.

Sir,—I was not until very lately aware that the profession were ignorant of the fact of vaccine virus being the Small Pox merely passed through the blood of the cow. It is now more than forty years since, I believe, I inoculated the first child in the county of Kent, with the vaccine lymph, and about that time I well remember old Dr. Dobell saying, that he believed it to be identical with Small Pox. He was a celebrated man for inoculation, and received patients into his house. He found his cows frequently attacked from the female patients occasionally milking the cows. I have no doubt the only safe virus is to be obtained in this way, and that when so obtained, and carefully used, is a certain preventative of the Small Pox. I believe the causes of failure so often heard of arise from using spurious or worn out matter, or perhaps, what is worse, matter that has not only become useless, but in some way amalgamated (if I may so use the expression) with other animal poison, and thus producing those horrid cases of cutaneous eruptions so often seen.

Your plan of providing lymph deserves the thanks and support of the whole profession. I for one shall be very ready to subscribe my mite in support of it.

I remain, Sir, yours very truly,
W. R. MOTT.

Old Steine, Brighton,
January 17th, 1841.

Sir,—I have pleasure in complying with your request, that I should certify to the facts which have resulted from the interesting experiment you have recently made by the inoculation of a cow with variolous matter, and I have to thank you for affording me the opportunity of observing the same. On the 21st of December last I saw, in company with Mr. Burrows and yourself, the cow in question, and noticed *one* well-developed vesicle, situated near the external labium, presenting the ordinary characteristics of a vaccine vesicle as it appears on the arm of a child on the eighth or ninth day of maturation, failing only in the circumjacent areola of inflammation.

I understood from you that this was the eighth day from inoculation, with matter taken from a Small Pox patient, attended by Mr. Burrows; that you had inserted the virus in two places, on the teats, and also on the spot which presented the only external result. The cow did not appear to suffer any constitutional disturbance.

On the 1st of January I saw your little boy, and also the child of another person, both of whom, I understood, had been vaccinated by you with lymph taken from the vesicle I noticed on the cow.

In your own child's case (this being the seventh day) the vesicle presented the usual progressive appearance, though in miniature. The other child's arm, which had been vaccinated two days later, did not look as though the virus had taken effect.

On the 5th of January I again saw the children, *i.e.* on the eleventh and ninth days respectively, when the appearances in both cases were, to my mind, thoroughly satisfactory; the vesicle on your own child's arm having obtained a full size, and with the circumscribed blush of redness etc., offering ample evidence of perfect maturation. The progress in the second case was equally satisfactory. On the 14th inst. I again saw your child's arm, when the small dry tamarind-stone-like crust was still adhering.

The annexed quotation from the Annual Report of the N. V. I.,* dated January, 1840, though in the main highly satisfactory, certainly does not hold out any inducement to such experiments as that which you have taken the trouble to make. But without disparagement to anything emanating from the meritorious efforts of Dr. Jenner, whose memory as a benefactor to the whole human race is deservedly revered, the opinions therein expressed of the superior efficacy of that virus which has for forty-three years been transmitted through the constitutions of successive generations (allowing for argument sake that it were uninfluenced, uncontaminated, and pure as when taken from its parent source), have, I believe, many opponents among those who have unhappily noticed the occasional failures of its protective influence. And when in their endeavour to account for such casualties, with good reason they revert to the liability to modification in the qualities of the vaccine virus, so extensively transmitted over the habitable globe, as to preclude the possibility of insuring it from commixture with lymph, or matter, in circulation from unauthenticated sources, and consequently the inert, the spurious, and genuine, can often only be appreciated by their results. And that even when in cases of apparently successful vaccination under the interested and watchful superintendence of medical men operating on their own offspring, it does not invariably afford permanent security. The renewal of the stock of lymph originated as in the present instance, and carefully watched in its early transmissions more especially, so that it is productive of such appearances in the progress of the vesicle, as by the combined experience of all competent judges, is deemed evidence of the constitution being placed under the protective influence of vaccine matter, will, I believe, have very many impartial, disinterested, and zealous advocates; and I sincerely hope your second experiment upon another cow may afford you results which will enable you to promulgate, at all events locally, the genuineness and efficacy of this recently originated stock of lymph, as also to maintain an interesting physiological fact. With best wishes for your success,

I am, Sir,
Your obedient servant,
THOMAS WILLIS.

* "The experience of another year has confirmed our conviction of the efficacy of vaccination as the best security against Small Pox, and has afforded us, moreover, proofs of the propriety, in the present state of our knowledge, of preferring vaccine matter, the produce of the original virus furnished by Dr. Jenner, which has now passed happily through successive generations of subjects in the course of forty-three years, and which forms the principal source of our supply, to any which may have been taken recently from the cow."

Brighton, 1, *St. James's Street,*
January 20th, 1841.

My dear Sir,—I have watched through the late stages of your own child's arm, and have used the virus on one of my own patients, which has turned so highly satisfactory that I have no hesitation in saying I should prefer this stock to any I have previously used.

Yours, truly,
S. PAINE.

No. 1, *Castle Square, Brighton,*
January 25th, 1841.

Dear Sir,—I have tried your vaccine virus in five cases, and am happy to tell you with the best success; the development of the pustules appears a day or two later than that of the old virus. I am so pleased with the experiment, and its effects, that I shall continue to vaccinate from your supply in preference to any other; and am,

Dear Sir, yours truly,
J. C. BURROWS.

Brighton, 20, *Prince's Street.*
February 12th, 1841.

Dear Sir,—Having vaccinated my little girl with lymph from your child's arm, and being present when your little patient was vaccinated from the cow, and having had also the opportunity of observing the disease through all its stages upon both children, I can but express my perfect confidence and preference to your vaccine.

I am, dear Sir, yours very truly,
R. P. PELLOWE.

7, *Pavilion Parade, Brighton,*
February 13th, 1841.

Sir,—I have myself vaccinated with the lymph which you recently procured from the cow, and I have seen and examined the pock arising from the use of the same by yourself and by others, and I am of opinion that the success of your experiment is full and complete. Had any of my *own* children required vaccination, I should have had no objection to the use of your lymph; indeed, I would have preferred it.

I am, Sir, yours very truly,
A. PLUMMER, M.D.

Horsham, March 8th, 1841.

Dear Sir,—I beg to add my best thanks for your polite attention to my request as to the vaccine matter, a short account of the result of the first case. The vesicle produced was, to my eye, more exactly regular in shape than we have been accustomed to see of late, corresponding entirely to all that has been formerly defined as the genuine Cow Pock. The areola, perfect on the ninth and tenth days, showed the *pearl on the rose*, and no mixture of more common inflammation obscured its specific character. So far as *one* case can do, the progress of this completely negatives the idea entertained, I hear, in some quarters, as to the greater severity of constitutional disease produced by the variolo-vaccine process. I should be inclined to say that the specific influence seems more distinctly marked, the general febrile disturbance being proportionably less, for I cannot think the protective power is governed by the latter in any degree, but that it is regulated by the former entirely. How far your present endeavour will confirm this view, a *series* of cases (which you may ere this have before you), must, of course, determine. I feel little doubt but that they will afford their confirmation, at the same time proving (if proof of so plain a thing could now be required) the identity of variola and vaccinia in the most striking manner.

I am, dear Sir,
With best thanks for your favours,
Yours respectfully,
W. T. COLEMAN.

Waterford, March 25th, 1841.

Dear Sir,—I fear you will consider my long delay in acknowledging the receipt of the vaccine virus as a poor return for your great kindness in sending it. My apology must be, that a combination of much professional and personal anxiety prevented due attention to the first cases in which I used the lymph. From later cases it appears to me to be quite normal in its stages and progress, though less active as to the amount of inflammation it excites, and with vesicles smaller than I have witnessed before. It developes its first inflammation on the third day at latest; on the fourth or fifth day it is perceptibly vesicated; the areola appears generally on the eighth day, and is on the decline on the twelfth day; the scabs are detached from the twentieth to the twenty-seventh day. The transference of the infection from the arm first vaccinated to the opposite on the fourth or fifth day has in some instances failed, but in all these cases some allowance is to be made for the state of health. Some of these children I operated on were suffering more or less from the irritation of teething. Should anything further strike me as worthy of remark I will communicate it.

I remain, dear Sir,
Yours, very faithfully and obliged,
JOHN ELLIOTT, M.D.

Bristol, March 29th, 1841.

Sir,—Having been informed by Sir James Clark (whose desire to promote useful professional objects is well known) respecting the supply of vaccine lymph you had procured by variolating a cow, I had no hesitation in making trial of it; and having now employed it through *seven* successive courses of inoculation, I am able to say that I feel quite satisfied with it. It differs a little from that in ordinary use, in producing, during the first week especially, vesicles not quite so circular, and which, though yielding perfectly pellucid lymph, when punctured, have a more purulent aspect than the old vesicle.

The areola, too, though appearing at the regular *time*, I have found to be less defined than that following the use of the other lymph.

These slight differences, however, I consider as no objection to it.

I believe that an attentive observer who has watched different kinds of lymph (the origin of which he is acquainted with), will detect slight variations in them. Jenner described his lymph, but minute differences may be found in lymph from other sources, equally protective from Small Pox. I think Dr. Gregory has lately stated that at the Small Pox Hospital virus from three different sources is in use there, each being distinguishable from the other by a practised eye. The crust remaining from your lymph, during the third and fourth week, appears to me particularly satisfactory, and quite characteristic of genuine Cow Pox. Your lymph, I think, much resembles that which Mr. Ceely procured from a cow inoculated with Small Pox, of which a most interesting account is given in the 8th volume of the *Transactions* of the Provincial Medical and Surgical Association, accompanied by a beautiful series of coloured engravings.

I should prefer the lymph you have introduced to any procured from the National Vaccine Establishment. That the virus furnished by that Institution was in no greater favour with others than with myself, I can testify from the numerous applications made to me, from every part of the kingdom, for a supply of the stock which I had procured from some cows near Berkeley, in 1838, and which is the principal source of the Cow Pox now used in this city. How the National Vaccine Establishment can ascertain, as stated in their recent report, that the matter they circulate "is obtained by successions from the original virus communicated by Dr. Jenner himself," I know not. In a number of the *Lancet* (I think for July, 1839) Mr. Leese, one of the vaccinating surgeons at a station connected with the establishment, says, that the source of his virus was from some cows diseased in 1836, and that he had furnished the parent establishment with 27,183 charges; and from a letter in the *Medical Gazette* for July 6th, 1839, page 529, from Mr. Adams, of Lymington, there is every reason for believing that the National Establishment were distributing, without acknowledgment, the supply which I had furnished them with from the Berkeley cows. I have read the pamphlet by Mr. B——, of Brighton. A cautious practitioner cannot be blamed for not at once warmly espousing every novelty that is started, but I am sorry to see any discouragement thrown upon judicious attempts to establish valuable medical facts, and promote professional objects of a useful character. The importance of proving the possibility of speedily converting the direful poison of Small Pox into a benign lymph, capable of protecting the human constitution from all the danger and malignancy of that dreadful disorder, cannot be too highly appreciated, especially when we view it in reference to distant parts of the globe, where on the breaking out of Small Pox the old stock of vaccine matter is not to be procured. Mr. Ceely has, to my mind, satisfactorily demonstrated this fact, and I think the public are indebted to you for instituting a similar set of experiments. To render your results as conclusive as Mr. Ceely's, it would be well for you to inoculate with Small Pox one or two of the children that have been vaccinated with your lymph. A friend in Somersetshire whom I furnished with some of your virus, writes to me a most favourable account of it. He says he never saw finer vesicles than those produced by it; that he regrets not having had it at the commencement of his public vaccinations; that he was supplying neighbouring practitioners with it, and that he trusted he should be able to keep it up.

He sends me some points charged on the 26th, five removes from that which I provided him with.

I am, Sir, your obedient servant,

J. B. ESTLIN.

Brighton, April 2nd, 1841.

Dear Sir,—A fortnight to-day I had an opportunity of seeing a child at your house vaccinated with some lymph which you had originally procured by inoculating a cow with Small Pox matter; it was the tenth day after the insertion of the virus. I never saw vaccination more perfect. The areola was quite distinct, the vesicle limpid, and exhibiting those characteristics which Dr. Jenner was wont to describe as "the pearl upon the rose." I have since used your lymph upon a patient of my own; the result was the most perfect and satisfactory of any I ever obtained.

To describe the appearances produced would be merely to describe the true Jennerian vesicle with which we are all familiar. You have preserved an exact account of the genealogy of your lymph. Mr. Burrows told me he gave you the variolous matter; Dr. Willis saw the vesicle produced upon the cow; your own child was the first which you vaccinated, and since that period you have kept an exact account of the pedigree up to the present time. Indeed, I think that yours is the most successful experiment upon this subject ever performed in this country, and that it strikingly illustrates the accuracy of Jenner's views of the *variola vaccina*, and happily confirms his opinion of its protective influence, you having obtained the same result as he did by a different series of experiments, after a lapse of forty years. Jenner had to grope his way through great darkness, but in spite of the obscurity, by dint of much labour, he was enabled to detect the object of his research; he plucked "the rose," he held it up to the light of day, and transmitted it an inestimable boon to posterity. He propagated it by transplantation, you have produced it by ingrafting; and by the similarity of the results we are enabled to welcome a benign influence, the gift of a beneficent Providence to man. Jenner showed us how to recognise it,—you and Mr. Ceely, by your experiments, have shown us how to produce it; but we had never known how to produce it unless Jenner had first shown us how to recognise it, thus converting the means of our destruction into the instrument of our preservation, a result which may be hailed as the loftiest and most beneficent triumph of the human intellect.

By these and the like experiments it has well been said, that the protective power of vaccination has been placed upon an imperishable basis. Henceforth all prejudice must be overcome, all doubt of the efficacy of vaccination must cease, all fear of its loss must subside, for the same experiments which have confirmed its virtues, have said *Esto perpetua*! and from Britain to the remotest corner of the habitable globe it will be proclaimed that wherever the pestilence of Small Pox spreads, there does it carry with it its own antidote, and also, that this truth has been elicited by British sagacity, and has been promulgated by British philanthropy.

But not only do these experiments seem thus important in their bearings, and thus happy in their results, with regard to one disease, but their influence with respect to Pathology in general, appears to me of surpassing interest.

Thus in the instance of the Small Pox, no chymist has been able to separate the elements of the disease, no anatomist has been able to dissect it, and to demonstrate wherein consists its different properties; a chymical analysis of the lymph yields only water and albumen, but the occult nature of the morbific matter has completely eluded our researches. But by the experiments which you and Mr. Ceely have instituted, although this morbific matter (if indeed it be matter) is not appreciable by the senses, you have been enabled to take it, and as if by a subtile process of alchymy, to submit it as it were to sublimation, to decompose it, to reject its noxious qualities, and to retain its prophylactic virtues.

Who shall say that when the laws which govern these changes are better known, and the process better understood, but that medical philosophers shall be able to analyze disease at pleasure, and to reject its hurtful, and retain its salutary, qualities as they will? and who shall say, but that the infant whose life has been even now preserved by means of the vaccine virus, shall one day become a medical philosopher, who shall be able to demonstrate, to the wonder and admiration of his cotemporaries, that herein consists the contagious property of the disease, therein consists its preventive virtue?

And is not this in accordance with the enterprising spirit of the age, and the progress of modern discovery?

Has not man been able to seize the terrible power of lightning, to make it subserve his purposes, and become his messenger to convey intelligence, with almost the rapidity of thought, to distant parts? Has he not been able to make the light permanently to fix the image of the human features upon a plate of metal? And if the medical philosopher should allow those features to become scarred by a loathsome disease, would not the fidelity of that process reprove him by demonstrating the deformity as depicted by the sunbeam? Onward, then, in the path of improvement till an antidote is found for every evil; and until every production is made to answer the end for which it was designed, in ministering to the necessities or in assuaging the sufferings of mankind.

Many of my medical friends have asked me, wherein is the new virus superior to the old, for if any proof were wanting of the efficacy of vaccination, it would be found in the tenacity with which medical men adhere to the old. For my own part, convinced as I am of the protective powers of the new virus, I unhesitatingly assert my preference for it before all others; not that the virtues of one moss rose are superior to the virtues of another moss rose,—they are both the same, and far be it from me to wish to sully the beauty or to assail the fair reputation of the old one; still I think I may be allowed by contrast to show the reasons of my preference for *that* one recently plucked from its native soil. There was, I think, a little ambiguity in the origin of the former, but the origin of the latter is undoubted; the genealogy of the former has been lost in antiquity, the genealogy of the latter has been well preserved. Notwithstanding the former has been in use for the last forty years, I do not think that it has lost its colour, or that its petals have faded; still, to my eye, the hues of the latter are more vivid and bright.

In the history of the latter, too, are involved the pleasing facts, of the confirmation of its efficacy, and the perpetuity of its source. In conclusion, I beg to express my warmest wishes that you may succeed in your undertaking, and that you may derive a more solid satisfaction, than the unavailing though hearty praise of. Sir,

Your obedient servant,
D. RICHARDSON

Aylesbury, April 3rd, 1845.

My dear Sir,—I owe you many apologies for not before thanking you for your very interesting, satisfactory, and obliging letter. It contains particulars which I should have regretted not to have possessed, and I shall have a special pleasure in communicating them and the whole of the matter relating to the subject, so as to ensure you the high credit you so richly deserve.

I was much pleased to find you related to Mr. Alsop, for it was the anecdote which I related in the note, and which I heard soon after coming into this place, that first gave me the desire to ascertain by direct experiment the truth of what really appeared to me so very doubtful. I have never yet had any satisfactory information beyond that detailed, to enable me to judge whether Mr. A. *vaccinated* or *variolated* the cows.

The only circumstance that confirmed my scepticism was a very natural one. The man's detail was certainly striking; he had no end to serve, no theory to support: but how came it that Mr. A. (*who I am told was intimately acquainted with Jenner*) had not furnished the latter with so satisfactory and direct a proof of his theory? Did you ever hear Mr. A. speak of the fact I related? What think you of the incident? I am glad to hear that you have again succeeded: on what part of the animal this time? I wish very much to try, on a large scale, the process recommended for variolating the cow by Dr. Basil Thiele. I fancy it may be done with not more ultimate expense than a series of uncertain operations in the ordinary way.

I now send you some new vaccine lymph on points charged from a milker's hand, late in May last, from the first and second remove from him, and consequently the last time, the third from the cow.

You may be able and perhaps desirous to compare its effects locally and constitutionally with your own lymph, on the same and on different subjects, preparatory to testing the latter with Small Pox through the instrumentality of your friends, as I have done with mine. In the enclosed lymph, I see nothing unusually severe except on very thin skins; although the milker's hand exhibits now rough ulcers, one on the hand deep enough to encase a bean. I have been requested to supply (of course gratuitously) variola vaccine lymph, for the expedition to New Holland. I have promised a small supply, as much as the two or three weeks will allow me conveniently to collect. Could you add to the stock by charging three or four times about twelve large store points with your lymph? Jointly, then, you and I might supply them with enough for dependence, till it could be reproduced. I have reproduced several times from my early removes, *dried on points*, as efficient lymph as it was at first, from one to nine months; from crusts, ten months. I have no doubt the lymph will keep longer still. I always use these points on a scarified surface; there is no mode equal in certainty to that, and I have tried many. I will furnish you with large points for the purpose mentioned, if you can aid me; and am,

Dear Sir,

Yours very truly,

ROBT. CEELY.

Watlington, April 7th, 1841.

Dear Sir,—I ought to have written to you sooner to thank you for the vaccine lymph which you sent me, and to acquaint you with the results. I sent three of the six points to my brother at Kingston, near Abingdon, and with the remainder vaccinated a healthy boy in four places, using one point twice; all the punctures took effect, and the progress and appearance of the vesicles were quite perfect. With the lymph taken from this subject, I have vaccinated five more; in four of these it succeeded, but the fifth having been previously vaccinated was not affected by it. I should have continued using the lymph, but a person has been appointed to vaccinate this district, and I have, I fear, kept the points charged from the last subject too long, owing to the failure. I will, however, try them when an opportunity occurs. The vesicles appeared to proceed more slowly for the first six days, than usual, but arrived at maturity at the proper time, and were of a very perfect form. I have long been of opinion that the cow pock matter had become contaminated by passing through so many subjects during half a century, and that we ought to obtain it as often as possible from its original source. Some facts which I have ascertained make it very probable that eruptive diseases, which have entirely *left the skin* at the time of vaccination, may yet be communicated by using lymph taken from this subject. Some time ago, wishing to vaccinate the child of a respectable person, I carefully selected and examined an apparently fine, healthy boy; no spot of eruption could be detected, yet the child vaccinated from this had a scaly eruption all over the body and *tinea capitis*, which has not quite yet disappeared (four years). I then ascertained from some neighbours of the boy that he had had a severe attack of *porrigo larvalis* a twelvemonth before, but which had entirely disappeared some months before I vaccinated him.

I am, dear Sir,

Very truly yours,

HENRY BARRET.

Haughley, Stowmarket,
June 7th, 1841.

Dear Sir,—I beg to thank you for your kindness in having sent me some of your variola vaccine, which I have found to succeed very well.

Mr. Estlin sent me some of his vaccine the day after I received a supply from you. I have continued to use both kinds, and have been very careful to keep them separate. I cannot see that there is any difference in the appearance of vesicles produced by either kind.

I have certainly found the lymph received both from you and Mr. Estlin almost invariably to succeed; and I had some difficulty in procuring a supply of lymph to go on with when I used the vaccine from the National Institution, several cases being unsuccessful, which I afterwards vaccinated successfully with your lymph.

I remain, dear Sir,
Yours, very obliged,
WILLIAM EBDEN.

Brighton, July 28th, 1841.

Dear Sir,—I have kept no account of the numbers vaccinated by me, since you supplied me with virus from your stock, but should suppose them to amount to about one hundred.

I have never failed in one case in producing the pure vaccine pustule, and I am so much satisfied with it, that I have discontinued the use of the virus which I had previously employed. You ask me if I have seen it brought in contact with Small Pox. I have so; and in a manner which fully proves its protective power. The case was this:—A lady, who had been confined a month, failed with Small Pox, and as measles were also in the house, the character of the disease was not ascertained until the second day, during which time the child remained with the mother and was nursed by her; as soon, however, as the disease was recognised, the infant was vaccinated, the pustules were good, and it has not had the Small Pox; and it is now five weeks since its exposure to it. The rest of the family were re-vaccinated, and all escaped. With many thanks for the supply of matter which you have so freely afforded me,

I am, dear Sir,
Yours very truly,
R. W. PHILPOTT.

Lewes, August 14th, 1841.

Dear Sir,—I am extremely obliged to you for your supply of vaccine virus, which I decidedly prefer to that I was in the habit of formerly procuring from the Old London Establishment,

I have vaccinated between 70 and 80 patients from the virus I have received from you, and have invariably seen perfect pustules produced by it.

I remain, dear Sir,
Yours truly,
GEO. SCRASE.

N.B.—As the above communication was written for you some time since, many other opportunities have occurred for me to notice the superior qualities of your vaccine.

The last supply I had from you, was to vaccinate my own little girl, and it succeeded admirably.

Brighton, September 6th, 1841.

Dear Sir,—I have delayed writing to you respecting my success with the vaccine virus you were kind enough to give me, until, after two or three removes, I could satisfy myself of its genuineness. I now, however, can inform you, that the result of my examination has been such as I could wish; and I trust it will be long preserved to us, and sincerely hope you will continue to receive that meed of praise which is so deservedly your due.

I remain, dear Sir,
Yours very truly,
T. R. SIMMONDS.

Brighton, October 11*th*, 1841.

My dear Sir,—I have for many years most anxiously desired to see some individual employ himself in the propagation of a new virus, by inoculating a cow with variolous ichor, believing, as I have always done, that the original source of Cow Pock was in reality derived from Small Pox.

In you, Sir, I view one to whom I am, as an individual of the medical profession, highly indebted for having produced a virus, which in numerous applications I have the pleasure to bear testimony of its most satisfactory results; and have the honour to be,

My dear Sir,
Your obliged and obedient servant,
HENRY SUTTON.

London, Brook Street,
November 26*th*, 1841.

My dear Sir,—I beg to thank you for your attention in making me acquainted with the progress of your experiments on the subject of vaccination with your new stock.

I hope you will continue to watch over the growth of your infant progeny; but I fear, with you, that few will be found to devote the time to the subject which it really requires. In truth, none but those who feel a degree of enthusiasm in the subject will be found to give it the attention it requires. It is thus with almost all discoveries—they are only brought out by men who feel an unusual interest in them, and cultivate the subject with a devotion which few feel. I think, however, that what has been done lately on the subject of vaccination by Mr. Ceely, Mr. Estlin, and yourself, will do good, and, indeed, has done much good, by calling the attention of the profession to the state of the vaccine virus. The profession and the public in general have, therefore, reason to be grateful to you all for your exertions.

I am, my dear Sir,
Yours truly,
JAS. CLARK.

February 14*th*, 1842.

Dear Sir,—I am so much pleased with the success of the Small Pox matter when taken from the cow, that I should exceedingly like to have more if you can spare any. I have inserted it into the arms of adults, both male and female, in the way you directed, and it has never failed to produce all the appearance of the true vaccine vesicle.

I have not put it into the arms of infants, thinking it would produce, possibly, more violent inflammation in its effects than the simple vaccine; but, as I said before, into the arms of adults. I have also tried Mr. Ceely's, but cannot speak of it at present. If you can send me more of your variolæ vaccinæ, (as I believe you term it,) I shall be much obliged, and glad to make you any remuneration.

I remain, dear Sir,
Very truly yours,
E. H. MAUL.

46, *Old Steine, Brighton,*
September 20th, 1842.

My dear Sir,—In an experiment so interesting to medical science, and which I believe has never succeeded in this country but with yourself and one other person, it is of high importance that you should furnish the clearest testimony to the members of the profession. It affords me much pleasure in being able to state that the cow was inoculated with Small Pox from one of my patients, that I watched the progress of the disease in the animal, also in your own little boy, vaccinated direct from the cow, and the result has, to my mind, satisfactorily established the identity of *variola* and *vaccine*. The vesicles produced by your vaccine are very fine, and perfectly characteristic with those of Dr. Jenner's; and I quite agree, with Mr. Estlin, of Bristol, in the opinion given in his letter to Sir J. Clark, respecting your vaccine,—"That no virus ought to be so much esteemed as that converted by the cow from Small Pox to the vaccine vesicle." I am glad to find you are circulating your stock of vaccine lymph widely, and I consider the public is much indebted to you.

I am, dear Sir,
Truly yours,
J. CORDY BURROWS.

P.S.—I observe in the last volume of the Transactions of our Medical and Surgical Association, that your vaccine lymph was found to be in admirable perfection after four months. I, therefore, doubt not but that which you sent to our Colonies and to Germany will be found effective.

Brighton, September 24th, 1842.

Dear Sir,—During the time of my being House Surgeon to the Brighthelmston Dispensary, I was induced to make trial of your vaccine by the recommendation of Sir M. J. Tierney, M.D., one of the Vice-Presidents. I vaccinated more than 200 patients at the Institution, and the results were very satisfactory; since which time I have continued to use it in my own practice.

I remain, dear Sir,
Very truly yours,
W. VERRALL.

Camden Crescent, Dover,
March 14th, 1844.

Sir,—I shall be much obliged by your sending me, as early as convenient, a supply of vaccine lymph, as the season is now favourable for vaccination. The last supply that you sent me, about a year ago, produced very fine vesicles, and I vaccinated in succession nearly 100 patients.

I remain, Sir,
Your obedient servant,
W. SANKEY.

Aylesbury, May 12th, 1844.

My dear Sir,—I beg you will accept my sincere thanks for your very gratifying communication received this morning, announcing your deserved success in again variolating the cow, and obtaining the vaccine disease (the vaccine modification of *variola*, as I still presume to call it). I assure you I am fully as much gratified as you can be, at your thus twice more succeeding in this difficult and precarious experiment; and I do say that your unwearied perseverance after so many failures is deserving of unqualified praise, although your former success must have assured you of eventual triumph.

I hope you will carefully note any circumstance that may differ as to time, season, mode of operation, character of constitution of the animal, or its integuments, or anything in the temporary condition of it: in fact, any circumstance that may have contributed in all probability to the result in these last cases, which may not have existed in former experiments.

I am not inclined to think we are likely soon to arrive at a knowledge of all the circumstances which favour success in this interesting experiment; but for that reason nothing is too minute to be recorded in the detail of the particulars attending a successful attempt.

Thank you for the two points you have sent me: I will soon employ them, and shall be glad to use some of the succeeding removes, when you can spare any that you approve of. Keep it carefully under your own eye at present, and let others see its effects under your operations, except you have careful and experienced and unprejudiced observers, willing to aid you in the use of it.

Be under no apprehension from the source of the variolous virus having been a *confluent* pustule. Any *opinion* to the contrary will be of no value, for Dr. Basil Thiele, of Kasan, (S. Russia,) has himself settled this point by direct experiments. He says, "The greater or less malignity of the epidemic Small Pox, and of the individual case from which the matter has been taken, *has no essential* influence upon the *vaccine* generated; for in a case in which the Small Pox eruption was confluent, became black, and the child died, a perfectly genuine vaccine was generated by the transmission."

I wish you success in the human transmissions, and when they are fully and completely established, pray draw up the cases, and if you don't publish them, you will be very blameable.

If you do not contemplate the publication yourself, I hope you will allow me to suggest a mode of disposing of them, to which I am sure you cannot object.

I am so desirous to hear of the complete success of your subsequent trials with the generated vaccine, and to see the local effects on the animals, (human and brute,) that I have a great inclination to run down and see you. When, think you, would be a proper day to see as much as possible in both these respects?—for I cannot be away more than two days from home.

I am better certainly than when I left Brighton, and have gone through a most fagging and harassing winter, and spring, without one day's rest; but I should like another five or six weeks' holiday soon at Brighton, but fear I cannot obtain it this year,—certainly not till autumn, if then.

With best wishes and many thanks, believe me,

My dear Sir,

Yours very truly,

ROBERT CEELY.

116, *Marine Parade, Brighton,*
June 4th, 1844.

Sir,—The virus which I procured from you, marked *one remove,* was employed to vaccinate a healthy child, aged five months.

Up to the fifth day so little local and general irritation appeared, as to lead to the supposition that the operation had failed; but on the eighth, the pustules were full-sized, charged with limpid lymph, and surrounded by a small areola. On the tenth day, the inflammation had spread nearly down to the elbow, the fever was considerable, and red blotches appeared on the back and lower limbs of the child.

The constitutional symptoms gradually subsided, together with the eruption just described.

The matter taken from one arm was employed to re-vaccinate six persons of different ages; in three, aged 7, 11, and 16, it succeeded. In these cases the inflammation began early, subsided after the eighth day, and did not reach any great height.

Should this statement be of use to you, pray employ it as you think proper.

With every desire to see you duly recompensed for your exertions in this matter,

I am, Sir,
Your obedient servant,
CHARLES MAITLAND, M.D.

Dover, March 15th.

Sir,—The very scanty supply, three points, were all used on a healthy child, and three fine vesicles produced, when, to my astonishment and annoyance, the lady refused to have any virus taken from the child's arm; under these circumstances you will, I hope, send me more. I enclose a statement of the result of the last two or three years' vaccinations; all the difference I have observed is in the larger size of vesicles.

Yours very faithfully,
W. SANKEY.

During 1843, fifty-seven patients were vaccinated from vaccine obtained from points of Mr. Badcock, of Brighton; of these, four were instances of re-vaccination, fifty-three of vaccination for the first time. In forty-seven of the fifty-three, four vesicles (corresponding to the number of punctures made) were formed. In three (the first three vaccinated) it was noted that the vesicles were very fine; one, that they were small (the fourth vaccinated). In another instance, vaccination from the points first obtained, had failed, and the four vesicles resulting from the second vaccination were destroyed by scratching. In the forty-two remaining cases, the vesicles formed were considered efficient, but there is no note of any peculiarity.

In three instances, three vesicles only were formed. In two instances there were only two vesicles. In another instance only one vesicle.

In 47—4 vesicles.
,, 3—3 vesicles.
,, 2—2 vesicles.
,, 1—1 vesicle.
——
53

Two separate supplies, in 1844, obtained from same sources, failed.

1845. Eighty-four cases from ichor from Brighton. Seventy-eight, first vaccination. Six, re-vaccination. Of seventy-eight:—

In 71—4 vesicles formed.
,, 2—1 vesicle.
,, 2—2 vesicles.
,, 3—3 vesicles.
——
78

In the instances where two vesicles formed, the vaccine matter was compared with other ichor by the two sorts being introduced into different arms of the same patient by two punctures. There was not any difference perceived in the two sets of vesicles.

Not a single case of Small Pox has occurred to test the protective power of the lymph; but upwards of twenty years since, patients under vaccination have been placed in contact with Small Pox and have not been infected.

Aylesbury, April 3rd, 1845.

My dear Sir,—I must beg pardon for not acknowledging the receipt, and long ago returning the memoranda which you kindly sent me; but, really, I have been so harassed by a continued series of urgent duties, that I have not been able to pay them that careful attention which I wish to do before I send them back. Your lymph has been extensively used in the neighbourhood from the last supply, vaccination having been practised in all directions, from the appearance of Small Pox. Many hundreds have been vaccinated and re-vaccinated with it, and I have heard my own opinion of its perfect efficiency confirmed, with much satisfaction, by those to whom I have distributed it. I have watched the operation of both stocks in many cases of my own patients, and have been perfectly satisfied with its effects in every particular; I really could not see any difference between the two stocks, on the same subjects, so I soon blended them.

I have been obliged to suspend my vaccination lately, from the occurrence of scarlatina and other impediments, and having used all my most recent points in some unproductive re-vaccinations, I have been unable to supply six applicants for it; one of them is Mr. J. G. Crosse, Surgeon, of Norwich, where, already, more than 200 deaths have occurred from Small Pox. He wants the enclosed points charged from the latest lymph from the cow. Could you conveniently do so for him? and could you spare me a few points also for other applicants? If you have not many to spare, I must use what you can spare, and again get a supply; for Small Pox has just occurred here, and I have some patients already requiring vaccination.

I return you your own points. A case of Small Pox has, I learn, just appeared here; if it be a natural and not a modified case, I will collect you some virus.

Believe me, my dear Sir,
Yours truly,
ROBT. CEELY.

Aylesbury, June 29th, 1845.

Dear Sir,—I have lately had an opportunity of testing with variolous infection, two children vaccinated with your last lymph, and have found them perfectly safe.

In almost every case in which I have used the last supplies, the patients have exhibited the primary constitutional symptoms on the sixth or seventh day, abundance of areola on the tenth day, and a full and satisfactory amount of the secondary fever; and have shown as fine vesicles as I ever wish to see. I intend to continue it.

A large number of patients now in the Vale of Aylesbury, therefore, have had to rejoice in your lymph; besides some hundreds in various other parts of the kingdom.

I am sorry that I must, for want of time, defer writing a longer letter; I trouble you now, because I thought you might have referred Mrs. W. to me, as she applied from Brighton.

Believe me, dear Sir,
Yours truly,
ROBT. CEELY.

SMALL POX AND COW POX.

AUZIAS-TURENNE.

I. *Communicated to the Academy of Medicine.*

1865.

II. *Courrier Médical du* 26 *Mai.*

1866.

[Reprinted in *La Syphilisation. Publication de l'œuvre du Docteur Auzias-Turenne, faite par les soins de ses amis.*]

TRANSLATED BY THE EDITOR.

SMALL POX AND COW POX.

OBSERVATIONS ON THE RELATIONS WHICH EXIST BETWEEN SMALL POX AND COW POX.

I.

Communicated to the Academy of Medicine, September 5, 1865.*

AS the question which the Lyons Commission undertook to solve has already been brought prominently before the Academy, it is unnecessary for me to make an historical preamble. Paris has said much, and although Lyons may not have listened to everything, or at least, may not have retained everything, nevertheless it has done much for the cause of science and truth.

The Lyons Commission, having at its disposal resources which offer themselves to those who know how to call them into existence and to profit by them, has multiplied inoculations of vaccine and varioline under diverse names; it has made various experiments and counter-experiments on animals belonging principally to the bovine and equine species, and on man.

Before proceeding to explain and to estimate what it has done, it will not be out of place to acquaint the reader with its preconceived ideas and its language. Which of us has not his own opinions—I had almost said prejudices—and his own way of expressing them? What is a regenerated virus? Is it not a virus which has been intensified by being passed through suitable organisms, human or animal: a virus which produces stronger and more certain effects, and is the agent of a more efficacious prophylaxis?

* *Apropos* of the following work: *Vaccine et Variole*, Nouvelle étude expérimentale sur la question de l'identité de ces deux affections, étude faite au nom de la Société des Sciences Médicales de Lyon, par une Commission composé de MM. Boudet, Chauveau, Delore, Dupuis, Gailleton, Horand, Lortet, P. Meynet et Viennois, Rapport par MM. Chauveau, Président de la Commission, Viennois Sécrétaire, P. Meynet, Sécrétaire adjoint.

Those ideas, as clear as they are simple, do not seem to have been sufficiently appreciated by the Lyons Commission. A regenerated vaccine would seem to the Commission to be whatever was retaken from the cow, whether weak or strong, and of whatever origin; the intensity of the virus derived from vesicular grease (*grease pustuleux*) appears to have been overlooked, and the most that was admitted was that the prophylactic virtue of the virus is in relation to its activity. It is true, that in order to recognise different degrees of intensity and efficacy in viruses, it was necessary to admit (and with some inconsistency perhaps) that one was imbued with the doctrines of syphilization.

The expressions *Cow Pox* and *Vaccine primitif* mean, further, in the language of the Lyons Commission, any description of virus derived from the cow. As for the name *Horse Pox*, it is well understood that it does not signify what it is alleged to mean, that is to say, Small Pox of the horse, but Cow Pox of the horse. What name, then, will be given to the true Small Pox, which the Lyons Commission make such a point of having communicated to the horse? This regrettable neologism will not prevent the name of its author from being honourably inscribed in the history of vaccination.

The results of the work of the Lyons Commission may be summed up under three headings.

1.—Cow Pox and Small Pox can be inoculated in bovines and equines; the first energetically, the second feebly.

2.—Whatever may be their successive transmissions, direct or crossed, these two diseases breed true on every soil.

3.—The protection from one by the other is assured in all cases.

This is not the place to guarantee the accuracy of this last proposition, which may more properly be discussed elsewhere. It is sufficient to remark that although pointing out the splendid development of the bovine vesicles, the Lyons Commission does not go so far as to consider the virus of unparalleled quality. On this point, therefore, there is nothing to take exception to.

With regard to the experimental proof supplied by M. Mathieu, that foot and mouth disease is not the same disease as Cow Pox, it will appear superflous to any one who has restricted himself to casual observation of this disease. It is the same with Sheep Pox, which requires only to be seen to convince that it bears no relation to Cow Pox.

This question of the nature of Sheep Pox, which the Lyons Commission proposed to examine and thoroughly work out, has been elucidated at various times by Camper,* in a remarkable chapter on the diseases common to animals and man; by Pessina,† by A. J. Chrestien ‡ of Montpellier, who, after having had Small Pox, inoculated himself with Sheep Pox with at least as much success as the Lyons Commission had in communicating Small Pox to animals; by Gohier § of Lyons, Voisin ‖ of Versailles, Legallois,¶ Dupuy,** M. Huzard, and several others ††

Thanks to the hereditary kindness and intelligence of M. Camille Leblanc, and to the active assistance of an excellent collaborator, M. Mathieu, it has lately been a subject of investigation by the writer.

Among the variolæ of animals, which can be transmitted to man, there may be mentioned as an example the Hog Pox (*variole de cochon*), of which Count Lauraguais having, it appears, witnessed a case of such transmission, and anticipating Jenner by nearly half

---

* *Œuvres d'histoire naturelle de physiologie et d'anatomie comparée*, t. ii., p. 327, il dit: "La clavelée n'a rien de commun avec la petite vérole, comme je m'en suis convaincu par l'inoculation de la matière variolique a des brebis, sur lesquelles elle n'a pas eu la moindre influence, et n'a même pas causé d'inflammation locale."

† *Bibliothèque Britannique*, "Sciences et Arts," t. xxi., pp. 316—320.—Voir aussi la page 398 du t. ix. du même Recueil.

‡ "Je me piquai au bras avec du pus de claveau; je me procurai une pustule qui fut accompagnée du douleur à la gorge et à la poitrine, assez vive, mais très courte, et qui avait pu être augmentée par l'affection morale. Du moment de la piqûre à l'exsiccation de la pustule, il ne s'écoula que trois jours. Dira-t-on que j'ai eu le claveau? " . . . J'inoculai, il y a plusieurs années deux moutons avec du levain variolique, ils eurent une maladie éruptive, qui aurait dû les garantir du claveau, si quelques traits de ressemblance établissaient l'identité dans les résultats. Ces animaux exposés dans les troupeaux infectés, contractèrent la maladie propre à leur espèce." (Opuscule SUR L'INOCULATION DE LA PETITE VÉROLE, avec quelques réflexions sur celles de la vaccine. . . . In-8°. de 240 pages. Montpellier et Paris, an ix.)—Lettre à De Carro dans le *Conservateur de la santé* du 10 brumaire an 11.

§ OBSERVATIONS ET EXPÉRIENCES—Suivies du précis de plusieurs essais sur la vaccination des bêtes à laine. In-8°. de 107 pages. Lyon: 1807.

‖ EXPOSITION DES PRINCIPAUX FAITS RECUEILLIS SUR L'ÉTAT ACTUEL DE LA VACCINATION DES BÊTES À LAINE. Versailles: 1812.

¶ *Réponse expérimentale à cette question: "La vaccine perd-elle son efficacité préservatrice après 20 ans d'insertion?"* Thèse de la Faculté de Médecine de Paris, 1828, p. 32.

** *Idem, Ibidem.*

†† *Rapport du Comité Central de Vaccine*, 1803, p. 410. Séance générale de la Société centrale établie pour l'extinction de la petite vérole en France par la propagation de la vaccine, tenue le 12 juin, 1806, *passim*. Rapport du Comité Central de Vaccine, an xi., 1803, p. 410. . . . Despaux: INSTRUCTION SUR LA VACCINE suivie de quelques Observations sur la Clavelée des Moutons (Paris: 1808). In-8°, 161 pages. Rapport du Comité Central de Vaccine sur les vaccinations pratiquées en France pendant les années 1808 et 1809. Paris—1811, p. 111.—Rapport sur les Vaccinations de 1810, Paris, 1812, p. 117 et suivantes.—Heurtrel d'Arboval: DICTIONNAIRE DE MÉDECINE ET DE CHIRURGIE VÉTÉRINAIRES, article "Variole."

a century, proposed to the Academy of Sciences to practise prophylactic inoculation on man.*

It is asserted that the discoverer of vaccination inoculated his own son in this way. This is neither the first nor the last time that our neighbours across the Channel have taught us to put our ideas into practice.

The following is a brilliant triumph of the Lyons Commission. It only remains to confirm it. Bovines and equines are susceptible of Small Pox; that is to say, of the mere shadow of Small Pox in the form of a papule existing at the place of inoculation. This papule—and this is the novelty and wonder of the discovery—protects these animals very efficaciously even from the action of the most virulent Cow Pox (p. 58 §2), which, for the Commission, is saying a good deal. Is this not almost asserting that spurious vaccination is able to protect from Small Pox, and from true Cow Pox? The important fact consists, then, in complete protection produced by an imperfect illness. Must we invert a famous proverb and say, "*Qui peut le moins, peut le plus?*"

But, on the contrary, it is far from demonstrated that a mild attack of a virulent malady, once undergone, can give absolute protection from a strong one. "He who is strongly syphilized," says Fernel, "gives something to the one who is less so, and raises him, so to speak, to his own virulent level." "He who has undergone a mild attack of Small Pox in infancy," says Rhazes, "may contract a second attack in youth, or maturity, by contact with stronger virus." It is, therefore, a law of viruses, foreseen and formulated by great minds centuries before it was definitely established and promulgated by syphilization.

The Lyons Commissioners, as well as all other human beings, if not all animals, must submit to this: *dura lex, sed lex.*

The successful transmission of Small Pox to a child, by an imperceptible amount of matter from the equine papule, in no way proves that the animals had been completely variolated. In the same way, vesicles are produced on the vaccinated and variolated, which are no more Small Pox than an abortive seed is a fruit; though they are capable of transmitting it to those who are able to contract the disease and revivify the virus.

It is to be regretted that the Commissioners did not, in their

* MÉMOIRE SUR L'INOCULATION, par M. le Comte de Lauraguais, lu a l'Académie des Sciences, dont il est membre, le 6 juillet, 1763, et approuvé par l'Académie (in 8°, Paris: 1763; pp. 18, 19, 20).

animals, examine the lymphatic glands connected with the seat of inoculation. Perhaps they might have discovered important changes, if we may judge by what takes place in most, if not in all, of the other virulent maladies, and in Small Pox itself when inoculated in man. The modifications which take place in the lymphatic glands deserve at least as much attention as the onset of fever, or the stage of development of a vesicle.

We now come to an assertion which, emanating from such talented observers as the Lyons Commissioners, does not fail to cause surprise: they affirm that the primary variolous eruption resembles, even to confusion, in a child, the vaccinal vesico-pustule. If we consult *Le Recueil des Travaux de la Société Médicale Allemande de Paris*, we shall find some differential characters which could not have escaped the sagacity of the Lyons doctors if they had merely turned over the pages of the writings of the compatriots and contemporaries of Jenner.

Without maintaining positively that bovines intensify the vaccine when transmitted to them, the Lyons Commission adopts the theory that these animals are the natural soil of Cow Pox. But this opinion will not continue to prevail over that of Jenner (which will be discussed later on), who considered the horse to be the source of vaccine lymph. Why was it that the inventor of vaccination suggested the strange idea that the equine virus must pass through the cow, in order to afford true protection against Small Pox? Genius has its weaknesses!

The Lyons Commission has a tendency to admit that the virus of the variolous mother-pustule does not possess so much intensity as that of a secondary pustule. The facts, which it states, appear at first sight to authorize this conclusion, but they are capable of a better interpretation than this.

Thus, on the 14th (pp. 68 and 69),* a subject was inoculated, and on the 22nd (*i.e.* on the *ninth day* after), virus was taken, from the pustule which had been produced, to inoculate another subject. The result proved that this virus was weak; but, some days earlier, and also, perhaps, some days later, a much stronger virus might have been collected at the same spot.

And for this reason:—In every primary virulent vesicle, there is a moment when the virus is accumulated (*foyer primitif*). Re-absorption soon dissipates it. Ordinarily it reappears there

* [Of the Report of the Lyons Commission.—E.M.C.]

more or less abundantly at the period of the general eruption (*foyer secondaire*).

It was during the time between these two stages, that the Lyons Commission collected the matter which it put to the test. It would have been certainly more successful had the virus been taken some days earlier, and perhaps also some days later.

Has it not fallen into the same error (suspected by Mons. J. Guérin) as the Chartres' Commission, which, some time ago, experimenting on the virus of anthrax, denied the inoculability of the serosity of the malignant pustule? But it cannot too often be repeated that viruses must be collected just at the right time—*i.e.* at the best possible hour, and before they are too much diluted by the fluids of the body.

The Lyons Commission was at one moment very near the truth which has escaped them. We read at page 78 of the *Report* that a pustule, which was retarded and contemporary with the general eruption, showed itself at the point of insertion. The Commissioners rightly recognized it as a pustule dependent on the general eruption. The fact is, that there is generally found at this point a secondary development, which may be mistaken, because its seat is the same as that of the primary symptom.

In this case it was distinct, the primary symptom having failed, as if to give a hint to the Commissioners. The Commissioners apparently had their minds occupied elsewhere.

The Lyons Commission denies that the horse has the power of regenerating the vaccine, and of distilling the best virus. It remains to be proved whether its decision is justified by the cases which it furnishes.

In a first experiment (page 38), equine virus was inoculated, which had been collected on the *tenth day*, if not later, in the form of a crust, which was mixed with water. The result obtained was nothing wonderful. But there is no reason for surprise, for a virus in the form of a crust taken so late, and mixed with water, is a virus, so to speak, thrice weakened: it could only take, even moderately, on an excellent soil. Besides, is the date of the formation of the different parts of a crust ever well known?

In a second and final experiment the virus was also taken too late. This precious agent can never be taken, let me repeat, soon enough.

Moreover, why is it that the horse does not always produce a good vaccine? For the same reason that man does not always produce a good varioline or a good syphiline, nor the sheep a good claveline. One reason that man does not always produce a good varioline or a good syphiline, or the sheep a good claveline, is because the one has been vaccinated or more or less completely syphilized, and the other clavelized. There is no reason to doubt that the horse often contracts, at an early age, vesicular grease under one form or another, which affects the mucous membranes, and is overlooked (*gourme*,* *étranguillon*,† etc., etc.). I bring this subject to the attention and study of veterinary surgeons. In this is found the cause of a considerable loss of the vaccinal receptivity of this animal. On the other hand, this manifests itself in its full development in those horses which, like the exotic animals of the *Jardin d'acclimatation*, have never suffered from the malady. This affords an explanation of the apparently contradictory results obtained by Numan, in his attempts to generate vaccine in the horse—attempts which puzzled and discouraged the experimenter.† Nature never contradicts herself, but we must understand her language.

The Lyons Commission is unwilling to admit the existence of generalized vaccinal eruptions, or vaccinides. It is not that it did not observe cases, but it explains them away. Theories are screens which intercept the truth when they are not the reflectors which illuminate it. "We have observed," says the Commission (page 37), "on our two asses, on different parts of the body, on the hind-quarters, a falling off of the hair and epidermis, with serous secretion, apparently following a marked vesication." There is the fact, but here is the explanation which obscures it: "As these animals already showed, at the time of inoculation, traces of depilation, we cannot say whether any relation existed between the vaccination and the symptom which we have just mentioned." Do *traces of depilation* generally resemble *a marked vesication*? Why was not the observation more precise? and does it not appear to be tainted with negligence?

At page 25, there is an example of what is very probably a vaccinide, followed of course by an explanatory comment: "However, on the child of M. Dupuis, one of your Commissioners, two

* Marinus, *Académie de Médecine de Belgique;* séance du 30 mai, 1857, pp. 51 et 52.—H. Bouley, *Académie de Médecine* du 23 août, 1864.

† Sacco, TRAITÉ DE LA VACCINATION, etc.: Traduction française par Daquin, 2e édition, 1813, pp. 313 et 393. Sacco, il est [illegible]ai ne mérite qu'une confiance restreinte.

‡ Marinus, *loc. cit.*

little hemispherical vesicles appeared on the areola of a vesicle, and a slight eruption of similar vesicles was observed on various parts of the body. . . . But evidently there is not in these eruptions, which are a sort of *strophulus volaticus* sometimes observed in the inoculations with ordinary vaccine, anything which resembles a generalization of Cow Pox."

On the contrary, we think that this *strophulus volaticus* can be shown to *resemble* Cow Pox, with the help of a reflector borrowed from analogy, which will fully illuminate it. Does it not as much resemble a generalization of Cow Pox, as the syphilitic roseola resembles the pseudo-chancre; as the large nummular tubercle of inoculated Sheep Pox resembles the generalized eruption of Sheep Pox; as the mother-pustule of Small Pox resembles the daughter-pustules; as the malignant pustule resembles anthracæmia; as the papule of inoculated measles resembles measles, or the red circle * of scarlet fever resembles scarlet fever?

The fact is that the general eruptive phenomena do not strictly take for their model the events which occur at the seat of inoculation. But more than this, these phenomena are not always identical. May not syphilis, the type of virulent maladies, present itself under forms sufficiently varied and dissimilar to embarrass the diagnosis of an accomplished physician?

Between syphilis and Cow Pox the analogy may be a long way followed up. The inoculation of Cow Pox—a malady with a fixed virus sufficiently well named Pox of the Cow (*Vérole de vache*)—may, for example, give rise to polymorphic vaccinides, and sometimes to disseminated pathognomonic vesico-pustules, just as the contagion of the mucous patch, symptom of a malady with an equally fixed virus, gives rise to various secondary eruptions, and sometimes to the appearance of disseminated mucous patches.† But, happily for the vaccinated, Cow Pox passes through a rapid evolution, and does not leave virulent remains for so long a time or so frequently as syphilis.

We may find fault with the Lyons Commission in some details. It has given, for example, on page 52, the following note:—"Does human vaccine, originating in the horse, behave in the same manner as vaccine from the cow? This is quite an open question, for possibly spontaneous Cow Pox and Horse Pox, as MM. Leblanc and Auzias-Turenne think, may not be absolutely

* DES FIÈVRES ÉRUPTIVES EN GÉNÉRAL, par François Gautier (Thèse de Paris, 1846), p. 30.

† Bazin, LEÇONS THÉORIQUES ET CLINIQUES SUR LES SYPHILIDES . . . rédigées par Le Fournier (Paris, 1859), p. 113, et suiv.

identical. The latter, Horse Pox, has been unfortunately wanting for the purpose of comparative experiments."

What would the Commission answer if it were asked where it found this statement, and what it means?

But the *Report* is too important, its language too measured and dignified, for it not to be allowed to entrench itself behind the adage: *De minimis non curat prætor.*

* * * * * *

[M. Auzias-Turenne then compliments the Commissioners on the result of their labours, and explains the object and spirit of his criticisms.—E. M. C.]

This discussion would not have completely attained its object were it not followed by some propositions summing up its general meaning.

I. Viruses vary in form, intensity, and qualities, owing to certain circumstances which ought never to be overlooked by investigators and all those who endeavour, in spite of a thousand difficulties, to utilize for the benefit of the public health these formidable, but at the same time valuable, natural agents.

II. To obtain active viruses their germs must, in the first place, amongst other conditions, be sown on suitable media, and they must be afterwards taken at the right time.

III. A mild attack of a virulent malady—described by the words *ébauchée*, abortive, spurious, etc.—does not afford complete protection from its own virus, if this be very active. It will, therefore, be understood that vaccination will perhaps have lost, temporarily, some of its credit, which will be ultimately regained by revaccination.

IV. Indeed, from this point of view, a mild attack, if repeated, may to a certain extent take the place of a more vigorous attack of the same illness, the quantity making up, in a way, for the quality. This is an important secret of prophylaxis and therapeutics.

V. At the same time, an organism may be vulnerable to the attacks of a virulent malady, for which it offers a suitable soil, when it has not undergone a complete evolution of the same.

VI. When a virulent eruptive disease is inoculated or contracted by accident, the initial lesion of the general eruption does not absolutely resemble that of the primary lesion—neither being equal to it, as a rule, in development, nor in virulency (vaccine, syphilis, etc.); it may be said that the initial symptom acquires in depth and in height what the general eruption gains in extent. The one seems to be the concentration, and the other the dissemination, of the virulent principle. The first represents the virus as it enters the organism, and the second the virus which has developed in it.

VII. Sometimes vesicular grease spreads in the horse to an extraordinary extent; sometimes, on the contrary, it appears as if abortive. In the latter case, the animal has often undergone, when very young, a mild form of vesicular grease, of which the horse is the true soil.

VIII. All things being equal, the horse—and all other animals, including man—should furnish the best vaccine at the vesicles of insertion, which, moreover, are ordinarily single.

IX. A horse inoculated with Small Pox may become an agent for its transmission in the same way as a vaccinated man, on whom the same malady has been inoculated. But this horse cannot be considered, any more than the man, to have had complete Small Pox. It is even more than doubtful whether the horse would be proof against Small Pox for as long a period as the vaccinated man would be.

X. Cow Pox differs from Small Pox in a great many characters, besides those which have long been recognized in science, or especially mentioned by the Lyons Commission. Indeed, it is possible by comparative examination of the vaccinal and variolous vesicles, to establish between them differences in form, volume, colour, circumference, surface, areola, base, surrounding erythema, structure, liquid, crust, cicatrix, number, and lastly, duration.*

XI. Foot and mouth disease, which is only an acute pemphigus, examples of which are found in man, is not produced by the same virus as Cow Pox.

XII. These two maladies, which are not at all similar, do not supplant each other in any organism.

XIII. Lastly, Sheep Pox, a virulent tuberculo-bullous and papulo-vesicular disease of sheep, is, in relation to Cow Pox (a disease of the horse), or to Small Pox (a disease of man), in the same position as foot and mouth disease. It differs from both in its origin as well as in the greater part of its characters and consequences.

* According to the statement of the Lyons Commission the mother-pustule of variola in the child exactly resembles the pustule of vaccina, while it differs considerably from it in animals. It seems that the Commission only observed on the latter an *abortive* variola.

II.

Small Pox and Cow Pox are not produced by the same Morbid Poison.

IN my studies of the virulent maladies, I am accustomed to take syphilis as a type and guide. As it progresses by definite stages its course can be observed. The phenomena which I have observed in this malady, I endeavour to detect in the evolution of other diseases. Here they are much more rapid, and in consequence much less apparent; nevertheless I nearly always succeed in discovering them. I assure myself, in every case, of their reality or of their absence; and this verification constitutes knowledge—a scientific conquest. To my mind, he who subordinates the study of other virulent maladies to that of syphilis, may be compared to a traveller who, proceeding by short stages, has time to take cognizance of the country through which he passes, instead of traversing it without observing anything—by rail.

However rapid, therefore, the virulent maladies may be in their course, their stages can be traced with the help of syphilis, which progresses slowly. Analogy is a valuable aid, but it must be carefully employed. It is an adventurous guide whose directions must be kept under a firm control.

But we must never take syphilis, for example, as a guide in the case of chronic constitutional maladies, or diatheses, like scrofula or cancer. These are not produced by a virus, nor do they accomplish a uniform evolution. They form, so to speak, part of the constitution. The virulent maladies, on the other hand, appear to spread more or less regularly through the organism, which they leave free, when it has been able to resist them without having been harassed with drugs.

To return to my subject: Are there two distinct viruses, a vaccine virus and a variolous virus?

This question—which is no new one, being contemporary with Jenner—ought, in my opinion, to be answered in the affirmative. In fact, what was Cow Pox when it was first brought forward? It was called Small Pox of cows. There was nothing astonishing in its affording protection from human Small Pox, of which it was believed to be a modification. Jenner himself took care not to oppose an argument which pleaded so strongly for his discovery. So this made its entry into the world under the guarantee of variolous inoculation. Moreover, vaccinal accidents, which are of little consequence at the present day, were imputed to syphilis, and, in the majority of cases, had nothing to do with it, so afraid were the early partizans of vaccination that it would be accused of leaving in the body some bestial ferment!

Further, who of us has not been attracted at the outset by this idea of unity. May we not say, reversing an adage: *Un peu de science nous en rapproche; beaucoup de science nous en éloigne?* It results from a superficial and an imperfect survey in which we are struck only by the resemblances. But an attentive examination will at once establish fundamental differences. The two viruses, or the two virulent diseases, are no more identical than, for instance, potash and soda are one and the same thing in the eyes of chemists.

I will not devote myself to an enumeration of the resemblances; they have been many times repeated, and are known to all. In the two cases, we have to do with a virus and a virulent malady, of which the course and effects are perceptibly identical. In order to be sure that a confusion is being made of two distinct things, a minute examination is required, of which the following is an outline:—

Firstly: Small Pox virus is at the same time infectious and contagious—*i.e.* it is communicable to man by means of the atmosphere as well as by inoculation. The latter is the only way of entrance in the case of Cow Pox, equally in man and the lower animals. M. Mathieu and I have multiplied proofs, negative ones it is true, of this assertion. We consider that the opposite opinion in point of fact is based on a misstatement.

Secondly: A reciprocal transformation of the two viruses, analogous to that which takes place between the virus of the syphilitic chancre and the false-chancre, has never been proved. Are we not able, indeed, thanks to the ingenious researches of M. Bidenkap, to produce in part, at least, this latter transformation?

But as regards Cow Pox and Small Pox it has never been found possible to produce this, or even to establish anything resembling it. In fact, whatever animals they may be to which Cow Pox is given, the vaccine which they give back is always the same, except as to degree of strength; and when we succeed in giving them the Small Pox it is invariably also varioline, and not vaccine, which they give us back.

Thirdly: *Vaccine*, all things being equal, has more energy than *varioline*. It cannot therefore be a mitigated form of it, any more than a modification of another kind. It takes, in fact, on a large number of animals. I do not know any species to which one cannot transmit Cow Pox if one can transmit Small Pox.

Variolous inoculation aborts always after an efficient vaccination, but a strong Cow Pox may have some effect after any kind of variola. In a word, an absolute immunity from Cow Pox implies still more decisively an immunity from Small Pox.

I acknowledge, however, that the importance of this characteristic is restricted because it is only a question of degree.

It is an argument to be used exclusively by those who have deeply investigated the matter, and whose convictions are already founded on other considerations. But in their eyes, it possesses great value—it appears to them as strongly confirmatory of the others.

Fourthly: If Cow Pox and Small Pox were the products of the same virus, one of these maladies would not momentarily retard, as it does, the evolution of the other.

As an example, inoculate Cow Pox in a subject who has already been inoculated with it three days previously. The last inoculation would soon equal the first in its development. The level would, so to speak, be established between them. They would progress together in concert, one being nearly as advanced as the other.

On the other hand, inoculate Cow Pox in a subject in which Small Pox is already incubating, and this Cow Pox will frequently be retarded in its progress, as if Nature were not capable of accomplishing two different pathological processes at the same time.

In the first case, the same thing is re-demanded from Nature. Far from disturbing her, she is stimulated anew, and in a certain way we come to her assistance.

In the second case, on the contrary, it is a question of two different processes. There is a tendency to call forth a diversion; a dispersion, not to say an antagonism, of force is imposed on Nature, which exhausts her resources and paralyzes her efforts.*

But this characteristic is also a subordinate one; forming part of a whole, it should not be made use of alone.

Fifthly: As the soils in which the two viruses develop, or which they select, are not absolutely the same, the animals which constitute these soils may be considered as the re-agents, or as a touchstone, of these viruses.

Cow Pox develops better in the young horse, and in one that

---

* The two viruses only develop together when they have simultaneously attacked the organism, and then it is not certain that it will be for the immediate benefit of the latter.

has not had strangles (*la gourme*), than under any other conditions: the lymph becomes stronger there, all things being equal. This is why I have proposed vaccination *ex equo* as being the best of the vaccinations *ex animalibus*; and I may mention that I predicted the failure of the recent Neapolitan importation.

Many other animals are susceptible of Cow Pox which do not so readily contract Small Pox. In the cow, we have a soil common to both. She can take Small Pox, but much less readily than Cow Pox.

This is a source of confusion and error, which has led to the belief that Small Pox of the cow was nothing else than Cow Pox.

Finally, man can contract Cow Pox and regenerate the vaccine better than the cow; here again is a soil common to both. But man is especially a soil proper to Small Pox, which hardly ever germinates completely in the horse. The affinity of Small Pox with man, and its almost absolute incompatibility with the horse, are characteristically differential.

Some animals, as the dog and ape, are susceptible of Small Pox; but the number is not great, and the same animals can contract Cow Pox still more readily.

Most of the differential characters of the two maladies can be deduced from a graphic study—that is to say, from a description of the vesicles. Amongst them there are some which are difficult to appreciate; some have only a subordinate importance. But others are of great value.

Some of these characters are, in fact, well marked, and they have, when taken together, a very complete significance. The attempt has sometimes been made to deceive me by showing me the vesicles of Cow Pox as those of Small Pox, and *vice versâ*; but I have never hesitated to distinguish one from the other at first sight, and thus to baffle a friendly trick.

The comparative examination of the vaccinal and variolous vesicles establishes differences between them in FORM, VOLUME, COLOUR, CIRCUMFERENCE, SURFACE, AREOLA, BASE, ERYTHEMA, STRUCTURE, LIQUID, CRUST, SCAR, NUMBER, and lastly, DURATION.

Form.—The primitive Small Pox vesicle is not so regular as the Cow Pox vesicle. From its first appearance, defects can be detected, particularly with a lens, which become much more apparent towards the *fourth and fifth days*,—about the *sixth* and *seventh* if we date from the inoculation. The vaccinal vesicle is regularly circular and depressed in the centre during its entire duration. It is not the same with the variolous proto-pustule, which shows itself, particularly at its first appearance, in the form of a smooth and flattened vesicle.

Volume.—The volume of the Cow Pox vesicle at first surpasses in every way that of the variolous proto-pustule. The size of the latter only increases later, by the confluence of small vesicles. It may then surpass, and generally does surpass, that of the Cow Pox vesicle.

Colour.—The vaccine vesicle has a decided colour; it is transparent, glistening, of a bluish white—azured and silvery, if one may so speak. No trace of blood or pus sullies its purity. The variolous proto-pustule, which is less clear and duller, has somewhat the appearance of dull mother-of-pearl. It only appears slightly bluish when examined with a large and strong lens—doubtless on account of the reflection of the adjacent parts, which creates the combination of colours. Very small islets of purulent matter in the middle of the lymph are only observed at first with a lens, but soon with the naked eye. The lymph is soon invaded, and then entirely replaced, by pus. Hence an appearance, almost from the commencement, which I consider pathognomonic. This is described from nature in one of my notes made in pencil, and therefore wanting in finish.

"The general colour results principally from the existence in the vesico-pustule of two kinds of matter disseminated in small globules, which can be made out fairly well with the naked eye, but more easily with a lens. Thus, there are white opaque points, and clear or translucent ones. They are not all of the same form or size: the smallest do not attain ·5 mm., the largest are several mm. in extent; the white points are pus, the clear ones serosity.

"I did not employ pressure on the vesico-pustules in order to ascertain whether the two kinds of matter were capable of blending, but their presence together produces a characteristic appearance. This arrangement exists in the small pustules bordering upon the mother pustule, and in those which are entirely independent of it, and even far removed."

Circumference.—The circumference of the vaccine pustule, although soft, regular, and rounded at the edges, is often raised some millimètres above the skin, whilst the circumference of the inoculated variolous vesicle is almost on a level with it.

Besides, the variolous pustule is surrounded by small pustules, which are sometimes quite distinct, and at other times more or less blended with it in such a way as to deface its edges. Moreover, it is never clearly defined. Combinations of intersecting lines make it triangular, quadrilateral, pentagonal, etc., and often shapeless. These supernumerary vesicles are sometimes rather distant from the arm which is their headquarters. They may even be observed on the fore-arm, shoulder, etc., but they never stray sufficiently from the seat of inoculation, to represent the general eruption. This does not generally exist; but it is in all cases consecutive to the secondary fever.

The considerable elevation of the edges of the vaccine vesicles and the number of these vesicles—which in most cases does not exceed, and sometimes is less than the number of the punctures—constitute, by comparison with what occurs in the case of the variolous proto-pustules, two essential characters, by which they can be easily distinguished by touch alone. I have trusted myself several times to this diagnostic refinement.

Surface.—The vaccine vesicle presents a gentle and regular slope from the edges to the centre, which is umbilicated. The variolous proto-pustule shows a surface with irregular depressions. The umbilication scarcely exists on it, and, only as if to preserve the mark of the puncture.

Areola.—The vaccinal areola is of a bright, deep, uniform red; it is regular, soft, and extended. The variolous aerola is unevenly red, dull, and without lustre; it is less regular, firmer, and usually smaller than the vaccine areola; but as it is moreover studded with small pustules, of which the greater part are abortive, these have their miniature confluent areolæ, which must also be taken into account.

Base.—The base of the variolous vesicle is hard, tense, and swollen, as if it were phlegmonous. It is deeper and less clearly circumscribed than that of the vaccine vesicle. The latter vesicle appears to be simply laid on the skin, the variolous vesicle seems to be formed in the cutis.

Erythema.—It is more common to see a large erythema (which must not be confounded with the areola) extending in the neighbourhood of the variolous proto-pustule, than in the neighbourhood of the vaccinal vesicle.

Structure.—The vaccinal vesicle shows cells, little pockets, which have been compared to the compartments of an orange. The variolous proto-pustule has generally only one cavity; but I have not had an opportunity of dissecting it, so as to prove whether, like secondary pustules, or deuto-pustules, it encloses a variolous disc.

Liquid.—Good vaccine is ropy, viscous, glutinous, and always serous. If pus be found in the vesicle, it is because there is no longer any vaccine in it. The variolous liquid has not these characters; it does not long remain serous; it rapidly becomes altogether purulent without losing its virulent properties.

On the *eighth day*, there is no longer any lymph to be collected in the variolous proto-pustule. The liquid of this proto-pustule can be used for inoculation for a much longer period than that of the vaccine vesicle, which posseses its greatest energy at the time when it can first be taken, in however small a quantity.

Crust.—The vaccine crust is thick, and ecthymatous—at first yellow, stalactiform, and transparent; then black, opaque, and compact; it is glistening, uniform, dry, firm, and adherent. The crust of the variolous proto-pustule is flat, impetiginoid; at first yellow, then a dirty black; porous; it is dull, dead, pitchy, soft, always opaque, easily detaches itself, and quickly re-forms.

Scar.—The granulation and the mode of cicatrization differ in the two pustules.

The scar of vaccination is more spread out, more depressed, deeper, more regular, whiter, and more characteristically crimped than that of the variolous proto-pustule. The latter is cut off by a little dull whiteness from the surrounding skin. It is, all things being equal, much less apparent than the ordinary scar of a deuto-pustule in the natural malady. This is due perhaps to the apparently phlegmonous engorgement by which the proto-pustule has been surrounded, and which has taken its place.

Number.—All variolous inoculations are followed by pustules. This is not so in the case of vaccinal inoculations; the variolous vesicle generally exhibits, as has been already said, small satellite pustules, which often blend with it and deform it. In vaccination we hardly ever meet with a single supernumerary pustule, and, moreover, this is never confluent with the mother-pustule. If the vaccinator intentionally make punctures which are quite contiguous, the neighbouring pustules which occasionally result do not tend to encroach on each other at their edges.

Duration.– Varioline has a rather shorter incubation than vaccine, but the variolous proto-pustule generally lasts longer than the vaccinal pustule.

I will not speak of the secondary fever, which is very intense in inoculated Small Pox, and is scarcely perceptible in most cases of vaccination,—in which, in contra-distinction to what occurs in Small Pox, a primitive fever can sometimes be observed,—nor of the profuse perspirations and rashes which occur at different parts of the body, following on variolous inoculation.

We must recognize positively that variola and vaccinia are quite distinct from each other.

We shall find in this certainty a considerable indemnification, for all well-established truth opens the horizon to other new truths.

Let us still follow analogy, but always with prudence.

If Cow Pox can take the place of her human sister Small Pox, and afford protection from her, may we not presume that other viruses will lend themselves to analogous substitutions? Let us profit by this information; let us seek for the vaccine of other virulent maladies, and principally of the more serious ones, without ever ceasing to follow, as we never cease to keep a watch over, our guide: Analogy.

Thus, every question set at rest, gives rise to several others to be solved; in whatever direction our conquests extend, we find immense territories to cultivate. Science is infinite, its domain is inexhaustible.

I have made the greater part of my researches on viruses in conjunction with M. Mathieu, veterinary surgeon, of Sèvres.

(*Courrier Médical du* 26 *Mai*, 1866.)

COW POX AT EYSINES (LAFORET).

(FIRST OUTBREAK.)

1881.

DUBREUILH.

[*Rapport sur le Concours de Vaccine de* 1881. *M. Ch. Dubreuilh, Rapporteur. Travaux du Conseil d'Hygiène Publique et de Salubrité du Département de la Gironde pendant l'année* 1881. *Tome* xxiii. *Bordeaux*, 1882.]

TRANSLATED BY THE EDITOR.

DISCOVERY OF COW POX IN THE GIRONDE.

ON November 17th, 1881, M. Landeau, physician at Eysines (Gironde), wrote the following letter to the Prefect of the Gironde:—"I have the honour to report to you a discovery, which I have just made, of a cow with vesicles of Cow Pox on the teats. On Sunday, the 13th inst., an inhabitant of the village of Laforêt, in the commune of Eysines, came to my house to consult me about an eruption, which had appeared four days previously on his hand, face, and neck. This eruption appeared in the form of several silvery vesicles; large, flattened, depressed in the centre, and surrounded by an erythematous areola, recalling to my mind an inoculation of vaccine lymph. When carefully questioned as to the exciting cause of this cutaneous affection, the man informed me that amongst his cows, there was one which was very difficult to milk, having had, for seven or eight days, large *boutons* on its teats, from which pus escaped. On going this morning to verify this interesting fact, I was convinced that he was suffering from Cow Pox, the true regenerating agent of vaccine. If you wish, Sir, to have the subject which has been brought under my observation examined by experienced persons, they will find me at their service."

This letter was sent to me by the Prefect on the evening of the 18th inst. On the morning of the 19th, I went to Dr. Pujos, chief physician of the *Bureau de Bienfaisance*, and begged him to be kind enough to accompany me to Eysines, in order to verify the fact. We were sorry not to find Dr. Landeau at home, but we proceeded to the village of Laforêt, to see the milker who asserted that he had been inoculated from his cow.

This man, aged thirty-one, told us that on November 11th, the first vesicle appeared on the ring finger of the left hand; on the 14th, other vesicles appeared on his hand and on his face. He had suffered from extreme lassitude and loss of appetite. These symptoms had led him to consult M. Landeau. We were only able to see the cicatrices of these vesicles. The cow which was suspected of having communicated Cow Pox to the milker, who milked her every day, was in the fields with six others. She was eleven years old; the vesicular eruption was very characteristic, scattered on the teats and udder. On the day of our visit, we found only crusts, resembling the crusts of the vesicles of Small Pox. Six of these crusts were detached, two were still soft and not so dry as the others; they were put between two slips of glass, and on our arrival at Bordeaux were entrusted to M. Duluc, the veterinary surgeon of the Department, who obligingly placed his services at our disposal. On November 26th, the first inoculation took place. The crusts from the Eysines cow were mixed, some with glycerine, others with a little tepid water. Dr. Pujos and I undertook this in the presence of several persons, who met at M. Duluc's house.

The same day I hastened to make this fact known to the *Société de médecine et de chirurgie*, begging them to appoint a Commission to control our experiments, and, if they should succeed, to follow the results.

First Inoculation.

On November 26th, M. Duluc inoculated with the Eysines vaccine, a Bordeaux heifer, nine months old, on the right side of the belly in the region of the teats. Previously this region had been soaped and shaved. He made eighteen punctures, consisting of an equal number of inoculations of the mixtures referred to above. The heifer was tied up to prevent her from licking the punctures, and she was frequently examined by the man appointed to look after the shed. Dr. Pujos and I went every day to study the effects of this inoculation.

There was scarcely the least derangement noticeable in the general condition of the animal. She fed well, had a lively aspect, and showed no symptom of fever, except slight pain and heat in the region inoculated. During the *first two days* nothing particular was remarked in the state of the punctures, but on the evening of the *third day*, a red areola was noticed round each of them, which indicated that inflammation was taking place there. During the *fourth day* swelling occurred, the cuticle being raised and giving hope of vesiculation; but this might, on the other hand, be nothing more than the result of the introduction of foreign matter under the cuticle. It was not until the evening of the same day, that the characters became more marked, and that an accumulation of serosity took place at several of the inoculated places; but this was not sufficiently abundant nor characteristic to show conclusively that it was a true variolous vesicle. It was not really until the *fifth day*, that we could be almost certain that we had to do with the transmission of Cow Pox. Nearly all the punctures were raised and perfectly circumscribed. A white ring surrounded the large crust resulting from the deep incision which had been made in order to introduce a large quantity of liquid.

By raising the crust and forcibly squeezing one of these vesicles with forceps, a white limpid serosity, with a yellowish tinge, escaped.

On Thursday, December 1st, the members of the Commission appointed by the *Société de médecine et chirurgie*, MM. Charles Dubreuilh, Donaud, Pujos, and Saint-Philippe, came to see the heifer, and were able to establish the fact that the vesicles, which had developed exactly on the *fourth and fifth days*, had reached on the *sixth day* the commencement of the stage of desiccation. The swelling had subsided, and the whitish ring surrounding the crust was already assuming a purulent character. Nevertheless, on squeezing these vesicles with forceps, a serous exudation was still found which was fit for inoculation.

It was decided by the members of the Commission that the inoculation of a second heifer should be undertaken.

Second Inoculation.

On Friday, December 2nd, M. Duluc proceeded to make the second inoculation on a Garonne heifer, four months old, in the following manner: Heifer No. 2 was thrown and held by two assistants; she was soaped and shaved on the right side of the belly. Heifer No. 1 was also thrown and held. After charging a grooved lancet, each vesicle was forcibly squeezed in order to express all the serosity.

M. Duluc made fifteen punctures on the second heifer: five only were made with the limpid serosity; the ten others were made with a mixture of sanguineous serosity and of matter more or less purulent, being all that was collected at the bottom of the vesicles which were well advanced towards desiccation.

The newly inoculated heifer was tied up in its stall, but during the night she broke the rope, and next morning was found walking about in the stable. It was noticed that she frequently licked herself on the seat of the punctures. It was easy to see that she had devoted a part of the night to this operation.

In fact, for the next five to six days the punctures showed nothing abnormal, except perhaps a tendency towards cicatrization and a little heat in the part; but on the *seventh day*—that is to say, on Friday, December 9th, two small vesicles made their appearance as the result of inoculation of the sero-sanguineous matter obtained by scraping the vesicles of the first heifer. They were situated quite close to the nipples; a slight inflammatory swelling could also be seen at the other punctures.

A heifer, eight months old, from a herd in the Bacalan marshes, was immediately obtained for inoculation.

Third Inoculation.

Sunday, December 11th, at 1 p.m., M. Duluc proceeded to inoculate the third heifer in the presence of about a dozen persons. The operation was carried out with the same precautions and in the same manner as in the case of the second heifer; the same assistants were employed. The two vesicles situated near the nipples of the second heifer had undergone further development, and furnished sufficient serosity for six punctures. For comparison M. Duluc made five more punctures with matter collected by squeezing the vesicles which were accidentally abortive. We had every reason to think that a satisfactory result could not be obtained with lymph collected from vesicles so little developed, and it was not until the Saturday—that is to say, the *sixth day* of the inoculation—that we found in the place of the eleven punctures, eleven perfectly developed vesicles. We collected the liquid of these vesicles in the presence of several colleagues; seven tubes were very rapidly filled with a slightly opaline liquid. They were enclosed in a larger glass tube, which was waxed and sealed.

M. Baillet, veterinary surgeon to the town, was kind enough to inoculate a heifer, from the abattoir, on Wednesday, 21st.

Fourth Inoculation.

A fourth heifer was inoculated on Monday, December 19th, with the vaccine from the third heifer. Eighteen punctures were made; the development of the vesicles began on the *third day*. The *fourth day* they were completely formed, with the characteristic umbilication.

Saturday, December 24th. Drs. Saint-Philippe, Layet, Pery, and Charles Dubreuilh, members of the Commission; Drs. Verdalle, Moreau, Dubourg, Martial-Durand, and Trocard, members of the *Société de médecine*, and M. Baillet, veterinary surgeon to the town, assembled at 10 a.m., at M. Duluc's establishment. The heifer was examined with the greatest care; the vesicles were perfectly formed, the liquid which escaped on pressure was not yet abundant; it was evident that they had not yet arrived at maturity.

Messrs. Trocard, Durand, and Dubourg, filled tubes in order to inoculate children. I myself inoculated a little girl who was brought to me—Suzanne Delau, three years old, living at 20, Place d'Aquitaine.

A fifth heifer was inoculated, aged five weeks.

The vaccine virus obtained from the third heifer had been inoculated in a heifer from the abattoir, by M. Baillet, veterinary surgeon to the town. Seven punctures were made on Wednesday, December 21st; other punctures were made concurrently on the same heifer with ordinary vaccine. On Sunday, December 25th, M. Duluc and I went to see the results of this inoculation; the seven punctures with the Eysines vaccine had commenced to inflame, forming little vesicles. On December 27th, Dr. Moussous, Professor of Midwifery, came with me to visit the heifer inoculated at the abattoir, and the fifth heifer which was at M. Duluc's. This distinguished Professor felt no doubt as to the nature of the eruption which he saw. Six tubes filled with Eysines vaccine were taken to vaccinate children at the St. André hospital.

M. Duluc and I, wishing to ascertain whether the Cow Pox eruption had given our heifers an immunity from a fresh inoculation, heifer No. 4 was taken to the abattoir, and on Wednesday, December 28th, was inoculated by M. Baillet with vaccine from a heifer which was intended to be used for the public vaccinations. No inflammatory process manifested itself.

Friday, December 30th, the *Conseil central d'hygiène et de salubrité* appointed a Commission to examine and control the results of inoculation with the Eysines Cow Pox. This Commission was composed of Drs. Lande, Métadier, Armaingaud, Donaud, and Peyronny (veterinary surgeon). They examined the fifth heifer, five months old, inoculated on Saturday, December 24th: there were twelve vaccinal vesicles, which were large and well developed.

A heifer, aged three months, of the Garonne breed, was inoculated in the presence of the Commission, and by one of its members. She was intended for the *Académie de médecine* of Paris. Thirty punctures were made on her.

Little Suzanne Delau, who had been vaccinated on December 24th, from heifer No. 4, was shown to the Commission. This child, who was rather ill-developed, had three vesicles on each arm, which were large, umbilicated, and surrounded by a very intense inflammatory areola. On Saturday, December 31st,

Dr. Armaingaud, member of the *Conseil d'hygiène*, came with me to M. Duluc's in order to observe the effect of the new virus on the children.

Simonnet, four months old; Moulinier, ten days old; Simon, three weeks old; Aubeau, one year old; Pescadores, two brothers, one sixteen months old, the other six years old, were inoculated on the left arm with the vaccine from little Delau, and on the right arm with Cow Pox from heifer No. 5.

At the meeting of the *Société de médecine et de chirurgie* on January 6th, 1882, Drs. Trocard and Durand gave very interesting details of the results of inoculations made on children with vaccine taken from heifer No. 4. All the vesicles had developed, and were very beautiful and characteristic. Dr. Durand inoculated simultaneously the virus in one arm and the Cow Pox in the other arm; he found that the vesicles produced by the latter virus were larger and had a more extensive inflammatory areola.

The inoculation practised by Dr. Moussous at the St. André Hospital on three children, was successful in only two of them; the third, a wretched little thing, was suffering from thrush. The success of the two first was absolutely certain. Like Dr. Durand, Dr. Moussous observed that all the vesicles were not of equal size, but this is always the case when first starting a new stock of vaccine lymph. I consider, added Professor Moussous, that we are dealing with an excellent vaccine, that we ought to do everything possible to collect it, and with it to renew the vaccine previously at our disposal.

Dr. Armaingaud had never seen a finer result than that in three out of the six children whom he had vaccinated.

Finally, on an observation of Professor Azam that it would be the duty of those who are concerned in the public interest, to cultivate this Cow Pox, which has originated here, the *Société de médecine et chirurgie* put to the vote the following resolution which, after discussion, was adopted unanimously. "The *Société de médecine et chirurgie* of Bordeaux having heard the statement of the facts concerning vaccination with the Cow Pox, recently discovered at Eysines by M. Landeau, as set forth by Drs. Ch. Dubreuilh, Moussous, Martial-Durand, Trocard, Armaingaud, etc.; and having examined several children who had been vaccinated with this virus, cultivated on heifers, express the hope that the Prefect of Gironde and the Mayor of Bordeaux will take the necessary steps to have this new vaccine cultivated, and distributed by every possible means."

Let us now follow up the heifer which was inoculated on

December 30th, before the Commission of the *Conseil central d'hygiène* of Gironde, and presented to the *Académie de médecine* of Paris by the kind assistance of Professor Depaul on Tuesday, January 3rd.

We have mentioned that this heifer had been inoculated by thirty punctures on the belly in the neighbourhood of the teats. The vesicles arising from these punctures had not yet attained their maximum development, but as four full days had elapsed since the inoculation, and as at this period the vaccine of the heifer possesses its full activity, Dr. Hervieux did not hesitate to utilise the vesicles for the meeting of the Academy on January 3rd.

In thirteen vaccinations made during the first month after birth, the vaccine taken from the fifth heifer inoculated at Bordeaux, succeeded twelve times, as completely as possible, for with the exception of one case where there were only three *boutons*, the other subjects exhibited six, seven, or eight beautiful vesicles. The vaccinations had been made by four punctures in each arm. The vesicles were large, very well developed, and possessed all the characters of genuine vaccine. To guard against any contingency, Dr. Hervieux had a heifer inoculated, on January 5th, with eighty-four incisions on the animal's belly, which had been previously shaved. Tuesday, January 10th, the vesicles of this heifer, the sixth from the cow at the village of Laforêt, were utilised by the *Académie de médecine* in the following manner :—

1st. To vaccinate those who presented themselves at the next public vaccination.

2nd. To collect a large quantity of vaccine for different destinations.

3rd. To inoculate a seventh heifer.

From the general statement of the operations made by Dr. Hervieux, in presence of the members of the Academy, recorded in his report read at the meeting of January 24th (see *Bulletin de l'Académie de médecine*, the following conclusions result :—

"1st. That the heifer sent to the Academy by M. Ch. Dubreuilh of Bordeaux, had in the neighbourhood of the teats about thirty vesicles, which exhibited on the *fourth and fifth days* of their development the characters of genuine Vaccine.

"2nd. That the matter extracted from these vesicles, either by punctures with a lancet or by squeezing with the forceps, and inoculated either into heifers or children, gave rise to a vesiculation completely identical with that of normal Vaccine.

"3rd. That, with very few exceptions, the inoculations produced as many positive results as there were children vaccinated, and very nearly as many as there were punctures.

"4th. That the transplantation of the vaccine from the Bordeaux heifer to heifers bought by us, was followed by complete success, since we had on each of them as many successful vesicles as there were incisions.

"5th. That we were thus able to substitute the Gironde vaccine for our official vaccine, both for the Tuesday series and the Saturday series.

"6th. That M. Chambon's vaccination station, which supplies all the hospitals of Paris, has also been able to renew its animal vaccine, and thus to assist in the propagation of the Gironde vaccine in our city.

"7th. That, in consequence of these facts, the Gironde vaccine deserves to be classed with the most celebrated vaccines, the vaccine of 1836, known as that of Pau, and the vaccine of 1866 of Beaugency.

"At the meeting, January 6th, Dr. Armaingaud, in the name of a Commission composed of MM. Métadier, Lande, Donaud, Dubreuilh, Peyronny, and Armaingaud, read before the *Conseil central d'hygiène* a report, in which he laid before you the practical results of the discovery of the Eysines Cow Pox, set forth its importance, and proposed to you means of utilising it for the benefit of the public health.'

"In consequence of this report, your Commission submits to you the following conclusions, which were adopted by the *Conseil d'hygiène*, and sent to the Prefect of Gironde:

"1st. To appropriate from the funds of the Department, an annual sum of, say 5,000 francs, for the preservation, cultivation, and propagation of the Eysines Cow Pox, by the successive and continuous inoculation from calf to calf.

"2nd. In case this sum could not be voted immediately by the *Conseil Général* at its extraordinary sitting in the month of January, would it not be possible, from the urgency of the case, to appropriate to this use the available portion of the fund intended for the premiums of vaccinated children, which, voted for two years by the *Conseil Général*, has not been employed up to the present time, and which will be still less needed under the new organisation which we are preparing?

"3rd. To bring officially to the notice of the public, by a préfectoral announcement published in the newspapers and posted up in the communes of the Department, the discovery of the Eysines Cow Pox, of which the genuineness has been proved by the *Conseil d'hygiène* of Gironde and accepted by the *Société de médecine et chirurgie* of Bordeaux, and by the *Académie de médecine* of Paris.

"Such, gentlemen, is the very much condensed history of the discovery of the Eysines Cow Pox.

"Eighteen heifers have been successively inoculated since the month of November; they have served to spread the new vaccine not only in Gironde, but over the whole of France and in foreign countries. We may even assert that this discovery has given a new start to vaccination. Paris began by giving it a welcome; and the departments have followed her example. More than three hundred tubes have been distributed in Bordeaux, in Gironde, and in the Departments of Gers, Lot-et-Garonne, Haute-Garonne, Basses- and Hautes- Pyrénées, Charente, Ariège, Finistère, and Isère, in Algeria; to Athens, Hayti, and London.

"The reporter of your Commission hopes he may be allowed to take from his correspondence some facts which are full of interest for the *Conseil d'hygiène*."

Dr. Brun-Buisson, of Voiron (Isère), writes me as follows :—

"Our little town and its neighbourhood have been ravaged for more than a year by an epidemic of Small Pox, of more than usual violence. The first cases appeared amongst the rag-pickers of a paper factory, which then received its rags from Italy. This source may have something to do with the especial virulence of the germs of this Small Pox, or perhaps the vaccine which we have been using may have lost its strength. A fact which made me entertain the latter supposition was that a great many children were attacked, and children who had been vaccinated within two, three, or four years. At the present moment, I have a niece attacked by the epidemic, and yet she had, six months ago, as a result of vaccination performed under the best conditions, three vesicles which have left very characteristic marks. I believe that, under these circumstances, you may render us a great service by forwarding some of the new to replace our old vaccine."

From another quarter, Dr. Bordot, *Médecin de colonisation* in Algeria, being charged by the Department of Algiers to establish a vaccine institute at Beni-Mestour, near Cheragas, writes to me: "I shall be happy to make the first attempts with the Eysines Cow Pox."

Hayti, ravaged by an epidemic of Small Pox (of which the *Moniteur*, brought to me by the consul of this small republic, shows the heavy mortality), begs for some of the new vaccine.

Twelve tubes have been immediately sent to the medical staff of Port-au-Prince.

Lastly, even the country of Jenner comes to the Gironde to ask for Cow Pox.

"You will render a great service to our National Vaccine Establishment," writes Dr. Buchanan to me, "if you will have the kindness to give us vaccine from one of the heifers you have inoculated with the spontaneous Cow Pox from Laforêt. I therefore beg you to send us some of this vaccine for use on the animals in our establishments in London."

Impressed with the importance of this great discovery, and with the benefits which ought to result from it on behalf of vaccination and the well-being of communities; upheld by the sympathetic encouragement of the medical profession, and of the learned societies, M. Duluc, veterinary surgeon to the Department and the reporter of your Commission, have, at our own expense, continued the cultivation of the Eysines Cow Pox for more than three months. It would be unfair not to point out to the *Conseil central d'hygiène* and to the Administration, the active and disinterested part taken by M. Duluc, in the preservation of the new vaccine. Associated in the work, he placed everything at my disposal and that of the distinguished colleagues who came to him to obtain the vaccine—zeal, devotion, and intelligence, and his establishment and assistants to take care of the heifers.

Also, in consequence of the immense success of the Gironde Cow Pox, and the sacrifices which have been made by those who have undertaken its cultivation, we hope that the *Conseil Général* of the Department will take into consideration the request made by the *Conseil d'hygiène central* to assist, by a generous and philanthropic grant, in the preservation, cultivation, and distribution, for a long time to come, of this new source of vaccine.

CH. DUBREUILH.

COW POX AT EYSINES

(SECOND OUTBREAK),

1883.

AND AT CÉRONS,

1884.

LAYET.

[*Rapports sur la Découverte du Second Vaccin d'Eysines, par Dr. A. Layet. Rapport au Conseil municipal sur le Service de Vaccinations et Revaccinations publiques pendant l'année* 1883. *Par M. A. Plumeau, adjoint au maire* 1884.

TRANSLATED BY THE EDITOR.

FIRST REPORT ON THE DISCOVERY OF THE SECOND EYSINES COW POX.

TO THE MAYOR.

SIR,

I propose in my own name and in that of M. Baillet, veterinary surgeon to the town, to render you an account of the experiments undertaken in the municipal service of vaccination, with a view to ascertaining the nature and character of the eruption observed on three cows on the farm of M. Lalanne at Eysines, and on the milkman and milkwoman who came into contact with these cows. This multiple eruption was discovered and announced to the Municipal Service of Vaccination by M. Ducamp, a doctor at Bruges. In his letter, M. Ducamp expressed the opinion that it might be a case of spontaneous Cow Pox. On receipt of this letter, which was placed in the hands of M. Durand, *Médecin-vaccinateur de service*, by M. Ducamp's son, on Thursday, March 22nd, 1883, at the Academy, during a public vaccination, you immediately appointed a Commission composed of Drs. Dupuy, Durand, Pujos, and Layet, and of the veterinary surgeons, Messrs. Baillet and Peyronny, who proceeded next day to M. Lalanne's farm in the village of Eysines.

The members of this Commission, in the first place, established the existence in the milkwoman, who milked the cows, of a vesicle without well-marked characters, situated on the upper lip at the opening of the right nostril, which had produced erysipelatous inflammation, with fever; a disorder which compelled the patient to keep in bed. On being questioned, she stated that she had inoculated herself with the disease by her fingers touching the part attacked. The milkman showed, on the dorsal aspect of both hands, a certain number of ulcerated sores, which caused swelling of the parts; sores which had lost all character of a specific eruption in consequence of repeated friction and washing.

The milkman did not hesitate to ascribe, as the cause of his malady, the repeated contact with the teats of three cows,

[illegible]

[illegible] the means of comparing the evolution of the real [illegible] with that of the supposed vaccine which was under investigation.

The following are the phenomena which were observed.— [illegible] which was intended for the municipal [illegible] normal course, the [illegible] was being experimented upon, vaccinated on March [illegible] at a quarter past three, with the liquid from the cows said [illegible] from spontaneous Cow Pox, showed at the end of eight days, at the seat of the punctures, only some slight [illegible] of the size of a pin's head. We must mention that [illegible] punctures [illegible] were made—11 with discharge from the cow first attacked, 5 from the second, and 6 from the third The slight inflammatory process to which the elevations were due, was observed alike in all the punctures. The word elevation, which we have here used, shows the undecided character of the eruption; but it was impossible not to see that a special inflammatory process of some kind was present.

[M. Layet then reports the result of microscopic examination of the blood of the inoculated heifers.—E.M.C.]

* * * * * * *

We were led to inoculate a second heifer with the lymph which exuded on pressing the little elevations above mentioned, whose want of character did not disturb our convictions. This second operation was performed on March 30th, 1883, by MM. Layet, Peyronny, and Baillet. We always employed for all these operations new lancets, and forceps previously scalded, or heated in the flame. Fourteen punctures were made on this second heifer. These punctures, having been made, the first heifer under examination, which had furnished the lymph, was then vaccinated with the vaccine of the Service. This, by means of which we sought to find out whether the immunity resulting from a first efficacious vaccination had been acquired, speedily caused the characteristic eruption; in the case of this heifer, therefore, there was no acquired immunity. The second experimental heifer to which the Eysines virus was transmitted, continued until the following Thursday, April 5th, without showing the least sign of eruption. On the evening of Thursday, slight reddish elevations, without any very determined characters, were seen. The next day, just as we were on the point of definitely doubting the vaccinal value of these elevations and of selling the animal for slaughter, a final examination showed at two of the inoculated points, two vesicles characteristic of Cow Pox. The next morning, April 7th, the nature of these vesicles was established by MM. Pujos, Plumeau, and Peyronny. In consequence of these observations, MM. Layet, Peyronny, and Baillet made fourteen punctures on a third heifer with liquid expressed from one of the *boutons* of the second experimental heifer. New lancets and previously heated forceps were again employed.

[M. Layet then details the result of microscopical examination of the blood of this heifer.— E.M.C.]

* * * * * * *

The fourteen punctures on the third heifer all gave rise to magnificent vaccine vesicles; and this result was verified by

SECOND REPORT OF THE EXPERIMENTS UNDERTAKEN BY THE MUNICIPAL VACCINATION SERVICE.

TO THE MAYOR.

SIR,

In accordance with the conclusions of the preceding Report, as to the necessity of confirming, by two final experiments, the results obtained in the Municipal Vaccination Service, one being to ascertain whether a heifer, from association with a vaccinated heifer with vaccine vesicles still developing, would be susceptible of infection, either by immediate contact, or by indirect transmission; and the second, the most important and the most irrefutable, to assure ourselves of the acquired immunity, on the one hand of the three Eysines cows, and on the other of the milkman and milkwoman infected by them, by vaccinating these three cows and the milkman and milkwoman: in accordance, as I have said, with the conclusions of this Report, the test asked for has been carried out; and it is the final result of the researches and the experiments undertaken, that I have the honour to submit to you to-day.

On Friday, April 20th, M. Baillet made, with a lancet, previously heated in the flame, fourteen simple punctures, that is to say, without vaccine, in a heifer which had come direct from the market. This heifer was placed in the same stall as the vaccinated heifer, and treated in the same way.

On Wednesday, April 25th,—the same day as that on which a Commission composed of Drs. Dupuy, Durand, Pujos, and Layet, M. Ducamp (of Bruges), and veterinary surgeons, Messrs. Baillet and Peyronny, had been called together to go to Eysines to the house of M. Lalanne, who, at the request of M. Ducamp, of Bruges, had consented to allow the cows, milkman and milkwoman, of his farm to be vaccinated—M. Baillet observed at the abattoir, on the experimental heifer, a vaccine vesicle, and at once came to inform me of it. M. Baillet declared, at the same time, to the Commission, that he had certainly used a lancet heated in a flame, but that he had made the punctures in this heifer without having previously washed his hands, a precaution [illegible] attacked by the eruption, and [illegible] belonging to the same [illegible] attacked, had not shown [illegible]

[illegible] been found for making a comparison [illegible] experiment.

The [illegible] and his wife received three punctures on each [illegible] were vaccinated by twelve to fourteen punctures on the left flank, that is to say, on the side on which they did *not* [illegible] lying down

M. Ducamp, of Bruges, undertook to watch the course of our experiments, and to let us know as soon as there was any result.

We now come to a point which it is well to notice ; it relates to the state of the cows, the milkman and the milkwoman at the time of our second visit. The milkwoman showed at the opening of the right nostril only a small crust on the point of becoming detached, and beneath it a fairly well marked scar could be seen. All inflammation had disappeared, but she told us that two or three days after we had seen her, that there had appeared on her body, under the right breast, two little vesicles, which Mme Lalanne, the proprietress of the farm, told her (and she repeated it to us) were absolutely similar to the vesicles of vaccination in infants. Another vesicle had also appeared below the right ankle, and the milkwoman told us that it was from scratching herself with her fingers that she must have given herself these vesicles. We asked to see them, and we observed the presence of fresh scars which were circular and very superficial, and very far from having the characters of the indelible mark of vaccination. Was it a case of a secondary vaccinal eruption ?

As to the milkman, nothing remained on his hands except sufficiently well-marked scars, traces of the ulcerations which we had observed.

On the cows, the eruptions had nearly disappeared. Nothing remained on the teats except some small shrivelled or flattened vesicles, and at the seat of the ulcerations very superficial white scars, contrasting with the blackish skin of the teats.

On Wednesday, May 2nd, M. Ducamp, of Bruges, wrote to me to inform me of the result of the vaccinations made on April 25th. I transcribe this letter word for word :—

"I visited the day before yesterday, and again to-day, the cows, the milkman and milkwoman. The day before yesterday the three cows which had the original vesicles, showed no trace of commencing vesiculation, nor did they to-day. *Griselle*, on the contrary, who had escaped the natural Cow Pox, had on the day before yesterday commencing vaccine vesicles, which are to-day very characteristic.

"As to the milkman and milkwoman, they have had for four to five days, a little redness at the level of the punctures, which has disappeared. This fact appears to be as convincing as possible ; but it would be well if the Commissioners would come and verify it, and give their own account of it ; I should personally be pleased if they would.

"DUCAMP."

On May 4th, at 9 a.m., a Commission, composed of MM. Layet, Pujos, Baillet, and Peyronny, went to Eysines, to M. Lalanne's farm, with the view of verifying the result announced by M. Ducamp.

This result is in truth most clear and convincing.

The three cows primarily attacked showed on examination nothing at the seat of inoculation except a smooth surface, without a trace of any eruption whatever.

The milkman and milkwoman showed nothing except the remains of simple punctures.

The *fourth cow*, on the contrary, the one used as a *control* experiment, exhibited at the seat of the inoculations fine characteristic vaccine vesicles, equal in number to the punctures which had been made.

I have informed you, Sir, of the whole series of researches undertaken by the Municipal Vaccination Service. The facts need no comment. Indeed, my intention is to abstain entirely from them, leaving it to everyone to draw the conclusions to which scientific truth must lead. I cannot, however, omit to call attention to some points which stand out prominently from all that precedes :—

1st. The extreme importance and utility which is more and more recognised, of a Service which, in addition to its function, which is essentially the preservation of the public health, has lent itself to researches and experiments, the importance of which no one can dispute.

2nd. The difficulty there is in guarding against all chances of error, when researches such as these in question are being made.

3rd. The necessity of having recourse to a final and irrefutable test : the comparative vaccination of cows supposed to have been attacked by Cow Pox, and of other cows not attacked, and so far as possible which belong to the same herd, that is to say, having lived under the same conditions without having shown any eruption.

Lastly, there are some points deserving consideration which concern at the same time, the *scientific* and the *practical side* of the question, which seem to me useful for future reference.

They relate :—

1st. To the absence of the *classical vaccinal characters* in the bullous eruption observed on the *teats* of the Eysines cows, and not on the *udder*.

2nd. To the *analogy* which exists between the *bullæ* of this vaccinogenic eruption and the vesicles (*ampoules perlées*) of true Horse Pox, to which M. Bouley has directed attention, and also between the ulcerations of this same vaccinogenic eruption and the ulcerations of Horse Pox.

3rd. To the *dissimilarity* of the eruption seen on the three Eysines cows by M. Ducamp, of Bruges, and that seen on the Laforêt cow, by M. Landeau, of Eysines, who discovered the first Cow Pox called Eysines. This dissimilarity is certified by Dr. Landeau and Dr. Pujos, who have seen both eruptions; hence the following conclusion:—*Are there several eruptive maladies of the bovine species which are capable of furnishing true vaccine?* Side by side with these conclusions, another has occurred to me which deserves especial attention. Allow me to lay it before you.

There is anything but agreement about what is called *spontaneous Cow Pox.* According to some, the vaccinogenic eruption is never spontaneous in the cow, but originates from Horse Pox. According to others, the eruption develops in the cow under special conditions of predisposition, or of preparation of her organism. In any case, Cow Pox is always supposed to manifest itself with its classical characters, in the form of an *umbilicated* vesicle.

The discovery of the *second Eysines Cow Pox* shows that the classical characters are not invariably present. I ask myself whether its absence may not be a proof in favour of the spontaneousness of the eruption in the cow, just like the bullous vesicle of Horse Pox, which is not umbilicated.

The umbilication would then be the essential character of a *transmitted* vaccinogenic eruption. Two kinds of Cow Pox would then be recognised in the cow: one, *really spontaneous,* analogous to Horse Pox in the horse, without umbilication and with all the characters of a bullous eruption; the other, the classical Cow Pox umbilicated, *owing to its transmission* from the horse to the cow. If this be the case, the Municipal Vaccination Service of Bordeaux, will have had the good fortune to discover really spontaneous Cow Pox.

DR. A. LAYET,
Medical Director of the Municipal Vaccination Service.

May 1883.

REPORT ON THE DISCOVERY OF A CASE OF SPONTANEOUS COW POX AT CÉRONS GIRONDE.

TO THE MAYOR.

SIR,

I have the honour to lay before you a special Report on the discovery, at Cérons, of a new case of spontaneous Cow Pox and on the renewal of the vaccine employed by the Municipal Vaccination Service. On December 25th, M. Lanusse, Administrator des Hospices, conveyed to you on the part of the Mayor of Cérons (Gironde) the news that M. Barbe, veterinary surgeon, and M. Pichausel, doctor at Podensac, had observed on an isolated cow, in the locality of Cérons, an eruption which they supposed to be Cow Pox.

On December 26th, at 8 a.m., M. Bailiet, veterinary surgeon to the town, and I, went to Cérons, where we were received by M. Dubroca (the Mayor), and MM. Barbe and Pichausel. The cow mentioned, showed, on the four teats and on the adjacent parts of the udder, a very considerable number of small vesicles, the greater part already dried up and covered with a black crust, some of them containing a liquid more or less milky. This eruption was very confluent, and did not exhibit *a single umbilicated vesicle*. Six or seven tubes were filled with the liquid of these vesicles, with all the precautions required in such a case. The cow was in milk, and the owner used her milk to feed a foster-child. During the period of the eruption, which was only observed on Tuesday, December 22nd, the condition of the child seemed to be affected by the modifications which occurred in that of the cow. Milk and blood from the cow were both taken for microscopical examination.

On returning to Bordeaux on the same day, December 26th, we immediately proceeded to inoculate a heifer bought at the time in the market, with the liquid collected at Cérons.

On December 31st, on this first heifer, on which about twelve punctures had been made, three vesicles were to be seen; one more advanced than the others showed the characters of the vaccine vesicle; at the place of the other punctures, there was only a slight redness.

A second heifer was inoculated with all the precautions indicated (a new lancet, sterilised forceps, etc., etc.), with lymph from two of these vesicles; thirteen punctures were made, and on January 4th, thirteen successes were seen on this heifer. Moreover, on examining the first heifer it was discovered that all the punctures had given rise to a more or less developed vesicle. The development had been retarded, but the result was only the more striking.

A third heifer was inoculated with the Cérons vaccine on January 5th. Forty punctures gave rise to forty characteristic vesicles.

The vaccine lymph expressed from these vesicles was pure and in abundance. This heifer has been used for the Service of Public Vaccination on Thursday, January 10th.

The following is an important fact:

On January 4th I wrote to M. Barbe, veterinary surgeon, to inform him of the success obtained, begging him to be good enough to write out his own observations. For, while we followed the result of our inoculations of the two first heifers at Bordeaux, M. Barbe noticed, on December 28th, that the two persons who milked the Cérons cow, had contracted on their hands the eruption with which the latter was attacked.

Here are, moreover, the principal points of the note which M. Barbe sent me, on January 6th, concerning the complete evolution of the eruption observed on the Cérons cow, and the transmission of this eruption to the two women who milked the cow:—

"On December 23rd last, on examining for the first time the cow belonging to M. E——, *garde-champêtre* of the commune of Cérons, I observed on the udder the presence of a peculiar eruption, which was localised to this organ, and the closest examination did not reveal anything on any other part of the body (buccal, pedal, or perinæal regions). This eruption, which is situated on the teats as much as on the udder, is characterised by a great number of elevations, which are small and of varying dimensions, of which the greater part are still reddish papules, hard to the touch, and without special character.

"Those which, more advanced in their development, have arrived at the secreting stage, are hemispherical and rather vesicular than pustular, and filled with a small quantity of whitish-yellow liquid; each vesicle is surrounded by an inflammatory, pale red areola. The volume of these vesicles varies from that of No. 2 shot to that of nearly No. 7. The larger ones are principally situated on the teats, and several of them, crushed in milking, are transformed into little sores which are quite superficial, reddish and granular at the bottom.

"From the preceding symptoms, I eliminate the diagnosis of foot and mouth disease, which, however, is raging in the neighbourhood. I consider that I can diagnose the vaccinogenic disease.

"The same day I told Dr. Pichausel, of Podensac, of my observation, and through the Mayor of Cérons made it known to the Municipal Vaccination Service of Bordeaux, which at once appointed a commission to study the fact in question.

"On the morning of the 24th, the animal was again examined. The vesicles of the day before had lost their contents, and were covered by a very thin reddish-yellow crust. A number of the papules of yesterday were now vesicles with all the characters described above.

"The two women (mother and daughter), who milked the cow, one aged forty-five, the other nineteen, although having numerous scratches on their hands, showed nothing abnormal on them.

"On the morning of the 25th, the same observations were made as before; the vesicles had lost their contents, which dried on the surface in the form of thin crusts, and the papules had become vesicles which developed in their turn during the day.

"On the morning of the 26th, Professor Layet, of the Faculty of Bordeaux, and M. Baillet, veterinary surgeon to the same town, collected in our presence, with all the necessary precautions, the liquid of those vesicles which still remained.

"On the morning of the 27th, the two women who milked the cow complained that during the night they had suffered from great itching between the fingers. On examining the seat of the irritation, little reddish elevations were seen which were hard to the touch, elevations which on the 28th and following days developed into vesicles analagous to those observed on the udder of the cow.

"On the morning of the 31st, when I saw her for the last time, the latter showed no longer any trace of the eruption.

"In the history of this eruption, one important fact is to be noted: this is, that the owners of the cow, not possessing any horses had not for a long time had anything to do with them; and, in spite of the investigations which I made, I could not find, in the neighbourhood, a single horse which showed the least trace of the eruption of Horse Pox.

"One more remark has still to be made on the *rapid course of this malady*: it was first remarked only on December 22nd, dated at the earliest from the 20th, and terminated on the 30th of the same month, thus accomplishing in ten days nearly all the phases of its development."

There is no need, Sir, to urge the clearness of the preceding remarks. For the second time, since its organisation, the Municipal Vaccination Service has had the good fortune to observe the characters of the eruption which constitutes spontaneous Cow Pox, and which, up to the present time, have not been determined. The results of researches and experiments concerning the discovery and cultivation of the second Eysines Cow Pox have already been sent to the *Académie de médecine*. I think that those which have reached us to-day ought again to be brought to its notice. We have here an absolute demonstration of the importance of this Service, and of the duty which it has been called upon to perform on behalf of science and public Hygiene. Bordeaux, in fact, for the past two years, has been protected from the epidemic manifestations of Small Pox, whilst this malady has been noted all round the city.

The few deaths from Small Pox which have been published and commented upon have been traced to their origin, and have been considered as cases of importation, which can no longer find, in our city, a favourable soil in which to propagate.

I am, etc.,

DR. A. LAYET,

Medical Director of the Municipal Vaccination Service.

January 1884.

OUTBREAK

OF

COW POX NEAR CRICKLADE (WILTSHIRE),

1887.

CROOKSHANK.

[*Published in part in the British Medical Journal, December*, 1887, *and July 7th and* 14*th*, 1888.]

ON AN OUTBREAK OF COW POX NEAR CRICKLADE (WILTSHIRE).

IN the course of an investigation in 1887, undertaken on behalf of the Agricultural Department of the Privy Council into the micro-pathology of a disease in cows in Wiltshire, and its relation, if any, to scarlet fever in man, I was led, on observing several cases of transmission of this cow disease to the hands of the milkers, to pursue another line of inquiry—the nature and origin of the disease in question.

Statements of Persons on the Farms.—On visiting the farms in Wiltshire I obtained as much local information as possible by questioning the bailiff, the milkers, and others employed on the farm. Two of the head cowmen were very intelligent men, and had had the care of cattle for very many years. I took down the statements which they made, in writing, and I will give them in full as they are not without interest.

Charles Pontinc, sixty-four years of age, had been employed with cows ever since he was a boy. In fact he had had about fifty years' experience of cows. He states that this disease only occurred in the same dairy, from his experience, at long intervals. Cow Pox had last occurred on these farms twenty-five years ago. It affected the cows then in the same way as the present outbreak, upsetting the arrangements of the farm owing to the severity of the disease in the cow, and to the milkers getting their hands inoculated. He states that the teats became red and swollen. A pimple was first noticed, and a kind of blister would rise up which was broken in milking. The depth of the sore which resulted, and the thickening and large size of the scab, he considered characteristic.

The outbreak twenty-five years ago, was pronounced by his father to be Cow Pox. His father told them, at the time, that the same disease had occurred at the farm about twenty-five years previously, and that he had caught the same eruption on his hands, while other milkers on the farm were at the same time affected in the same way. His father was "cut for the Cow Pox" afterwards, but it did not take. His father, he adds, had not been previously vaccinated, as they did not vaccinate all children in those days as they do now.

This was the third outbreak of Cow Pox he had seen. He was familiar with the common diseases of cows. Cows frequently suffered from chapped teats. This affection, he thought, was due to the cows getting their teats wet and dirty, or scratched by brambles. There was also a complaint very common in the spring which was much milder than Cow Pox; it often occurred when the cows went out to grass; blisters formed which broke and dried up readily. This disease was of no consequence, but Cow Pox was a serious trouble, owing to the difficulty in milking the cows, and the disorder it caused among the milkers.

Foot and mouth disease he had seen three or four times; the cows were lame, and their mouths were affected, so that they had to be fed with a horn. Altogether it was a very different disease from Cow Pox.

Chapped teats and blistered teats were easily cured. By rubbing the teats with grease or oil, the sores quickly healed. There was another disease which they called "bad quarters," but this was quite different, for there were no sores on the teats. There were a few cases every year; it was generally owing, he thought, to the cows catching cold. He had two or three cases under his care at the present time, but they were not more numerous this year than in previous years. He thought it was a good thing for the milkers to get the Cow Pox from the cows. He had heard his father say, and had always believed himself, that those who had had the Cow Pox, would not have the Small Pox,—or would not get it so badly, and some thought they were more healthy after it.

William Winchcomb, fifty-eight years of age, also had nearly all his life had the care of cows. He was quite familiar with this disease. It was what they always called the Cow Pox. He said that twenty years ago Cow Pox broke out on another estate. The cows were affected with the same eruption which the cows on these farms had. He and his fellow milkers caught the eruption on their hands. He had escaped this time, and had no fear in milking the cows, as he believed he would not catch it again.

During this outbreak some cows with the disease were mixed with his herd, and he is quite sure that the healthy ones caught the eruption owing to his milking them. The eruption only appeared on the teats, that is to say, on the part which is grasped by the hand in milking. The cows appeared to be in good health, but they gave less milk. He gave the same account as Pontine of the various stages of the eruption.

Locality of the Wiltshire Outbreak.—There is considerable interest attached to the fact that the farms I inspected are situated a few miles from Cricklade. They are close to the borders of Gloucestershire, and about twenty-five miles from Berkeley. They are, therefore, within that district which was easily within Jenner's reach, a district which he described in his day as one in which Cow Pox was particularly prevalent.*

Time of Year.—The outbreak commenced about the end of September and lasted until about the middle of December.

Origin of the Outbreak.—I made close inquiries as to the origin of the outbreak, but beyond ascertaining with certainty that the disease appeared first at one farm, and was conveyed from this to other farms, all evidence was negative. The milkers were unable to say whether it commenced in one particular cow or whether it broke out in several simultaneously.

There were no horses on this farm, nor could I obtain the history of any horses suffering from Horse Pox on the neighbouring farms. The only information which could be obtained, and was very suggestive, was that the milkers were in the habit of receiving their friends from neighbouring farms on Sundays. The friends would assist in the milking, to get the work done as quickly as possible on these occasions. As it was reported that the same disease had occurred that summer on a neighbouring farm, it is quite possible that it was introduced by one of the milkers' friends.

Mode of Dissemination.—When the disease made its appearance at farm W, the bailiff, attributing it to the farm being for some reason unhealthy, decided to remove the cows to other farms. The herd was therefore divided into two, and some of the animals were sent to farm X, and the rest to farm Y. From these cows the disease was communicated to the healthy cows, and, as this interchange was repeated, not only of the cows, but of the milkers, the disease was communicated to all the separate farms W, X, Y, and Z.

In all cases the disease was limited to the teats, being conveyed

* The very first case of casual Cow Pox which was put to the variolous test came from Cricklade, and quite possibly from one of the very farms on which the recent outbreak has occurred, these particular dairy farms having been in existence for several generations. See vol. i., p. 105.

eruption to study, and I had to rely for the early history on the description given me by the milkers.

On visiting a byre at the time that the cows were brought in to be milked, it was very striking, on passing through the sheds, to see one animal after another affected with the eruption; an important characteristic of this affection was thus impressed on the mind—the tendency to spread through the whole herd.

On examining the eruption carefully, the degree of severity was found to differ very much in different animals. In a few cases the condition was most distressing, both to the cow and to the observer. In such cases the teats were encrusted with huge dark-brown or black crusts, which, when roughly handled by the milker, were broken and detached, exposing a bleeding, suppurating, ulcerated base. Such ulcers varied in size from a shilling to a florin, and in form were circular, ovoid, or irregular (Plate X. Vol. i.). Weeks afterwards, when the animals had recovered, the sites of these ulcers were marked by irregular scars.

All the milkers agreed as to the general characters of the malady, laying particular stress on the teats being red, swollen, and painful when handled. Vesicles would then appear on the teats, two, three, four, or more on each teat. They were soon broken in milking, and irritated into sores, which became covered with thick crusts. From four to six weeks elapsed before they had entirely healed. Other more observant milkers insisted that before the teats were red and swollen, spots or pimples first appeared which "came to a head like a blind boil." This head increased if it were not broken (which might be the case if it were situated between the bases of the teats), until it formed a "dismal-white blister" of the size of a fourpenny piece, or even larger.

General Symptoms in the Cow.—As to the general condition of the cows nothing abnormal was observed. They appeared in the best of health, and in only one particular was any difference from their condition in health stated to exist. This was, that in the majority of the cases there could be no doubt that the milk supply was diminished. This might in an individual animal escape the notice of inexperienced milkers, but the total amount of milk supplied by the herd was considerably below the average. By a rough estimation the bailiff calculated that the diminished supply of milk, taking all the herds together, had entailed a loss of about £50.

History of the Eruption Communicated to the Milkers.—The most striking characteristic of this outbreak was the communicability of the disease to the milkers. At first I only had the opportunity of studying the characters of the eruption in its later stages, but on a subsequent visit I was fortunate enough to meet with a recent case, and was thus able to follow the successive stages. This milker had vesicles which presented most typically all the characters of casual Cow Pox, and was therefore taken to London and kept under observation. I will describe this case more fully than the others, but I will first of all enumerate the various cases in the order in which they first presented themselves to me, giving their history as much as possible in the patients' own words.

Case I.—John Rawlins, milker, informed me that he was the first to catch the eruption from the cows. He states that it came as a hard, painful spot, which formed "matter" and then a "big scab." He had been inoculated about seven weeks ago. He pointed to the scar which remained on his right hand. This scar presented the characters of an irregular cicatrix, indicating considerable loss of substance. He states that he had also two places on his back, where he supposes he had inoculated himself by scratching. He had continued milking ever since, but had had no "fresh places."

Case II.—William Hibbert, senr., milker. He states that he was inoculated from the cows about the same time as John Rawlins. They were the two milkers of the herd in which Cow Pox first made its appearance. The eruption appeared in one place on each hand. He pointed to two irregular scars as the remains of the eruption.

Case III.—Joseph Lanfear, milker, states that he also caught the disease from the cows. On his right hand "a spot appeared which formed a blister, then discharged matter and produced a bad sore." Lumps formed at the bend of his elbow and in his armpit. He lost his appetite, felt very poorly, and was obliged to leave off work for two or three days and stay at home.

He states that about a fortnight or three weeks afterwards, after milking a very bad case, a sore on his left hand resulting from a wound with a rusty nail, became inflamed, and another "place broke out" at the tip of one of his fingers, but he was not poorly, nor did the lumps appear in his left armpit.

Case IV.—William King works on the farms, but was put on as a milker to take the place of one of the others with bad hands. After his fifth or sixth milking, that is to say about three days after first milking the cows, pimples appeared on his hands, which became "blistered and then ran on to bad sores." He pointed to three irregular scars on the first and third fingers and palm of the right hand. Lumps appeared in his elbow and in his armpit, but he did not feel very poorly in consequence.

CASE V.—James Febry, milker, states that about a month ago he noticed spots which appeared on both hands. His fingers swelled and were painful. He says it came first like a pimple and felt hard. Then it "weeped out" water in four or five days. There were red marks creeping up to his arm. There was a sort of throbbing pain, and he could not sleep at night.

When I saw him, I found on the right hand a scar, but on the left hand there was an ulcer about the size of a shilling covered with a thick black crust. The crust was partially detached and exposed a granulating ulcer. It was in this stage the exact counterpart of the ulcers on the cow's teats.

CASE VI.—William Hibbert, jun., milker, states that he had both hands bad about a month ago. First the index finger of the left hand, and then on the knuckle and between the first and second fingers of the right hand.

He says that "it came up like a hard pimple, and the finger became swollen and red. After a few days it 'weeped out' water and then matter came away." Both his arms were swollen, but his left arm was the worst.

About a fortnight after, he noticed kernels in his armpits, which were painful and kept him awake at night. His arms became worse, he could not raise them, and he had to give up milking. He also had had a "bad place" on the lower lip.

On examination, I found that the axillary glands were still enlarged and tender. He volunteered the statement that the places were just like the sore teats. (Plate XVII., Fig. 4, Vol. i.)

CASE VII.—John Harding, the bailiff's son, also milked the cows. He had a sore on the upper lid of his right eye and on his left hand. In both cases he had been previously scratched by a cat, and the scratches were inoculated from the cow's teats. The right hand also had been inoculated. The eruption broke out a fortnight ago. His hands were swollen, red, and hot. He felt very poorly and went to bed. Little spots like white blisters appeared on the back of his right hand. His mother remarked that they "rose up exactly as in vaccination." Thick dark-brown scabs formed. He was very ill for two or three days, but did not send for a doctor. He had painful lumps at the bend of his arm and in the armpit. He gave up milking and had not taken to it since.

On examining him the thick crusts on his right hand were identical with the stage of scabbing in ordinary vaccination.

[illegible] gradually diminished [illegible] black, and finally [illegible] an irregular depressed scar [illegible] was found [illegible]

[illegible] after exposure to [illegible], the vesicle was at its height on the seventh or eighth day, and a typical tamarind-stone crust fell off on the twenty-first day after infection, leaving a depressed, irregular cicatrix.

A vesicle also formed on the thumb of the left hand. Two days after the pimple appeared on his cheek, the lad says that he noticed a pimple on his thumb, and this, on my visit on December 2nd, presented a greyish flattened vesicle, about the size of a sixpence. On the following day its vesicular character was much more marked, and a little central crust had commenced to form. (Plate XVII., Fig. 1, Vol. i.) On the Sunday, especially towards the evening, the margins became very tumid, giving it a marked appearance of central depression. On Monday, December 5th, I punctured the vesicle at its margin with a clean needle, and from the beads of lymph which exuded I filled a number of capillary tubes. This lymph was used the following morning for retro-vaccinating four calves.

On Wednesday, December 7th, suppuration had commenced; the vesicle contained a turbid fluid, and the areola was well marked. (Plate XVII., Fig. 2, Vol. i.) On December 9th the crust had assumed a peculiar slate-coloured hue, and, on pressing it, pus welled up through a central fissure. (Plate XVII., Fig. 3, Vol. i.) The areola had increased, and there was considerable inflammatory thickening. The lymphatic glands in the armpit were enlarged and painful. Though there was deep ulceration, which left a permanent scar, the ulceration did not assume quite so severe a character as in some of the other milkers. Possibly this may be accounted for to some extent by the fact that the pock was covered with a simple dressing, instead of being subjected to the irritation and injury incidental to working on the farm.

Revaccination of the Milkers.—The bailiff's son (Case VII.) was shown at the Pathological Society of London on January 17th, nine weeks after he had been inoculated from the cows. On the afternoon of the same day (Tuesday), he was vaccinated with lymph taken direct from a child's arm. This child had beautifully correct vesicles, first remove from the calf.

On the second and third days there was topical redness at the places inoculated, but this rapidly subsided.

On the following Monday the boy returned to the farm, where he was able to report and demonstrate the failure of the vaccination. The news rapidly spread over the farm, and, as a result, his companion milkers volunteered, and others consented, to be submitted to the same test. The question then arose as to how this could be accomplished. I had intended to take lymph in tubes and vaccinate the men myself, but this idea was dismissed because I felt that as they would be cases of revaccination, it was advisable to obtain the services of a successful public vaccinator; and, secondly, it was necessary to avoid any fallacies which might arise from the use of stored lymph. Under these circumstances, I determined to apply to the local public vaccinator to vaccinate and report on the matter. Mr. Langley, of Cricklade, kindly consented, if I would select seven cases, to vaccinate them direct from children selected with typical vaccinal vesicles.*

The six men available were:—William Plowman, James Febry, William Hibbert, junr., William King, Joseph Lanfear, John Rawlins. Lastly, William Winchcomb, who had escaped inoculation from the cows, accompanied us. The vaccination took place on February 1st; the results were carefully watched, and are shown in the certificate which I received from Mr. Langley:—

Name.	Age.	Vaccine Cicatrices.	Result of Revaccination.
William Plowman	23	1, left arm	None.
James Febry ...	18	3, right arm	None.
William Hibbert, Junr.	17	3, left arm	None.
William King ...	22	3, left arm	None.
Joseph Lanfear ...	24	2, left arm ... ...; 2 (of revaccination at 15), right arm	None.
John Rawlins ...	55	3, right arm	None.
William Winchcomb	58	None (states he was vaccinated in infancy)...	One place, apparently true vaccine vesicle.

I hereby certify that I vaccinated the above men with the results here stated.

(Signed) Noah Beldon Langley, Public Vaccinator,
Cricklade District, Cricklade and Wootton Bassett Union.

Winchcomb's case is of extreme interest. I had anticipated, as he had escaped inoculation from the cows, that he would not take. He, however, was vaccinated with success, so that his escape while milking the cows could not be attributed to his having had the Cow Pox, when a milker twenty years previously. He was one of three who escaped, and one of the two remaining, (Pontine) attributed his escape to the fact of his having had Cow

* I desire to express my thanks most cordially to Mr. A. and his bailiff for allowing me to make these arrangements, so interrupting to the work of the farms, and to Mr. Langley for undertaking the task of revaccination.

Pox twenty-five years previously, while the other who escaped (Febry, senr.), had never contracted Cow Pox at all.

It was not only interesting, under the circumstances, that the vaccination of Winchcomb should have taken so well, but it afforded evidence of the active property of the lymph, and he constituted a contrary experiment to the six milkers, who had suffered from the casual Cow Pox, and in whom revaccination was without result. To make the experiment of revaccination as complete as possible, I determined to vaccinate the two milkers who had not been able to accompany me to Cricklade. These were Hibbert, senr., aged forty-two; Charles Pontine, aged sixty-four.

They had both been vaccinated in infancy. Hibbert, senr., had on his arm three small pigmented patches, and Pontine three marks. I employed Dr. Warlomont's lymph from three tubes. There was considerable topical irritation, in Hibbert in one place, which gradually disappeared; while in Pontine all three places developed into angry looking wounds with unhealthy discharge, an appearance which at first, considering the age of the patient, caused me considerable anxiety.

To sum up, there were in all eight milkers, varying in age from seventeen to fifty-five, who had contracted Cow Pox on their hands from milking the cows. Seven had been vaccinated in infancy, but not since; one had been revaccinated on entering the navy at fifteen. They were all revaccinated after complete recovery from the casual Cow Pox (that is to say, from three to four months afterwards), and were all completely protected. On the other hand, two of the three milkers who had escaped infection from the casual Cow Pox were also vaccinated, with the result in Winchcomb of typical revaccination, in Pontine of very considerable local irritation.

Jenner was of opinion that Cow Pox did not protect against Cow Pox, but there can be no doubt, from these experiments, that Cow Pox does protect against itself, for a time, though the duration of that time does not appear, even at the present day, to be satisfactorily determined.*

* Un fait des plus intéressants que le service municipal de la vaccine à Bordeaux a mis le premier en lumière, c'est la nécessité des revaccinations dans les écoles primaires. Chez les écoliers vaccinés avec succès dans la petite enfance, les revaccinations peuvent déjà donner à partir de six ans 38 per cent. de succès: sur près de 8,000 écoliers de six a quatorze ans, la moyenne des succès obtenus a été de 41 per cent. Ces revaccinations d'écoliers comparées aux revaccinations chez des adultes nous ont amené aux remarques suivantes: La durée de l'immunité est variable suivant les individus; elle est variable aussi suivant les âges.—LAYET.

As I have already stated, Pontine and Winchcomb both attributed their escape when the cows were attacked to their having caught the Cow Pox, one twenty and the other twenty-five years ago, but as Winchcomb was revaccinated with success, and as Febry, senr. (who had never had the Cow Pox), also remained free from the disease, the escape of these men must be attributed to some other cause. Possibly the skin on the hands of these veteran milkers was not in such a favourable condition for receiving the virus.

Retro-vaccination of Calves.—I have mentioned that on Monday, December 5th, I collected lymph from a vesicle on the hand of William Plowman, and the following morning, without loss of time, I retro-vaccinated four calves at the Royal Veterinary College. This boy, it will be remembered, stated that he first noticed a pimple on his thumb on Tuesday, so that, allowing two days for incubation, the lymph was taken from his thumb about the eighth day. In all cases, the belly of the calves was shaved, and the skin sponged and cleansed with warm water, and wiped dry with a clean cloth. The vaccination was made with a new scalpel. The skin was put on the stretch by an assistant, and a number of scratches and cross-scratches were made, as in the ordinary process of vaccination of infants, as superficially as possible, to avoid hæmorrhage.

The following are the details of the results which were obtained:

First Series of Retro-vaccinated Calves.—*Calf* 1, a small red calf, was vaccinated in six places. Next day a little dried serum had collected at the points of inoculation. The scratches were slightly reddened. The serum rubbed off in the course of a day or two, and there was no result.

Calf 2, a large red calf, was inoculated in six places. On the third day each place was promising. On the fourth day, Friday, December 9th, each place was tumid, reddened, and vesiculating. On the following day, these appearances were more marked; the areola had considerably increased. There was infiltration extending around the inoculated spot for a distance of half an inch, and the discharge from the vesicle was turbid. On Monday, the 12th, brown crusts had formed, and, on pressure, pus appeared at the edges from underneath the crusts. The temperature of this calf, during the experiment, was as follows: December 6th, $102\frac{3}{5}$; 7th, $101\frac{2}{5}$; 8th, 102; 9th, 102; 10th, $102\frac{1}{5}$; 11th, $103\frac{2}{5}$; 12th, 102; 13th, $101\frac{4}{5}$; 14th, $101\frac{2}{5}$; 15th, $101\frac{3}{5}$.

Calf 3 was a small red calf. This calf was vaccinated in six places. No result followed the vaccination except topical irritation.

Calf 4, a blue-roan calf, was suffering from a severe attack of ringworm, consisting of thick eczematous-looking crusts on the side of the face and neck, along the back, and especially at the root of the tail. Similar results to those in Calf 2 occurred in all of ten places which were retro-vaccinated. The temperature of this calf was as follows:—December 6th, $102\frac{1}{5}$; 7th, $102\frac{4}{5}$; 8th, $102\frac{3}{5}$; 9th, $102\frac{2}{5}$; 10th, $101\frac{3}{5}$; 11th, $102\frac{2}{5}$; 12th, 102; 13th, $102\frac{2}{5}$; 14th, $101\frac{4}{5}$; 15th, $101\frac{3}{5}$.

Thus, in two out of four calves, there were typical vaccinal vesicles. In both animals the crusts gradually thickened, and, on December 16th, there were still thick dark-brown crusts and some remaining induration.

The large red calf (No. 2), on December 20th, was sent to the Animal Vaccine Station of the Local Government Board, as it had been proposed to ascertain the result of a revaccination with lymph derived from the Eysines Cow Pox, as soon as the animals had recovered from the retro-vaccination.

On Thursday, December 28th, the places of inoculation were represented by depressed permanent scars. The calf was vaccinated by the Director in three places by linear incisions, two of which bled freely, and by myself in three places, by scarification by the method originally employed. Lymph was taken direct from the arm of a child selected with typical vesicles. The child had been vaccinated with calf-lymph at the institution.

On the second and third day there was slight redness at the three incisions, but no trace of vesiculation. At the three places inoculated by myself there was a collection of dried serum, with similar topical irritation.

On Monday, January 2nd, the incisions had completely dried up, being marked by small, dry linear scabs, and in the scarified places the dry serum crumbled away to the touch. Thus, the revaccination of Calf 2 had totally failed.

On December 30th, the blue-roan calf also presented a number of permanent depressed cicatrices. This calf, being the one which was suffering severely from ringworm,* had been retained at the Royal Veterinary College. Calf-lymph, obtained from Dr. Warlomont, was copiously applied in three places thoroughly scarified, the contents of two tubes being mixed and rubbed into each scarification.

On the next day there was slight topical redness on each place of inoculation.

* The highly contagious character of this eruption so common in calves was on the same day demonstrated on the person of the man who looked after the animals. His left arm was covered with a characteristic rash.

Monday, December 12th. On arriving at the Royal Veterinary College I found that the pocks of the original calves were suppurating; I nevertheless determined to ascertain what the result of inoculation would be. Three calves were therefore inoculated in the following way:—After detaching a brown crust some of the pus was collected on a scalpel and rubbed by scarification into the belly of two of the calves and inoculated by puncture in the vulva of the third.

Calf A, Series 2, was inoculated in six places in the belly. At each place there were positive results, but vesiculation was scarcely visible, and suppuration had commenced very early. On the evening of the fourth day, December 15th, this calf was shown by request at a special meeting of the Pathological Society. Each place of inoculation was pustular and covered with a brown scab. On Friday, December 16th, the crusts were raised, there was a well-marked inflammatory redness, and considerable thickening. On examining the crusts, there was pus underneath and an ulcer, with a slight tendency to bleed at the edges when pressed. On Saturday, December 17th, the inflammatory areola was less marked on each. Monday, December 19th, the crusts were thickening and areola disappearing, and there was a considerable amount of purulent discharge on squeezing the ulcer. On Tuesday, December 20th, this calf was also sent to the Animal Vaccine Station.

Similar results occurred in *Calf B.*, and no result in *Calf C.* Calves A and B, series 2, were, on recovery, revaccinated with success.

Third Remove of Calves.—Before the departure of Calf A, I inoculated by linear incisions two small steers in some thirty places with pus from one of these pustular pocks. On Thursday, 22nd, the third day, there was vivid redness of the incision, and slight tumidity. On December 23rd suppuration had occurred. Thus again we had a similar result of early suppuration. One of the calves looked dull, refused food, and died on January 2nd. From the *post-mortem* examination there could be no doubt that the calf died of septicæmia.

Thus the result of retro-vaccinating with the humanised lymph was successful in two out of the four calves; an eruption being produced with all the typical vaccinal characters, but running rather a rapid course,* while the result obtained in the second and

* Thus corresponding with the experience of Ceely, who has pointed out that in retro-vaccination from the milker's hands the results are doubtful and depend greatly on the animals selected. "Those of a light colour and with

third series was in accordance with what is well known to occur if lymph be not taken at the right stage for carrying on successive vaccinations.*

These results serve to illustrate what is well known in Animal Vaccine stations—the liability to rapid degeneration of vaccine lymph, if not taken on the right day, for carrying on calf-to-calf vaccination. Thus, starting with perfectly correct vesicles, if the lymph from these vesicles be not taken from selected vesicles at the right stage, in the course of two or three removes the lymph may be entirely lost. It will then become necessary to return to stock in order to start again a fresh series of vaccinations. It is on this account that, in order to carry on calf-to-calf vaccination, typical vesicles are selected, usually on the morning of the fifth day, and well-conditioned animals employed as subjects for the operation.

Diagnosis of Cow Pox.

In the diagnosis of Cow Pox it is necessary to bear in mind the existence of the following diseases of the teats and udders of cows:—

Chapped Teats.—Sores on the teats may result from slight injuries, such as scratches from brambles while the cows are out at pasture. Cowmen state that a similar condition arises from the cows soiling their teats in muddy ponds and being afterwards exposed to dry winds. A similar condition may occur as a result of inflammation of the udder soon after calving; this shows itself in the form of excoriations or sores, or small cracks or chaps on the teats, which are very troublesome (Youatt).

---

thin skins were generally preferred, but often without avail, scarcely one-half of the operations succeeding." Again, in speaking of some of his experiments, Ceely says: "The above experiments will serve to show the greater difficulty of vaccinating the cow with humanised than with primary lymph, and that, when successful, a much milder disease is the result. Take an abundance of lymph from one of the finest and most protective vesicles ever seen, and if you succeed in retro-vaccinating the cow you may perhaps be able to charge only a very few points from a vesicle which excites but trifling topical inconvenience. Vaccine lymph it is obvious, therefore, in passing from the cow to man indicates a change which renders it less acceptable and less energetic on being returned to many individuals of the class producing it; some refuse it altogether."

* The postponement of the carrying on of the successive inoculations was probably the main cause of the production of vaccine which is regarded as non-protective. Bryce, in his treatise on the Cow Pox, has laid particular stress upon this point: "The fluid contained in the vesicle in the advanced stages of Cow Pox has undergone a certain change, whereby it is rendered unfit for propagating this affection so as to give security from true Small Pox, and this change is said to be marked by the puriform appearances which the fluid then assumes. . . . The areola is fully formed, and this is said to be a mark that the virus begins to be less active, therefore improper for use." It must also be remembered that the calves were retro-vaccinated with the lymph of a revaccination.

Blister Pock, the White Vesicle or White Pock.—Variolæ vaccinæ bullosæ (Gunzel), bullatæ (Osiander), albæ (Jenner), vesiculosæ, pemphigoides; Wasser oder Windpocken (Hering).—This disease is communicable from the cow to the milker if the hand be not quite sound, and is conveyed by the milker to other cows. Jenner describes a case in a milkmaid: "On the fingers of each of the girl's hands there appeared several large white blisters. She supposes about three or four on each finger. The hands and arms inflamed and swelled, but no constitutional indisposition followed."

Hering points out that the structure of the vesicle is characteristic. There is only a simple raising of the epidermis, and in twenty-four hours the vesicle has reached the size of a pea or bean. The contents are sometimes absorbed and the vesicles are then found empty. Ceely also speaks of the vesicles as being subepidermic, and distinguished from Cow Pox in that the cellular character is wanting. When communicated to man, according to the same authority, the vesicle may resemble in appearance the vaccine vesicle; "but, on examination with a lancet, it is found neither cellular nor possessed of the fluid contents. It is in a state of desiccation, and has retained this appearance and its integrity so long, on account of the thickness of the epidermis."

Aphtha Epizootica—Fièvre Aphtheuse—"Foot-and-Mouth Disease" on the Teats.—This disease may be mistaken for Cow Pox if a medical man on discovering vesicles on the cow's teats makes a diagnosis without entering any further into the clinical history. It is most important, therefore, when milch cows are affected with vesicles on the teats, that a careful examination should be made for any eruption in the mouth or on the feet.

The best description of this eruption in milch cows is given by Rayer. The number of vesicles may vary from six to forty. They appear first about the size of a large pin, and enlarge till they form flattened circular vesicles. The vesicles dry up about the tenth or eleventh day, and a brownish thin crust forms and is detached about the sixteenth or eighteenth day of the malady. If subjected to the tractions of the milkers, a superficial excoriation of a brownish red colour results, and covered with a crust consisting largely of dried blood. But these ulcerations do not degenerate into phagedænic ulcers like those which occur in Cow Pox. The disease is said to be communicable to man when the milk is drunk while still warm from the cows. Vesicles make their appearance on the lips and tongue.

Cattle Plague.—The eruption of cattle plague may occur on the udder and teats, as well as on other parts of the body. The disease is analogous to human Small Pox. From the general characters of this affection, there is no difficulty in distinguishing it from other eruptive diseases of the teats. There is no cattle plague at present in this country, as it has been effectually stamped out.

Yellow-Pock is a disease described by Nissen as an eruption yellow from its first appearance, and continuing so. It is accompanied with an extremely unpleasant—almost putrid—smell, and soon degenerates into ulcerations, from which pus and blood exude. The disease is communicable from one cow to another, and to man; * boils and ulcers resulting.

Bluish or Black Pock has been described by Ceely, as forming bluish or black, or livid vesications on the teats and udders, followed by thin dirty brown or black irregular crusts and some degree of impetigo on the interstices near the bases of the teats.

Warts.—These, according to Ceely, are of two kinds, "long narrow pendulous and linear-shaped prolongations, easily removed, and often detached, the other short, thick, compact, broad elevations, lighter in colour generally than the ground from which they rise, of various sizes, from that of a pea to that of a horse-bean, frequently very numerous on the teats, where they are found bleeding and partially detached."

Other Eruptions.—Ceely has described "suppuration of the cutaneous follicles at the base of the teats; small hard knots, cutaneous or subcutaneous, in the same locality, about the size of a vetch, a pea, or even larger, which often remain indolent for a time, at length become red, vesicate, enlarge, suppurate, and burst after attaining not infrequently the size of a walnut or more, occasionally affecting the hands of the milker, and often the other cows milked in the same shed by the same hands; and an eczematous eruption, with intertrigo on the udder and near the roots of the teats." These diseases, like chapped teats and warts, could scarcely be mistaken for Cow Pox.

---

* Ceely met with a case which he describes as follows:—"Not long since I saw a wife and five children labouring under a pustular disease of six weeks' standing, and infected by the father, who had caught the disease from the cow, which was in a terrible condition. It was of the character of ecthyma, but communicable, affecting the face, trunk, and limbs, and could be propagated by inoculation."

CATALOGUE OF WORKS

PUBLISHED BY

H. K. LEWIS

136 GOWER STREET, LONDON, W.C.

Established 1844.

SIR WILLIAM AITKEN, KNT., M.D., F.R.S.
Professor of Pathology in the Army Medical School.

ON THE ANIMAL ALKALOIDS, THE PTOMAINES, LEUCOMAINES, AND EXTRACTIVES IN THEIR PATHOLOGICAL RELATIONS. Crown 8vo, 2s. 6d.

E. CRESSWELL BABER, M.B. LOND.
Surgeon to the Brighton and Sussex Throat and Ear Dispensary.

A GUIDE TO THE EXAMINATION OF THE NOSE, WITH REMARKS ON THE DIAGNOSIS OF DISEASES OF THE NASAL CAVITIES. With Illustrations, small 8vo, 5s. 6d.

G. GRANVILLE BANTOCK, M.D., F.R.C.S. EDIN.
Surgeon to the Samaritan Free Hospital for Women and Children.

I.

ON THE USE AND ABUSE OF PESSARIES. Second Edit., with Illustrations, 8vo, 5s.

II.

ON THE TREATMENT OF RUPTURE OF THE FEMALE PERINEUM IMMEDIATE AND REMOTE. Second Edition, with Illustrations, 8vo, 3s. 6d. [*Just published.*

III.

A PLEA FOR EARLY OVARIOTOMY. Demy 8vo, 2s.

FANCOURT BARNES, M.D., M.R.C.P.
Physician to the Chelsea Hospital for Women; Obstetric Physician to the Great Northern Hospital, &c.

A GERMAN-ENGLISH DICTIONARY OF WORDS AND TERMS USED IN MEDICINE AND ITS COGNATE SCIENCES. Square 12mo, Roxburgh binding, 9s.

A. HUGHES BENNETT, M.D.

Member of the Royal College of Physicians of London; Physician to the Hospital for Epilepsy and Paralysis, Regent's Park, and Assistant Physician to the Westminster Hospital.

I.

A PRACTICAL TREATISE ON ELECTRO-DIAGNOSIS IN DISEASES OF THE NERVOUS-SYSTEM. With Illustrations, 8vo, 8s. 6d.

II.

ILLUSTRATIONS OF THE SUPERFICIAL NERVES AND MUSCLES, WITH THEIR MOTOR POINTS; a knowledge of which is essential in the Art of Electro-Diagnosis. (Extracted from the above). 8vo, paper cover, 1s. 6d.; cloth, 2s.

E. H. BENNETT, M.D., F.R.C.S.I.

Professor of Surgery, University of Dublin.

AND

D. J. CUNNINGHAM, M.D., F.R.C.S.I.

Professor of Anatomy and Chirurgery, University of Dublin.

THE SECTIONAL ANATOMY OF CONGENITAL CŒCAL HERNIA. With coloured plates, sm. folio, 5s. 6d. [*Now ready.*

DR. THEODOR BILLROTH.

Professor of Surgery in Vienna.

GENERAL SURGICAL PATHOLOGY AND THERA-PEUTICS. In Fifty-one Lectures. A Text-book for Students and Physicians. With additions by Dr. ALEXANDER VON WINIWARTER, Professor of Surgery in Luttich. Translated from the Fourth German edition with the special permission of the Author, and revised from the Tenth edition, by C. E. HACKLEY, A.M., M.D. Copiously illustrated, 8vo, 18s.

DRS. BOURNEVILLE AND BRICON.

MANUAL OF HYPODERMIC MEDICATION. Translated from the Second Edition, and Edited, with Therapeutic Index of Diseases, by ANDREW S. CURRIE, M.D. Edin., &c. With Illustrations, crown 8vo, 6s. [*Now Ready.*

G. H. BRANDT, M.D.

I

ROYAT (LES BAINS) IN AUVERGNE, ITS MINERAL WATERS AND CLIMATE. With Frontispiece and Map. Second edition, crown 8vo, 2s. 6d.

II.

HAMMAM R'IRHA, ALGIERS. A Winter Health Re-sort and Mineral Water Cure Combined. With Frontispiece and Map, crown 8vo, 2s. 6d.

GURDON BUCK, M.D.

CONTRIBUTIONS TO REPARATIVE SURGERY: Showing its Application to the Treatment of Deformities, produced by Destructive Disease or Injury; Congenital Defects from Arrest or Excess of Development; and Cicatricial Contractions from Burns. Illustrated by numerous Engravings, large 8vo, 9s.

MARY BULLAR & J. F. BULLAR, M.B. CANTAB., F.R.C.S.

RECEIPTS FOR FLUID FOODS. 16mo, 1s.

DUDLEY W. BUXTON, M.D., B.S., M.R.C.P.
Administrator of Anæsthetics at University College Hospital and the Hospital for Women, Soho Square.

ANÆSTHETICS THEIR USES AND ADMINISTRA-TION. Crown 8vo, 4s. [*Ready.*
[LEWIS'S PRACTICAL SERIES.]

ALFRED H. CARTER, M.D. LOND.
Member of the Royal College of Physicians; Physician to the Queen's Hospital, Birmingham; late Examiner in Medicine for the University of Aberdeen, &c.

ELEMENTS OF PRACTICAL MEDICINE. Fifth Edition, crown 8vo, 9s. [*Just published.*

P. CAZEAUX.
Adjunct Professor in the Faculty of Medicine of Paris, &c.
AND
S. TARNIER.
Professor of Obstetrics and Diseases of Women and Children in the Faculty of Medicine of Paris.

OBSTETRICS: THE THEORY AND PRACTICE; including the Diseases of Pregnancy and Parturition, Obstetrical Operations, &c. Seventh Edition, edited and revised by ROBERT J. HESS, M.D., with twelve full-page plates, five being coloured, and 165 wood-engravings, 1081 pages, roy. 8vo, 35s.

FRANCIS HENRY CHAMPNEYS, M.A., M.B. OXON., F.R.C.P.
Obstetric Physician and Lecturer on Obstetric Medicine at St. George's Hospital: Examiner in Obstetric Medicine in the University of London, &c.

EXPERIMENTAL RESEARCHES IN ARTIFICIAL RESPIRATION IN STILLBORN CHILDREN, AND ALLIED SUBJECTS. Crown 8vo, 3s. 6d.

W. BRUCE CLARKE, M.A., M.B. OXON., F.R.C.S.
Assistant Surgeon to, and Senior Demonstrator of Anatomy and Operative Surgery at, St. Bartholomew's Hospital; Surgeon to the West London Hospital; Examiner in Surgery to the University of Oxford.

THE DIAGNOSIS AND TREATMENT OF DISEASES OF THE KIDNEY AMENABLE TO DIRECT SURGICAL INTERFERENCE. Demy 8vo, with Illustrations, 7s. 6d.

JOHN COCKLE, M.A., M.D.
Physician to the Royal Free Hospital.

ON INTRA-THORACIC CANCER. 8vo, 4s. 6d.

ALEXANDER COLLIE, M.D. ABERD., M.R.C.P. LOND.
Medical Superintendent of the Eastern Hospitals.

ON FEVERS: THEIR HISTORY, ETIOLOGY, DIAGNOSIS, PROGNOSIS, AND TREATMENT. Illustrated with Coloured Plates, crown 8vo, 8s. 6d. [LEWIS'S PRACTICAL SERIES.]

WALTER S. COLMAN, M.B. LOND.
Formerly Assistant to the Professor of Pathology in the University of Edinburgh.

SECTION CUTTING AND STAINING: A Practical Guide to the Preparation of Normal and Morbid Histological Specimens. Crown 8vo, 3s. [*Now ready.*

ALFRED COOPER, F.R.C.S.
Surgeon to the St. Mark's Hospital for Fistula and other Diseases of the Rectum.

A PRACTICAL TREATISE ON THE DISEASES OF THE RECTUM. Crown 8vo, 4s. [*Just published.*

W. H. CORFIELD, M.A., M.D. OXON.
Professor of Hygiene and Public Health in University College, London.

DWELLING HOUSES: their Sanitary Construction and Arrangements. Second Edit., with Illustrations. Cr. 8vo, 3s. 6d.

EDWARD COTTERELL, M.R.C.S. ENG., L.R.C.P. LOND.
Late House Surgeon, University College Hospital.

ON SOME COMMON INJURIES TO LIMBS; their Treatment and After-treatment, including Bone-setting (so-called). With Illustrations, small 8vo, 3s. 6d.

CHARLES CREIGHTON, M.D.

I.

ILLUSTRATIONS OF UNCONSCIOUS MEMORY IN DISEASE, including a Theory of Alteratives. Post 8vo, 6s.

II.

CONTRIBUTIONS TO THE PHYSIOLOGY AND PATHOLOGY OF THE BREAST AND LYMPHATIC GLANDS. New Edition with additional chapter, with wood-cuts and plate, 8vo, 9s.

III.

BOVINE TUBERCULOSIS IN MAN: An Account of the Pathology of Suspected Cases. With Chromo-lithographs and other Illustrations, 8vo, 8s. 6d.

H. RADCLIFFE CROCKER, M.D. LOND., B.S., F.R.C.P.

Physician, Skin Department, University College Hospital.

DISEASES OF THE SKIN: THEIR DESCRIPTION, PATHOLOGY, DIAGNOSIS, AND TREATMENT. With 76 Illustrations, 8vo, 21s. [*Now ready.*

EDGAR M. CROOKSHANK, M.B. LOND., F.R.M.S.

Professor of Bacteriology, King's College, London.

I.

MANUAL OF BACTERIOLOGY: being an Introduction to Practical Bacteriology. Illustrated with Coloured Plates from original drawings, and numerous Coloured Illustrations embodied in the text. Second Edition revised and enlarged, 8vo, 21s.

II.

PHOTOGRAPHY OF BACTERIA. Illustrated with 86 Photographs reproduced in autotype, and wood engravings, royal 8vo, 12s. 6d.

RIDLEY DALE, M.D., L.R.C.P. EDIN., M.R.C.S. ENG.

EPITOME OF SURGERY. Large 8vo. [*In the press.*

HENRY DAVIS, M.R.C.S. ENG.

Teacher and Administrator of Anæsthetics to St. Mary's and the National Dental Hospitals.

GUIDE TO THE ADMINISTRATION OF ANÆSTHETICS. Fcap. 8vo, 2s.

J. THOMPSON DICKSON, M.A., M.B. CANTAB.

Late Lecturer on Mental Diseases at Guy's Hospital.

THE SCIENCE AND PRACTICE OF MEDICINE IN RELATION TO MIND, the Pathology of the Nerve Centres, and the Jurisprudence of Insanity, being a course of Lectures delivered at Guy's Hospital. Illustrated by Chromo-lithographic Drawings and Physiological Portraits. 8vo, 14s.

HORACE DOBELL, M.D.
Consulting Physician to the Royal Hospital for Diseases of the Chest, &c.

I.

ON DIET AND REGIMEN IN SICKNESS AND Health and on the Interdependence and Prevention of Diseases and the Diminution of their Fatality. Seventh Edition, 8vo, 10s. 6d.

II.

AFFECTIONS OF THE HEART AND IN ITS NEIGH-BOURHOOD. Cases, Aphorisms, and Commentaries. Illustrated by the heliotype process. 8vo, 6s 6d.

JOHN EAGLE.
Member of the Pharmaceutical Society.

A NOTE-BOOK OF SOLUBILITIES. Arranged chiefly for the use of Prescribers and Dispensers. 12mo, 2s. 6d.

JOHN ERIC ERICHSEN.
Ex-President of the Royal College of Surgeons; Surgeon Extraordinary to H.M. the Queen, etc.

MODERN SURGERY; its Progress and Tendencies. Being the Introductory Address delivered at University College at the opening of the Session 1873-74. Demy 8vo, 1s.

DR. FERBER.

MODEL DIAGRAM OF THE ORGANS IN THE THORAX AND UPPER PART OF THE ABDOMEN. With Letter-press Description. In 4to, coloured, 5s.

J. MAGEE FINNY, M.D. DUBL.
King's Professor of Practice of Medicine in School of Physic, Ireland; Clinical Physician to St Patrick Dun's Hospital.

NOTES ON THE PHYSICAL DIAGNOSIS OF LUNG DISEASES. 32mo, 1s. 6d. [*Now ready.*

AUSTIN FLINT, JR., M.D.
Professor of Physiology and Physiological Anatomy in the Bellevue Medical College, New York; attending Physician to the Bellevue Hospital, &c.

I.

A TEXT-BOOK OF HUMAN PHYSIOLOGY; De-signed for the Use of Practitioners and Students of Medicine. New edition, Illustrated by plates, and 313 wood engravings, large 8vo, 28s.

II.

THE PHYSIOLOGY OF THE SPECIAL SENSES AND GENERATION; (Being Vol. V. of the Physiology of Man). Roy. 8vo, 18s.

J. MILNER FOTHERGILL, M.D.

Member of the Royal College of Physicians of London; Physician to the City of London Hospital for Diseases of the Chest, Victoria Park, &c.

I.

A MANUAL OF DIETETICS: Large 8vo, 10s. 6d.

II.

THE HEART AND ITS DISEASES, WITH THEIR TREATMENT; INCLUDING THE GOUTY HEART. Second Edition, entirely re-written, copiously illustrated with woodcuts and lithographic plates. 8vo. 16s.

III.

INDIGESTION AND BILIOUSNESS. Second Edition, post 8vo, 7s. 6d.

IV.

GOUT IN ITS PROTEAN ASPECTS. Post 8vo, 7s. 6d.

V.

HEART STARVATION. (Reprinted from the Edinburgh Medical Journal), 8vo, 1s.

ERNEST FRANCIS, F.C.S.

Demonstrator of Practical Chemistry, Charing Cross Hospital.

PRACTICAL EXAMPLES IN QUANTITATIVE ANA-lysis, forming a Concise Guide to the Analysis of Water, &c. Illustrated, fcap. 8vo, 2s. 6d.

ALFRED W. GERRARD, F.C.S.

Examiner to the Pharmaceutical Society; Teacher of Pharmacy and Demonstrator of Materia Medica at University College Hospital.

ELEMENTS OF MATERIA MEDICA AND PHAR-MACY. Crown 8vo, 8s. 6d. [*Just published.*

HENEAGE GIBBES, M.D.

Lecturer on Physiology and on Normal and Morbid Histology in the Medical School of Westminster Hospital; etc.

PRACTICAL HISTOLOGY AND PATHOLOGY. Third Edition, revised and enlarged, crown 8vo, 6s.

C. A. GORDON, M.D., C.B.

Deputy Inspector General of Hospitals, Army Medical Department.

REMARKS ON ARMY SURGEONS AND THEIR WORKS. Demy 8vo, 5s.

JOHN GORHAM, M.R.C.S.

TOOTH EXTRACTION: a Manual on the proper mode of extracting Teeth. Second Edition, fcap. 8vo, 1s.

JOHN W. S. GOULEY, M.D.

Surgeon to Bellevue Hospital.

DISEASES OF MAN: Data of their Nomenclature, Classification and Genesis. Crown 8vo, 14s.

W. R. GOWERS, M.D., F.R.C.P., M.R.C.S.

Physician to University College Hospital, &c.

DIAGRAMS FOR THE RECORD OF PHYSICAL SIGNS. In books of 12 sets of figures, 1s. Ditto, unbound, 1s.

J. B. GRESSWELL, M.R.C.V.S.

Provincial Veterinary Surgeon to the Royal Agricultural Society.

VETERINARY PHARMACOLOGY AND THERAPEUTICS. With an Index of Diseases and Remedies. Fcap. 8vo, 5s.

SAMUEL D. GROSS, M.D., LL.D., D.C.L. OXON.

Professor of Surgery in the Jefferson Medical College of Philadelphia.

A PRACTICAL TREATISE ON THE DISEASES, INJURIES, AND MALFORMATIONS OF THE URINARY BLADDER, THE PROSTATE GLAND, AND THE URETHRA. Third Edition, revised and edited by S. W. GROSS, A.M., M.D., Surgeon to the Philadelphia Hospital. Illustrated by 170 engravings, 8vo, 18s.

SAMUEL W. GROSS, A.M., M.D.

Surgeon to, and Lecturer on Clinical Surgery in, the Jefferson Medical College Hospital, and the Philadelphia Hospital, &c.

A PRACTICAL TREATISE ON TUMOURS OF THE MAMMARY GLAND: embracing their Histology, Pathology, Diagnosis, and Treatment. With Illustrations, 8vo, 10s. 6d.

[illegible]

ALEXANDER HARVEY, M.D. [illegible]

FIRST LINES OF THERAPEUTICS: [illegible]

[illegible] AS [illegible] THE [illegible] Fcap. 8vo. [illegible]

ALEXANDER HARVEY, M.D.

Emeritus Professor of Materia Medica in the University of Aberdeen, &c.

AND

ALEXANDER DYCE DAVIDSON, M.D., F.R.S. EDIN.

Late Regius Professor of Materia Medica in the University of Aberdeen.

SYLLABUS OF MATERIA MEDICA FOR THE USE OF STUDENTS, TEACHERS AND PRACTITIONERS. Based on the relative values of articles and preparations in the British Pharmacopœia. Eighth Edition, 32mo, 1s. 6d.

K. M. HEANLEY.

Matron of Boston Cottage Hospital.

A MANUAL OF URINE TESTING. Compiled for the use of Matrons, Nurses, and Probationers. Post 8vo, 1s. 6d.

GRAILY HEWITT, M.D.

Professor of Midwifery and Diseases of Women in University College, Obstetrical Physician to University College Hospital, &c.

OUTLINES OF PICTORIAL DIAGNOSIS OF DISEASES OF WOMEN. Folio, 6s.

C. HIGGENS, F.R.C.S.

Ophthalmic Surgeon to Guy's Hospital; Lecturer on Ophthalmology at Guy's Hospital Medical School.

MANUAL OF OPHTHALMIC PRACTICE.
Crown 8vo. [*Just ready.*
[LEWIS'S PRACTICAL SERIES.]

BERKELEY HILL, M.B. LOND., F.R.C.S.

Professor of Clinical Surgery in University College; Surgeon to University College Hospital and to the Lock Hospital.

THE ESSENTIALS OF BANDAGING. With directions for Managing Fractures and Dislocations; for administering Ether and Chloroform; and for using other Surgical Apparatus; with a Chapter on Surgical Landmarks. Sixth Edition, revised and enlarged, Illustrated by 144 Wood Engravings, crown 8vo, 5s.

BERKELEY HILL, M.B. LOND., F.R.C.S.

Professor of Clinical Surgery in University College; Surgeon to University College Hospital and to the Lock Hospital.

AND

ARTHUR COOPER, L.R.C.P., M.R.C.S.

Surgeon to the Westminster General Dispensary.

I.

SYPHILIS AND LOCAL CONTAGIOUS DISORDERS. Second Edition, entirely re-written, royal 8vo, 18s.

II.

THE STUDENT'S MANUAL OF VENEREAL DISEASES. Being a Concise Description of those Affections and of their Treatment. Fourth Edition, post 8vo, 2s. 6d.

C. R. ILLINGWORTH, M.D. ED., M.R.C.S.

THE ABORTIVE TREATMENT OF SPECIFIC FE- BRILE DISORDERS BY THE BINIODIDE OF MERCURY. Crown 8vo, 3s. 6d.

SIR W. JENNER, Bart., M.D.
Physician in Ordinary to H.M. the Queen, and to H.R.H. the Prince of Wales.

THE PRACTICAL MEDICINE OF TO-DAY: Two Addresses delivered before the British Medical Association, and the Epidemiological Society, (1869). Small 8vo, 1s. 6d.

C. M. JESSOP, M.R.C.P.
Associate of King's College, London; Brigade Surgeon H.M. British Forces.

ASIATIC CHOLERA, being a Report on an Outbreak of Epidemic Cholera in 1876 at a Camp near Murree in India. With map, demy 8vo, 2s. 6d.

GEORGE LINDSAY JOHNSON, M.A., M.B., B.C. CANTAB.
Clinical Assistant, late House Surgeon and Chloroformist, Royal Westminster Ophthalmic Hospital, &c.

A NEW METHOD OF TREATING CHRONIC GLAU- COMA, based on Recent Researches into its Pathology. With Illustrations and coloured frontispiece, demy 8vo, 3s. 6d.

NORMAN KERR, M.D., F.L.S.
President of the Society for the Study of Inebriety; Consulting Physician, Dalrymple Home for Inebriates, etc.

INEBRIETY: its Etiology, Pathology, Treatment, and Jurisprudence. Crown 8vo, 12s. 6d. [*Just published.*

RUSTOMJEE NASERWANJEE KHORY, M.D. BRUX.
Member of the Royal College of Physicians.

THE PRINCIPLES AND PRACTICE OF MEDICINE. Second Edition, revised and much enlarged, 2 vols., large 8vo, 28s.

NORMAN W. KINGSLEY, M.D.S., D.D.S.
President of the Board of Censors of the State of New York; Member of the American Academy of Dental Science, &c.

A TREATISE ON ORAL DEFORMITIES AS A BRANCH OF MECHANICAL SURGERY. With over 350 Illustrations, 8vo, 16s.

E. A. KIRBY, M.D., M.R.C.S. ENG.

Late Physician to the City Dispensary.

I.

A PHARMACOPŒIA OF SELECTED REMEDIES, WITH THERAPEUTIC ANNOTATIONS, Notes on Alimentation in Disease, Air, Massage, Electricity and other Supplementary Remedial Agents, and a Clinical Index; arranged as a Handbook for Prescribers. Sixth Edition, enlarged and revised, demy 4to, 7s.

II.

ON THE VALUE OF PHOSPHORUS AS A REMEDY FOR LOSS OF NERVE POWER. Sixth Edition, 8vo, 2s. 6d.

J. WICKHAM LEGG, F.R.C.P.

Assistant Physician to Saint Bartholomew's Hospital, and Lecturer on Pathological Anatomy in the Medical School.

I.

ON THE BILE, JAUNDICE, AND BILIOUS DISEASES. With Illustrations in chromo-lithography, 719 pages, roy. 8vo, 25s.

II.

A GUIDE TO THE EXAMINATION OF THE URINE; intended chiefly for Clinical Clerks and Students. Sixth Edition, revised and enlarged, with Illustrations, fcap. 8vo, 2s. 6d.

III.

A TREATISE ON HÆMOPHILIA, SOMETIMES CALLED THE HEREDITARY HÆMORRHAGIC DIATHESIS. Fcap. 4to, 7s. 6d.

ARTHUR H. N. LEWERS, M.D. LOND., M.R.C.P. LOND.

Assistant Obstetric Physician to the London Hospital; Examiner in Midwifery and Diseases of Women to the Society of Apothecaries of London; Physician to Out-patients at the Queen Charlotte's Lying-in Hospital, etc,

A PRACTICAL TEXTBOOK OF THE DISEASES OF WOMEN. With Illustrations, crown 8vo, 8s. 6d. [*Now ready.*

[LEWIS'S PRACTICAL SERIES.]

DR. GEORGE LEWIN.

Professor at the Fr. Wilh. University, and Surgeon-in-Chief of the Syphilitic Wards and Skin Disease Wards of the Charité Hospital, Berlin.

THE TREATMENT OF SYPHILIS WITH SUBCUTA-NEOUS SUBLIMATE INJECTIONS. Translated by DR. CARL PRŒGLE, and DR. E. H. GALE, late Surgeon United States Army. Small 8vo, 7s.

DR. V. MAGNAN.

Physician to St. Ann Asylum, Paris; Laureate of the Institute.

ON ALCOHOLISM, the Various Forms of Alcoholic Delirium and their Treatment. Translated by W. S. GREENFIELD, M.D., M.R.C.P. 8vo, 7s. 6d.

A. COWLEY MALLEY, B.A., M.B., B.CH. T.C.D.

PHOTO-MICROGRAPHY; including a description of the Wet Collodion and Gelatino-Bromide Processes, together with the best methods of Mounting and Preparing Microscopic Objects for Photo-Micrography. Second Edition, with Photographs and Illustrations, crown 8vo, 7s. 6d.

PATRICK MANSON, M.D., C.M.

Amoy, China.

THE FILARIA SANGUINIS HOMINIS; AND CER- TAIN NEW FORMS OF PARASITIC DISEASE IN INDIA, CHINA, AND WARM COUNTRIES. Illustrated with Plates and Charts. 8vo, 10s. 6d.

PROFESSOR MARTIN.

MARTIN'S ATLAS OF OBSTETRICS AND GYNÆCO- LOGY. Edited by A. MARTIN, Docent in the University of Berlin. Translated and edited with additions by FANCOURT BARNES, M.D., M.R.C P., Physician to the Chelsea Hospital for Women; Obstetric Physician to the Great Northern Hospital; and to the Royal Maternity Charity of London, &c. Medium 4to, Morocco half bound, 31s. 6d. *nett.*

WILLIAM MARTINDALE, F.C.S.

Late Examiner of the Pharmaceutical Society, and late Teacher of Pharmacy and Demonstrator of Materia Medica at University College.

AND

W. WYNN WESTCOTT, M.B. LOND.

Deputy Coroner for Central Middlesex.

THE EXTRA PHARMACOPŒIA with the additions in- troduced into the British Pharmacopœia, 1885, with Medical References, and a Therapeutic Index of Diseases and Symptoms. Fifth Edition, revised with numerous additions, limp roan, med. 24mo, 7s. 6d.

WILLIAM MARTINDALE, F.C.S.
Late Examiner of the Pharmaceutical Society, &c.

COCA, COCAINE, AND ITS SALTS: their History, Medical and Economic Uses, and Medicinal Preparations. Fcap. 8vo, 2s.

MATERIA MEDICA LABELS.

Adapted for Public and Private Collections. Compiled from the British Pharmacopœia of 1885. The Labels are arranged in Two Divisions:—

Division I.—Comprises, with few exceptions, Substances of Organized Structure, obtained from the Vegetable and Animal Kingdoms.

Division II.—Comprises Chemical Materia Medica, including Alcohols, Alkaloids, Sugars, and Neutral Bodies.

On plain paper, 10s. 6d. *nett.* On gummed paper, 12s. 6d. *nett.*

*** Specimens of the Labels, of which there are over 450, will be sent on application.

S. E. MAUNSELL, L.R.C.S.I.
Surgeon-Major, Medical Staff.

NOTES OF MEDICAL EXPERIENCES IN INDIA PRINCIPALLY WITH REFERENCE TO DISEASES OF THE EYE. With Map, post 8vo, 3s. 6d.

J. F. MEIGS, M.D.
Consulting Physician to the Children's Hospital, Philadelphia.

AND

W. PEPPER, M.D.
Lecturer on Clinical Medicine in the University of Pennsylvania.

A PRACTICAL TREATISE ON THE DISEASES OF CHILDREN. Seventh Edition, revised and enlarged, roy. 8vo, 28s.

Wm. JULIUS MICKLE, M.D., F.R.C.P. LOND.
Medical Superintendent, Grove Hall Asylum, London, &c.

I.

GENERAL PARALYSIS OF THE INSANE.
Second Edition, enlarged and rewritten, 8vo, 14s.

II.

ON INSANITY IN RELATION TO CARDIAC AND AORTIC DISEASE AND PHTHISIS. Crown 8vo, 3s. 6d.

KENNETH W. MILLICAN, B.A. CANTAB., M.R.C.S.

THE EVOLUTION OF MORBID GERMS: A Contribu-bution to Transcendental Pathology. Cr. 8vo, 3s. 6d.

ANGEL MONEY, M.D., M.R.C.P.
Assistant Physician to the Hospital for Children, Great Ormond Street, and to University College Hospital.

TREATMENT OF DISEASE IN CHILDREN: IN-CLUDING THE OUTLINES OF DIAGNOSIS AND THE CHIEF PATHOLOGICAL DIFFERENCES BETWEEN CHILDREN AND ADULTS. Crown 8vo, 10s. 6d.
[LEWIS'S PRACTICAL SERIES.]

E. A. MORSHEAD, M.R.C.S., L.R.C.P.
Assistant to the Professor of Medicine in University College, London.

TABLES OF THE PHYSIOLOGICAL ACTION OF DRUGS. Fcap. 8vo, 1s.

A. STANFORD MORTON, M.B., F.R.C.S. ED.
Surgeon to the Royal South London Ophthalmic Hospital.

REFRACTION OF THE EYE: Its Diagnosis, and the Correction of its Errors. Third Edition, with Illustrations, small 8vo. 3s.

C. W. MANSELL MOULLIN, M.A., M.D. OXON., F.R.C.S. ENG.

Assistant Surgeon and Senior Demonstrator of Anatomy at the London Hospital; formerly Radcliffe Travelling Fellow and Fellow of Pembroke College, Oxford.

SPRAINS; THEIR CONSEQUENCES AND TREATMENT. Crown 8vo, 5s. [*Now ready.*

PAUL F. MUNDÉ, M.D.

Professor of Gynecology at the New York Polyclinic; President of the New York Obstetrical Society and Vice-President of the British Gynecological Society, &c.

THE MANAGEMENT OF PREGNANCY, PARTURITION, AND THE PUERPERAL STATE, NORMAL AND ABNORMAL. Square 8vo, 3s. 6d. [*Just published.*

WILLIAM MURRELL, M.D., F.R.C.P.

Lecturer on Materia Medica and Therapeutics at Westminster Hospital; Examiner in Materia Medica to the Royal College of Physicians of London, etc.

MASSAGE AS A MODE OF TREATMENT. Third Edit., with Illustrations, crown 8vo, 4s. 6d. [*Just published.*

II.

WHAT TO DO IN CASES OF POISONING. Fifth Edition, royal 32mo, 3s. 6d.

III.

NITRO-GLYCERINE AS A REMEDY FOR ANGINA PECTORIS. Crown 8vo, 3s. 6d.

DR. FELIX von NIEMEYER.

Late Professor of Pathology and Therapeutics; Director of the Medical Clinic of the University of Tübingen.

A TEXT-BOOK OF PRACTICAL MEDICINE, WITH PARTICULAR REFERENCE TO PHYSIOLOGY AND PATHOLOGICAL ANATOMY. Translated from the Eighth German Edition, by special permission of the Author, by George H. Humphrey, M.D., and Charles E. Hackley, M.D. Revised Edition, 2 vols., large 8vo, 36s.

GEORGE OLIVER, M.D., F.R.C.P.

I.

THE HARROGATE WATERS: Data Chemical and Therapeutical, with notes on the Climate of Harrogate. Addressed to the Medical Profession. Crown 8vo, with Map of the Wells, 3s. 6d.

II.

ON BEDSIDE URINE TESTING: a Clinical Guide to the Observation of Urine in the course of Work. Third Edition, revised and enlarged, fcap. 8vo, 3s. 6d.

SAMUEL OSBORN, F.R.C.S.

Assistant-Surgeon to the Hospital for Women; Surgeon Royal Naval Artillery Volunteers.

I.

AMBULANCE LECTURES: FIRST AID. With Illustrations, fcap. 8vo, 1s. 6d.

II.

AMBULANCE LECTURES: NURSING. With Illustrations fcap. 8vo, 1s. 6d.

ROBERT W. PARKER.

Surgeon to the East London Hospital for Children, and to the Grosvenor Hospital for Women and Children.

I.

TRACHEOTOMY IN LARYNGEAL DIPHTHERIA, AFTER TREATMENT AND COMPLICATIONS. Second Edition. With Illustrations, 8vo, 5s.

II.

CONGENITAL CLUB-FOOT; ITS NATURE AND TREATMENT. With special reference to the subcutaneous division of Tarsal Ligaments. 8vo, 7s. 6d.

JOHN S. PARRY, M.D.

Obstetrician to the Philadelphia Hospital, Vice-President of the Obstetrical and Pathological Societies of Philadelphia, &c.

EXTRA-UTERINE PREGNANCY; Its Causes, Species, Pathological Anatomy, Clinical History, Diagnosis, Prognosis and Treatment. 8vo, 8s.

E. RANDOLPH PEASLEE, M.D., LL.D.

Late Professor of Gynæcology in the Medical Department of Dartmouth College; President of the New York Academy of Medicine, &c., &c.

OVARIAN TUMOURS: Their Pathology, Diagnosis, and Treatment, especially by Ovariotomy. Illustrations, roy. 8vo, 16s.

G. V. POORE, M.D., F.R.C.P.

Professor of Medical Jurisprudence, University College; Assistant Physician to, and Physician in charge of the Throat Department of, University College Hospital.

LECTURES ON THE PHYSICAL EXAMINATION OF THE MOUTH AND THROAT. With an Appendix of Cases. 8vo, 3s. 6d.

R. DOUGLAS POWELL, M.D., F.R.C.P., M.R.C.S.

Physician Extraordinary to H.M. the Queen; Physician to the Middlesex Hospital, and Physician to the Hospital for Consumption and Diseases of the Chest at Brompton.

DISEASES OF THE LUNGS AND PLEURÆ, INCLUD- ING CONSUMPTION. Third Edition, entirely rewritten and enlarged. With coloured plates and wood engravings, 8vo, 16s.

URBAN PRITCHARD, M.D. EDIN., F.R.C.S. ENG.

Professor of Aural Surgery at King's College, London; Aural Surgeon to King's College Hospital; Senior Surgeon to the Royal Ear Hospital.

HANDBOOK OF DISEASES OF THE EAR FOR THE USE OF STUDENTS AND PRACTITIONERS, With Illustrations, crown 8vo, 4s. 6d.

[LEWIS'S PRACTICAL SERIES.]

CHARLES W. PURDY, M.D. (QUEEN'S UNIV.)

Professor of Genito-Urinary and Renal Diseases in the Chicago Polyclinic, &c., &c.

BRIGHT'S DISEASE AND THE ALLIED AFFECTIONS OF THE KIDNEYS. With Illustrations, large 8vo, 8s. 6d.

CHARLES HENRY RALFE, M.A., M.D. CANTAB., F.R.C.P. LOND.
Assistant Physician to the London Hospital; Examiner in Medicine to the University of Durham, etc., etc.

A PRACTICAL TREATISE ON DISEASES OF THE KIDNEYS AND URINARY DERANGEMENTS. With Illustrations, crown 8vo, 10s. 6d.

[Lewis's Practical Series.]

AMBROSE L. RANNEY, A.M., M.D.
Professor of the Anatomy and Physiology of the Nervous System in the New York Post-Graduate Medical School and Hospital; Professor of Nervous and Mental Diseases in the Medical Department of the University of Vermont.

THE APPLIED ANATOMY OF THE NERVOUS SYSTEM. Being a Study of this portion of the Human Body from a standpoint of its general interest and practical utility in Diagnosis, designed for use as a text-book and a work of reference. Second Edit., 179 illustrations, large 8vo, 21s.

[Just published.

H. A. REEVES, F.R.C.S. EDIN.
Senior Assistant Surgeon and Teacher of Practical Surgery at the London Hospital; Surgeon to the Royal Orthopaedic Hospital.

BODILY DEFORMITIES AND THEIR TREATMENT: A HANDBOOK OF PRACTICAL ORTHOPÆDICS. With numerous Illustrations, crown 8vo, 8s. 6d.

[Lewis's Practical Series.]

RALPH RICHARDSON, M.A., M.D.
Fellow of the College of Physicians, Edinburgh.

ON THE NATURE OF LIFE: An Introductory Chapter to Pathology. Second Edition, revised and enlarged. Fcap. 4to, 10s. 6d.

W. RICHARDSON, M.A., M.D., M.R.C.P.

REMARKS ON DIABETES, ESPECIALLY IN REFERENCE TO TREATMENT. Demy 8vo, 4s. 6d.

SYDNEY RINGER, M.D., F.R.S.
Professor of the Principles and Practice of Medicine in University College; Physician to, and Professor of Clinical Medicine in, University College Hospital.

I.

A HANDBOOK OF THERAPEUTICS. Twelfth Edition, thoroughly revised, 8vo, 15s.

[Just ready.

II.

ON THE TEMPERATURE OF THE BODY AS A MEANS OF DIAGNOSIS AND PROGNOSIS IN PHTHISIS. Second Edition, small 8vo, 2s. 6d.

FREDERICK T. ROBERTS, M.D., B.SC., F.R.C.P.

Examiner in Medicine at the Royal College of Surgeons; Professor of Therapeutics in University College; Physician to University College Hospital; Physician to Brompton Consumption Hospital, &c.

I.

A HANDBOOK OF THE THEORY AND PRACTICE OF MEDICINE. Seventh Edition, with Illustrations, in one volume, large 8vo, 21s. [*Just published.*

*** *Copies may also be had bound in two volumes cloth for 1s. 6d. extra.*

II.

THE OFFICINAL MATERIA MEDICA. Second Edition, entirely rewritten in accordance with the latest British Pharmacopœia, fcap. 8vo, 7s. 6d.

R. LAWTON ROBERTS, M.D., M.R.C.S.

Honorary Life Member of, and Lecturer and Examiner to, the St. John Ambulance Association.

ILLUSTRATED LECTURES ON AMBULANCE WORK. Third Edition, copiously Illustrated, crown 8vo, 2s. 6d. [*Just ready.*

A. R. ROBINSON, M.B., L.R.C.P., AND L.R.C.S. EDIN.

Professor of Dermatology at the New York Polyclinic.

A MANUAL OF DERMATOLOGY. With 88 Illustrations, large 8vo, 21s.

D. B. St. JOHN ROOSA, M.A., M.D.

Professor of Diseases of the Eye and Ear in the University of the City of New York; Surgeon to the Manhattan Eye and Ear Hospital; Consulting Surgeon to the Brooklyn Eye and Ear Hospital, &c., &c.

A PRACTICAL TREATISE ON THE DISEASES OF THE EAR, including the Anatomy of the Organ. Sixth Edition, Illustrated by wood engravings and chromo-lithographs, large 8vo, 25s.

ROBSON ROOSE, M.D.

Fellow of the Royal College of Physicians in Edinburgh.

I.

GOUT, AND ITS RELATIONS TO DISEASES OF THE LIVER AND KIDNEYS. Fifth Edition, crown 8vo, 3s. 6d.

II.

NERVE PROSTRATION AND OTHER FUNCTIONAL DISORDERS OF DAILY LIFE. Crown 8vo, 10s. 6d. [*Just published.*

J. BURDON SANDERSON, M.D., LL.D., F.R.S.

Jodrell Professor of Physiology in University College, London.

UNIVERSITY COLLEGE COURSE OF PRACTICAL EXERCISES IN PHYSIOLOGY. With the co-operation of F. J. M. Page, B.Sc., F.C.S.; W. North, B.A., F.C.S., and Aug. Waller, M.D. Demy 8vo, 3s. 6d.

W. H. O. SANKEY, M.D. LOND., F.R.C.P.

Late Lecturer on Mental Diseases, University College and School of Medicine for Women, London; Formerly Medical Superintendent (Female Department) of Hanwell Asylum; President of Medico-Psychological Society, &c.

LECTURES ON MENTAL DISEASE. Second Edition, with coloured plates, 8vo, 12s. 6d.

JOHN SAVORY.

Member of the Society of Apothecaries, London.

A COMPENDIUM OF DOMESTIC MEDICINE AND COMPANION TO THE MEDICINE CHEST: Intended as a source of easy reference for Clergymen, Master Mariners, and Travellers, and for Families resident at a distance from professional assistance. Tenth Edition, sm. 8vo, 5s. [*Now ready.*

DR. B. S. SCHULTZE.

Professor of Gynæcology; Director of the Lying-in Hospital and of the Gynæcological Clinic at Jena.

THE PATHOLOGY AND TREATMENT OF DISPLACEMENTS OF THE UTERUS. Translated by J. J. Macan, M.R.C.S. and edited by A. V. Macan, M.B., M.Ch., Master of the Rotunda Lying-in Hospital, Dublin. With 120 Illustrations, medium [*Now ready.*

JOHN V. SHOEMAKER, A.M., M.D.
Professor of Skin Diseases in the Medico-Chirurgical College and Hospital of Philadelphia; Physician to the Philadelphia Hospital for Diseases of the Skin.

A PRACTICAL TREATISE ON DISEASES OF THE SKIN. Coloured Plates and other Illustrations, large 8vo, 24s.

WM. JAPP SINCLAIR, M.A., M.D.
Honorary Physician to the Manchester Southern Hospital for Women and Children, and Manchester Maternity Hospital.

ON GONORRHŒAL INFECTION IN WOMEN. Post 8vo, 4s. [*Just published.*

ALDER SMITH, M.B. LOND., F.R.C.S.
Resident Medical Officer, Christ's Hospital, London.

RINGWORM: Its Diagnosis and Treatment. Third Edition, enlarged, with Illustrations, fcap. 8vo, 5s. 6d.

J. LEWIS SMITH, M.D.
Physician to the New York Infants' Hospital; Clinical Lecturer on Diseases of Children in Bellevue Hospital Medical College.

A TREATISE ON THE DISEASES OF INFANCY AND CHILDHOOD. Fifth Edition, with Illustrations, large 8vo, 21s

---

FRANCIS W. SMITH, M.B., B.S.

THE SALINE WATERS OF LEAMINGTON. Second Edit., with Illustrations, crown 8vo, 1s. *nett.*

JAMES STARTIN, M.B., M.R.C.S.
Surgeon and Joint Lecturer to St. John's Hospital for Diseases of the Skin.

LECTURES ON THE PARASITIC DISEASES OF THE SKIN. VEGETOID AND ANIMAL. With Illustrations, crown 8vo, 2s. 6d.

LEWIS A. STIMSON, B.A., M.D.
Surgeon to the Presbyterian and Bellevue Hospitals; Professor of Clinical Surgery in the Medical Faculty of the University of the City of New York, &c.

A MANUAL OF OPERATIVE SURGERY. Second Edition, with three hundred and forty-two Illustrations, post 8vo, 10s. 6d. [*Just published.*

ADOLF STRÜMPELL.

Director of the Medical Clinic in the University of Erlangen.

A TEXT-BOOK OF MEDICINE FOR STUDENTS AND PRACTITIONERS. Translated from the latest German edition by Dr. H. F. VICKERY and Dr. P. C. KNAPP, with Editorial Notes by Dr. F. C. SHATTUCK, Visiting Physician to the Massachusetts General Hospital, etc. Complete in one large vol., imp. 8vo, with 111 Illustrations, 28s. [*Just published.*

JUKES DE STYRAP, M.K.Q.C.P., ETC.

Physician-Extraordinary, late Physician in Ordinary, to the Salop Infirmary; Consulting Physician to the South Salop and Montgomeryshire Infirmaries, etc.

THE MEDICO-CHIRURGICAL TARIFFS PREPARED FOR THE LATE SHROPSHIRE ETHICAL BRANCH OF THE BRITISH MEDICAL ASSOCIATION. Fourth Edition, fcap. 4to, revised and enlarged, 2s. *nett.*

C. W. SUCKLING, M.D. LOND., M.R.C.P.

Professor of Materia Medica and Therapeutics at the Queen's College, Physician to the Queen's Hospital, Birmingham, etc.

ON THE DIAGNOSIS OF DISEASES OF THE BRAIN, SPINAL CORD, AND NERVES. With Illustrations, crown 8vo, 8s. 6d.

JOHN BLAND SUTTON, F.R.C.S.

Lecturer on Comparative Anatomy, Senior Demonstrator of Anatomy, and Assistant Surgeon to the Middlesex Hospital; [illegible] Lecturer Royal College of Surgeons, England.

LIGAMENTS: THEIR NATURE AND MORPHOLOGY. With numerous Illustrations, post 8vo, 4s. 6d.

HENRY R. SWANZY, A.M., M.B., F.R.C.S.I.

Examiner in Ophthalmic Surgery in the Royal University of Ireland, and to the Conjoint Board [illegible] Royal College of Surgeons [illegible] Surgeon to the National Eye and Ear Infirmary [illegible] Surgeon to the Adelaide Hospital, Dublin.

A HANDBOOK OF THE DISEASES OF THE EYE AND THEIR TREATMENT. Second Edition, Illustrated with wood-engravings, colour tests, etc., small 8vo, 10s. 6d. [*Just published.*

EUGENE S. TALBOT, M.D., D.D.S.

Professor of Dental Surgery in the Woman's Medical College; Lecturer on Dental Pathology and Surgery in Rush Medical College, Chicago.

IRREGULARITIES OF THE TEETH AND THEIR TREATMENT. With 152 Illustrations, royal 8vo, 10s. 6d.

JOHN DAVIES THOMAS, M.D. LOND., F.R.C.S. ENG.

Physician to the Adelaide Hospital, S. Australia.

I.

HYDATID DISEASE, WITH SPECIAL REFERENCE TO ITS PREVALENCE IN AUSTRALIA. Demy 8vo, 10s. 6d.

II.

HYDATID DISEASE OF THE LUNGS. Demy 8vo, 2s.

HUGH OWEN THOMAS, M.R.C.S.

I.

DISEASES OF THE HIP, KNEE, AND ANKLE JOINTS, with their Deformities, treated by a new and efficient method. Third Edition, 8vo, 25s.

II.

CONTRIBUTIONS TO SURGERY AND MEDICINE:—

PART 1.—Intestinal Obstruction; with an Appendix on the Action of Remedies. 10s.

„ 2.—The Principles of the Treatment of Joint Disease, Inflammation, Anchylosis, Reduction of Joint Deformity, Bone Setting. 5s.

„ 3.—Fractures, Dislocations, Diseases and Deformities of the Bones of the Trunk and Upper Extremities. 10s.

„ 4.—The Collegian of 1666 and the Collegians of 1885; or what is recognised treatment? Second Edition, 1s.

„ 5.—On Fractures of the Lower Jaw. 1s.

„ 6.—The Principles of the Treatment of Fractures and Dislocations. 10s.

8.—The Inhibition of Nerves by Drugs. Proof that Inhibitory Nerve-Fibres do not exist. 1s.

(Parts 7, 9 and 10 are in preparation).

J. ASHBURTON THOMPSON, M.R.C.S.

Late Surgeon at King's Cross to the Great Northern Railway Company.

FREE PHOSPHORUS IN MEDICINE WITH SPECIAL REFERENCE TO ITS USE IN NEURALGIA. A contribution to Materia Medica and Therapeutics. An account of the History, Pharmaceutical Preparations, Dose, Internal Administration, and Therapeutic uses of Phosphorus; with a Complete Bibliography of this subject, referring to nearly 200 works upon it. Demy 8vo, 7s. 6d.

J. C. THOROWGOOD, M.D.

Assistant Physician to the City of London Hospital for Diseases of the Chest.

THE CLIMATIC TREATMENT OF CONSUMPTION AND CHRONIC LUNG DISEASES. Third Edition, post 8vo, 3s. 6d.

EDWARD T. TIBBITS, M.D. LOND.

Physician to the Bradford Infirmary; and to the Bradford Fever Hospital.

MEDICAL FASHIONS IN THE NINETEENTH CENTURY, including a Sketch of Bacterio-Mania and the Battle of the Bacilli. Crown 8vo, 2s. 6d.

H. H. TOOTH, M.A., M.D., M.R.C.P.

Assistant Demonstrator of Physiology at St. Bartholomew's Hospital.

THE PERONEAL TYPE OF PROGRESSIVE MUSCULAR ATROPHY. 8vo, 1s.

FREDERICK TREVES, F.R.C.S.

Hunterian Professor at the Royal College of Surgeons of England; Surgeon to and Lecturer on Anatomy at the London Hospital.

THE ANATOMY OF THE INTESTINAL CANAL AND PERITONEUM IN MAN. Hunterian Lectures, 1885. 4to, 2s. 6d.

D. HACK TUKE, M.D., LL.D.

Fellow of the Royal College of Physicians, London.

THE INSANE IN THE UNITED STATES AND CANADA. Demy 8vo, 7s. 6d.

LAURENCE TURNBULL, M.D., PH.G.
Aural Surgeon to Jefferson Medical College Hospital, &c., &c.

ARTIFICIAL ANÆSTHESIA: A Manual of Anæsthetic Agents, and their Employment in the Treatment of Disease. Second Edition, with Illustrations, crown 8vo, 6s.

DR. R. ULTZMANN.

ON STERILITY AND IMPOTENCE IN MAN. Translated from the German with notes and additions by ARTHUR COOPER, L.R.C.P., M.R.C.S., Surgeon to the Westminster General Dispensary. With Illustrations, fcap. 8vo, 2s. 6d.

W. H. VAN BUREN, M.D., LL.D.
Professor of Surgery in the Bellevue Hospital Medical College.

DISEASES OF THE RECTUM: And the Surgery of the Lower Bowel. Second Edition, with Illustrations, 8vo, 14s.

RUDOLPH VIRCHOW, M.D.
Professor in the University, and Member of the Academy of Sciences of Berlin, &c., &c.

INFECTION-DISEASES IN THE ARMY, Chiefly Wound Fever, Typhoid, Dysentery, and Diphtheria. Translated from the German by JOHN JAMES, M.B., F.R.C.S. Fcap. 8vo, 1s. 6d.

ALFRED VOGEL, M.D.
Professor of Clinical Medicine in the University of Dorpat, Russia.

A PRACTICAL TREATISE ON THE DISEASES OF CHILDREN. Third Edition, translated and edited by H. RAPHAEL, M.D., from the Eighth German Edition, illustrated by six lithographic Plates, part coloured, royal 8vo, 18s.

A. DUNBAR WALKER, M.D., C.M.

THE PARENT'S MEDICAL NOTE BOOK. Oblong post 8vo, cloth, 1s. 6d.

JOHN RICHARD WARDELL, M.D. EDIN., F.R.C.P. LOND.
Late Consulting Physician to the General Hospital Tunbridge Wells.

CONTRIBUTIONS TO PATHOLOGY AND THE PRACTICE OF MEDICINE. Medium 8vo, 21s.

W. SPENCER WATSON, F.R.C.S. ENG., B.M. LOND.
Surgeon to the Great Northern Hospital; Surgeon to the Royal South London Ophthalmic Hospital.

I.

DISEASES OF THE NOSE AND ITS ACCESSORY CAVITIES. Profusely Illustrated. Demy 8vo, 18s.

II.

EYEBALL-TENSION: Its Effects on the Sight and its Treatment. With woodcuts, p. 8vo, 2s. 6d.

III.

ON ABSCESS AND TUMOURS OF THE ORBIT. Post 8vo, 2s. 6d.

FRANCIS H. WELCH, F.R.C.S.
Surgeon Major, A.M.D.

ENTERIC FEVER: as Illustrated by Army Data at Home and Abroad, its Prevalence and Modifications, Ætiology, Pathology and Treatment. 8vo, 5s. 6d.

W. WYNN WESTCOTT, M.B.
Deputy Coroner for Central Middlesex.

SUICIDE; its History, Literature, Jurisprudence, and Prevention. Crown 8vo, 6s.

JOHN WILLIAMS, M.D., F.R.C.P.
Professor of Midwifery in University College, London; Obstetric Physician to University College Hospital; Physician Accoucheur to H.R.H. Princess Beatrice, etc.

CANCER OF THE UTERUS: Being the Harveian Lectures for 1886. Illustrated with Lithographic Plates, royal 8vo, 10s. 6d.
[*Just published.*

E. T. WILSON, B.M. OXON., F.R.C.P. LOND.
Physician to the Cheltenham General Hospital and Dispensary.

DISINFECTANTS AND HOW TO USE THEM. In Packets of one doz. price 1s.

DR. F. WINCKEL.

Formerly Professor and Director of the Gynæcological Clinic at the University of Rostock.

THE PATHOLOGY AND TREATMENT OF CHILD-BED: A Treatise for Physicians and Students. Translated from the Second German edition, with many additional notes by the Author, by J. R. CHADWICK, M.D. 8vo, 14s.

EDWARD WOAKES, M.D. LOND.

Senior Aural Surgeon and Lecturer on Aural Surgery at the London Hospital; Surgeon to the London Throat Hospital.

I.

ON DEAFNESS, GIDDINESS AND NOISES IN THE HEAD.

VOL. I.—POST-NASAL CATARRH, AND DISEASES OF THE NOSE CAUSING DEAFNESS. With Illustrations, cr. 8vo, 6s. 6d.

VOL. II.—ON DEAFNESS, GIDDINESS AND NOISES IN THE HEAD. Third Edition, with Illustrations, cr. 8vo. [*In preparation.*

II.

NASAL POLYPUS: WITH NEURALGIA, HAY-FEVER, AND ASTHMA, IN RELATION TO ETHMOIDITIS. With Illustrations, cr. 8vo, 4s. 6d. [*Now ready.*

DAVID YOUNG, M.C., M.B., M.D.

Licentiate of the Royal College of Physicians, Edinburgh; Licentiate of the Royal College of Surgeons, Edinburgh; Fellow of, and late Examiner in Midwifery to the University of Bombay; etc.

ROME IN WINTER AND THE TUSCAN HILLS IN SUMMER. A CONTRIBUTION TO THE CLIMATE OF ITALY. Small 8vo, 6s.

HERMANN VON ZEISSL, M.D.

Late Professor at the Imperial Royal University of Vienna.

OUTLINES OF THE PATHOLOGY AND TREATMENT OF SYPHILIS AND ALLIED VENEREAL DISEASES. Second Edition, revised by M. VON ZEISSL, M.D., Privat-Docent for Diseases of the Skin and Syphilis at the Imperial Royal University of Vienna. Translated, with Notes, by H. RAPHAEL, M.D., Attending Physician for Diseases of Genito-Urinary Organs and Syphilis, Bellevue Hospital, Out-Patient Department. Large 8vo, 18s. [*Just published.*

Clinical Charts For Temperature Observations, etc. Arranged by W. RIGDEN, M.R.C.S. 50s. per 1000, 28s. per 500, 15s. per 250, 7s. per 100, or 1s. per dozen.

Each Chart is arranged for four weeks, and is ruled at the back for making notes of cases; they are convenient in size, and are suitable both for hospital and private practice.

THE NEW SYDENHAM SOCIETY'S PUBLICATIONS.

President.—Sir Spencer Wells, Bart., F.R.C.S.
Honorary Secretary.—Jonathan Hutchinson, Esq., F.R.S.
Treasurer.—W. Sedgwick Saunders, M.D., F.S.A.

Annual Subscription, One Guinea.

[illegible]

[illegible]

[illegible]

PERIODICAL WORKS PUBLISHED BY H. K. LEWIS.

THE NEW YORK MEDICAL JOURNAL. A Weekly Review of Medicine. Annual Subscription, One Guinea, post free.

THE THERAPEUTIC GAZETTE. A Monthly Journal, devoted to the Science of Pharmacology, and to the introduction of New Therapeutic Agents. Edited by Drs. H. C. Wood and R. M. Smith. Annual Subscription, [illegible], post free.

THE GLASGOW MEDICAL JOURNAL. Published Monthly. Annual Subscription, [illegible], post free. Single numbers, [illegible] each.

LIVERPOOL MEDICO-CHIRURGICAL JOURNAL, including the Proceedings of the Liverpool Medical Institution. Published twice yearly, [illegible] each number.

THE INDIAN MEDICAL JOURNAL. A Journal of Medical and Sanitary Science specially devoted to the interests of the Medical Services. Annual Subscription, [illegible], post free.

TRANSACTIONS OF THE COLLEGE OF PHYSICIANS OF PHILADELPHIA. Volumes [illegible], 8vo, [illegible] each.

MIDDLESEX HOSPITAL. REPORTS OF THE MEDICAL, SURGICAL, AND Pathological Registrars [illegible]. Demy 8vo, [illegible] each volume.

*** Mr. Lewis is in constant communication with the leading publishing firms in America, and has transactions with them for the sale of his publications in that country. Advantageous arrangements are made in the interests of Authors for the publishing of their works in the United States.

Mr. Lewis's publications can be procured of any Bookseller in any part of the world.

London: Printed by H. K. Lewis, [illegible] Gower Street, W.C.

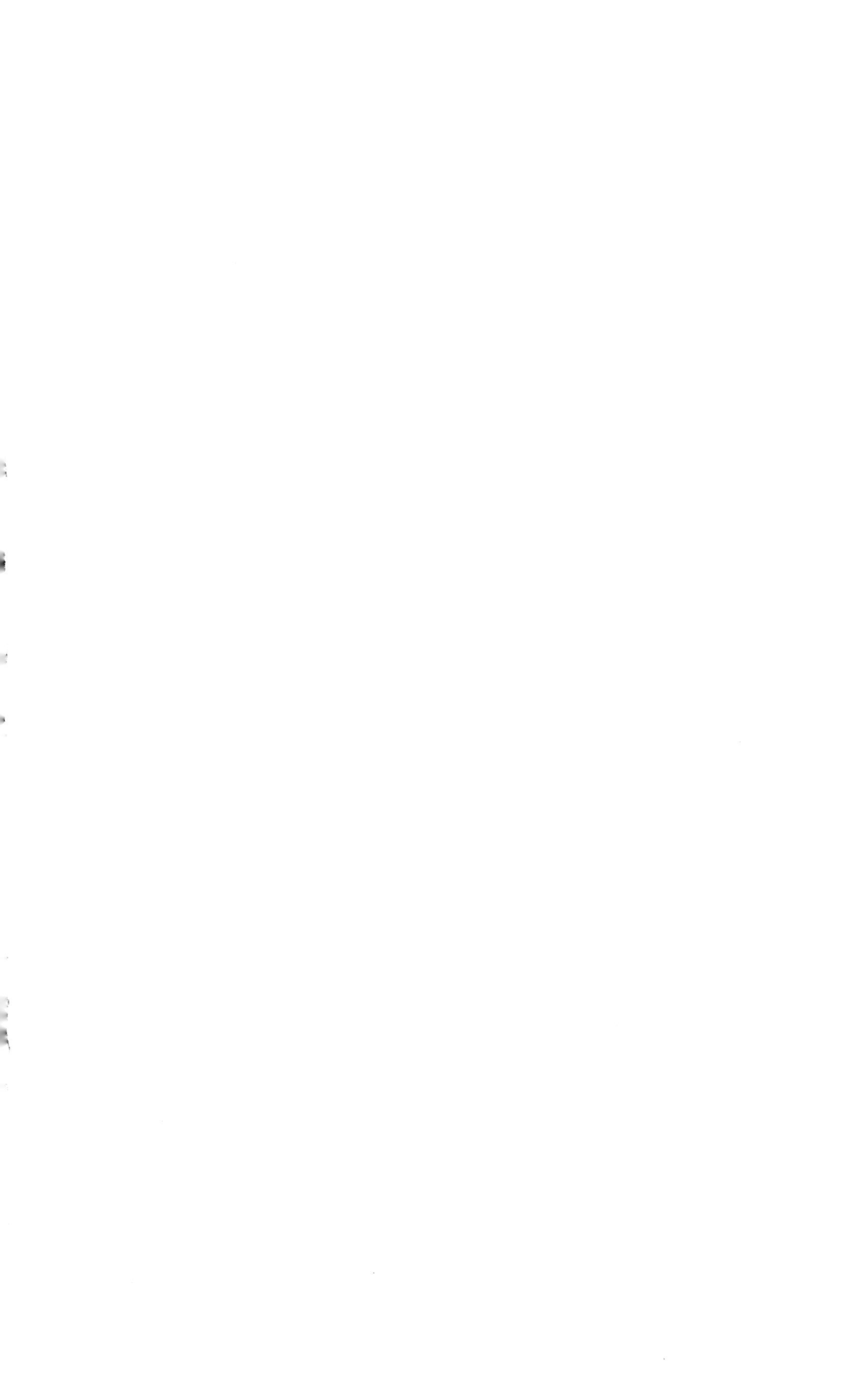

CPSIA information can be obtained
at www.ICGtesting.com
Printed in the USA
LVHW040208130420
653218LV00006B/750